THYROID NEOPLASMS

Editor

Bryan Haugen

*Division of Endocrinology,
Metabolism, and Diabetes
Denver, CO, USA*

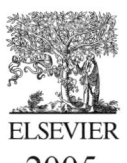

ELSEVIER

2005

AMSTERDAM – BOSTON – HEIDELBERG – LONDON – NEW YORK – PARIS
SAN DIEGO – SAN FRANCISCO – SINGAPORE – SYDNEY – TOKYO

ELSEVIER B.V.
Radarweg 29
P.O. Box 211
1000 AE Amsterdam
The Netherlands

ELSEVIER Inc.
525 B Street, Suite 1900
San Diego
CA 92101-4495
USA

ELSEVIER Ltd
The Boulevard, Langford Lane
Kidlington
Oxford OX5 1GB
UK

ELSEVIER Ltd
84 Theobalds Road
London WC1X 8RR
UK

First edition 2005

Library of Congress Cataloging in Publication Data
A catalog record is available from the Library of Congress.

British Library Cataloguing in Publication Data
A catalogue record is available from the British Library.

ISBN: 0 444 50952 6
ISSN: 1569-2566

∞ The paper used in this publication meets the requirements of ANSI/NISO Z39.48-1992 (Permanence of Paper).

Printed in The Netherlands.

Contents

Preface

Thyroid neoplasms are quite common (5–10% detected by palpation, 30–50% detected by imaging studies) and the incidence of thyroid cancer is 25,000/year, making this the eighth most common malignancy diagnosed in women in the United States. Fortunately, many patients do well with standard therapy and careful monitoring, but the estimated annual number of deaths due to thyroid cancer is 1500 in the United States alone.

In the past 10 years, tremendous advances have been made in our knowledge of the development of thyroid cancer, molecular markers in the diagnosis of thyroid nodules, technology in ultrasound, positron emission tomography (PET), laboratory measurements, and general approaches (e.g., surgery, radioiodine, and monitoring) to patients with thyroid cancer. I have enlisted the expertise of many leaders in the field of thyroid neoplasia to update us on these advances. This book is quite unique in that it encompasses the topic of thyroid neoplasm from basic biology to practical clinical approaches.

In one book, the reader can explore basic biology of thyroid cancer, review potential molecular markers in thyroid neoplasms, and learn about new therapies on the horizon for advanced thyroid carcinoma, while learning the latest approaches to ultrasonography, radioiodine therapy, and monitoring uses for thyroglobulin, radioiodine and PET that can be directly applied to clinical practice. We have also included two chapters on unique topics. The first chapter discusses the biology of and approaches to patients with medullary thyroid carcinoma, with special emphasis on monitoring and management of recurrent disease. The second chapter covers thyroid neoplasms in children and special approaches to this population.

The significant advances in the understanding of the basic biology of thyroid tumors as well as in clinical approaches to patients with this common neoplasm are the foundation of this book. This book provides the reader a single text as a reference to explore and understand these important advances in molecular, cellular, and clinical endocrinology.

Bryan R. Haugen, MD
Associate Professor of Medicine and Pathology
Director, Thyroid Tumor Program
University of Colorado at Denver and Health Sciences Center

List of contributors

Yuri E. Nikiforov

Department of Pathology and Lab Medicine
University of Cincinnati
College of Medicine
Cincinnati, Ohio

Nikolaos Stathathos

Section of Endocrinology
Washington Hospital Center
Washington, DC

Matthew D. Ringel

Divisions of Endocrinology, Oncology and
Human Cancer Genetics
The Ohio State University
Columbus, Ohio

H. Jack Baskin

Florida Thyroid Clinic
Orlando, Florida

Richard T. Kloos

Departments of Internal Medicine and Radiology
Divisions of Endocrinology, and Metabolism &
Nuclear Medicine
The Ohio State University
Columbus, Ohio

Carole Spencer

University of Southern California
Edmondson Building
Los Angeles, California

Shireen Fatemi

Southern California Permanante Medical Group
Panorama City, California

Richard J. Robbins

Endocrine and Nuclear Medicine Services
Departments of Medicine and Radiology
Memorial Sloan-Kettering Cancer Center
New York, New York

Chee-Yeung Chan

Endocrine and Nuclear Medicine Services
Departments of Medicine and Radiology
Memorial Sloan-Kettering Cancer Center
New York, New York

R. Michael Tuttle

Endocrine and Nuclear Medicine Services
Departments of Medicine and Radiology
Memorial Sloan-Kettering Cancer Center
New York, New York

Steven M. Larson

Endocrine and Nuclear Medicine Services
Departments of Medicine and Radiology
Memorial Sloan-Kettering Cancer Center
New York, New York

Sai-Ching Jim Yeung

Department of General Internal Medicine
Ambulatory Treatment and Emergency Care and
Department of Endocrine Neoplasia and
Hormonal Disorders
The University of Texas MD Anderson Cancer
Center
Houston, Texas

Jeffrey F. Moley

Washington University
St Louis, Missouri

Wellington Hung

Division of Pediatric Endocrinology and
Metabolism
Department of Pediatrics
Georgetown University Medical Center
Washington, DC

Chapter 1

Gene rearrangements in thyroid cancer

Yuri E. Nikiforov

Department of Pathology and Laboratory Medicine, University of Cincinnati, Cincinnati, Ohio, USA

1. Introduction

Activation of oncogenes through chromosomal rearrangement is a well-known mechanism of tumorigenesis. It can involve two types of rearrangement: translocation, when a portion of one chromosome is transferred to another chromosome and inversion, when two breaks occur within a single chromosome with inverted reincorporation of the segment. Rearrangements are typically found in hematopoietic tumors and certain types of sarcomas, but not in epithelial cancers. Thyroid cancer represents an exception from this general rule and is commonly associated with such large-scale genetic abnormalities. The most common rearrangements, *RET*/PTC in papillary cancer and *PAX8–PPARγ* in follicular tumors, are discussed in this chapter.

2. *RET*/PTC Rearrangement

2.1. *The* RET *proto-oncogene*

The *RET* proto-oncogene is located on chromosome 10q11.2 and encodes a cell membrane receptor tyrosine kinase [1,2]. The receptor consists of three domains: an extracellular domain with a ligand-binding site, a transmembrane domain, and an intracellular domain that includes a region with protein-tyrosine kinase activity. The ligands for RET receptor have been identified as neurotrophic factors of the glial cell-line derived neurotrophic factor (GDNF) family, including GDNF, neurtulin, artemin, and persephin [3]. Binding of a ligand causes the receptors to dimerize, leading to autophosphorylation of the protein on tyrosine residues and initiation of intracellular signaling cascade.

Wild-type *RET* is expressed in neuronal and neural-crest-derived tissues including thyroid parafollicular C-cells, but not in thyroid follicular cells. Point mutations of *RET* in C-cells are responsible for sporadic and familial medullary thyroid

ADVANCES IN MOLECULAR AND CELLULAR ENDOCRINOLOGY
VOLUME 4   ISSN 1569-2566/DOI 10.1016/S1569-2566(04)04001-3

carcinomas, and for the inherited cancer syndromes MEN2A and MEN2B, whereas 'loss of function' of RET is involved in Hirschsprung's disease [4]. In thyroid follicular cells, *RET* can be activated by fusion to different constitutively expressed genes. The product of this rearrangement is a chimeric oncogene named *RET*/PTC (PTC for papillary thyroid carcinoma).

2.2. *Structure of* RET/PTC *oncogenes*

Since the original report on *RET* activation by rearrangement in papillary thyroid carcinomas (PTCs) [5], three major types of the rearrangement have been identified: *RET*/PTC1, *RET*/PTC2 and *RET*/PTC3 (Fig. 1). All of them are derived from the fusion of the tyrosine kinase domain of *RET* to the 5′ portion of different genes. Breakpoints in the *RET* gene are almost always located in intron 11, so that the 3′ portion of *RET* fused to the activating genes encodes the tyrosine kinase domain but lacks the transmembrane and extracellular domains. *RET*/PTC1 is formed by fusion to the *H4* (also known as D10S170) gene [5], and *RET*/PTC3 is a product of *RET* fusion with the *ELE1* (*RFG* or *ARA70*) gene [6,7]. *RET*/PTC1 and *RET*/PTC3 are paracentric inversions since both genes participating in the rearrangement are located on chromosome 10q [8,9]. In contrast, *RET*/PTC2 is formed by reciprocal translocation between chromosomes 10 and 17, resulting in *RET* fusion to the 5′-terminal sequence of the regulatory subunit *RIα* of the cyclic AMP-dependent protein kinase A [10].

Recently, seven novel types of *RET*/PTC have been described (Fig. 1). Most of them (*RET*/PTC5, *RET*/PTC6, *RET*/PTC7, *RET*/KTN1, *RET*/RFG8, and *RET*/PCM-1) were found in papillary carcinomas from patients with a history of radiation exposure [11–15], while one novel type was identified in a sporadic (i.e., not associated with radiation) papillary carcinoma (*RET*/ELKS) [16]. All novel types of *RET*/PTC are the result of translocation and formed by fusion of the tyrosine kinase domain of *RET* to heterologous genes located on different chromosomes.

2.3. *Consequences of* RET/PTC *fusion and activation in thyroid cells*

The genes fused with *RET* are constitutively expressed in thyroid follicular cells and drive the expression of the chimeric *RET*/PTC oncogene. In addition, these partners provide a dimerization domain essential for ligand-independent activation of the RET tyrosine kinase [17,18]. In fact, all *RET* fusion genes encode putative dimerization domains, typically one or more coiled-coil domains (Fig. 1) [18]. It allows ligand-independent dimerization of the chimeric protein and autophosphorylation of the truncated RET receptor. Indeed, it has been demonstrated that Tyr-1015 and Tyr-1062, which are autophosphorylated in the wild-type RET only upon ligand binding, are constitutively phosphorylated in the RET/PTC chimeric protein [19]. The ligand-independent activation of the RET tyrosine kinase is considered essential for the transformation of thyroid cells [20].

Another important role of the genes fused with *RET* is in determining a subcellular localization of the chimeric protein that lacks the transmembrane domain and

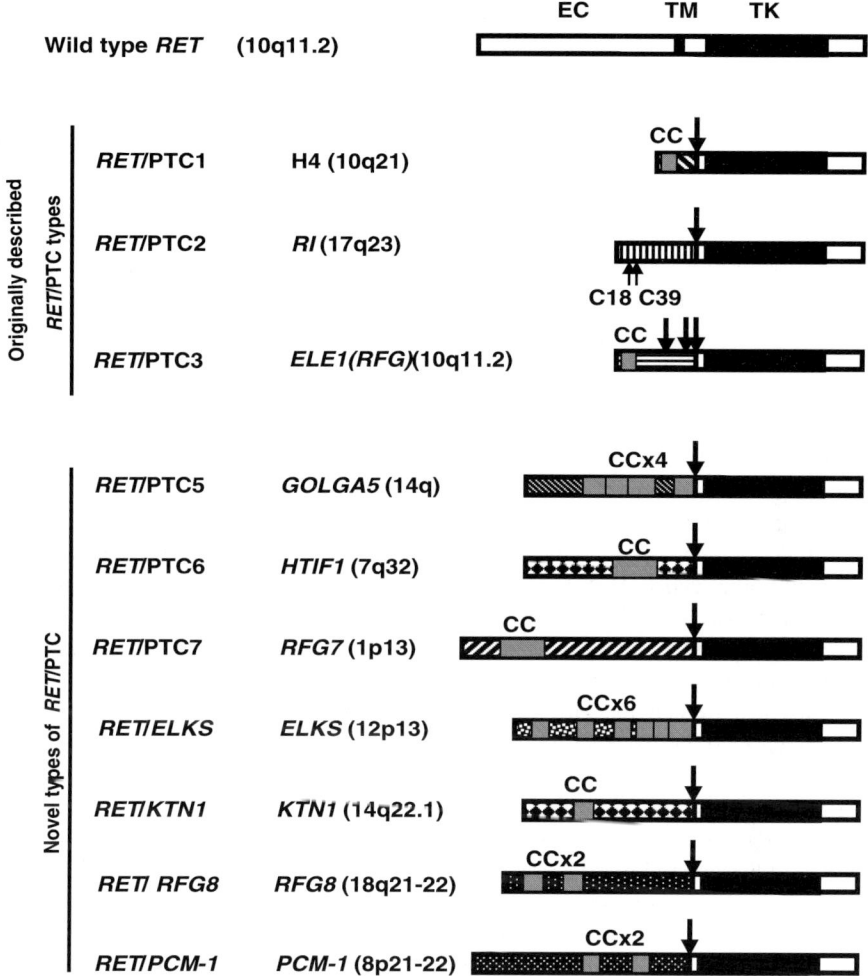

Fig. 1. Schematic representation of the wild-type *RET* gene: three initially described types of *RET*/PTC (*RET*/PTC1, *RET*/PTC2, and *RET*/PTC3) and seven novel *RET*/PTC types. Each type of rearrangement results from the fusion of the tyrosine kinase domain of *RET* to the 5′ portion of different genes that are constitutively expressed in thyroid follicular cells. All *RET* fusion genes encode one or more putative dimerization domains (CC, coiled-coil domain, C18 and C39, cystine residues forming disulfide bonds during dimerization) essential for ligand-independent activation of the truncated RET receptor. The breakpoint location is shown by arrows. Chromosomal location of the *RET* gene and its fusion partners is shown in parantheses. EC, extracellular domain; TM, transmembrane domain; TK, tyrosine kinase domain of *RET*.

cannot be anchored to the cell membrane. In RET/PTC3 protein, for instance, the N-terminal coiled-coil domain of ELE1 (RFG) not only mediates oligomerization of the receptor and chronic kinase activation, but also is responsible for the compartmentalization of the chimeric protein at plasma membrane level, where most of the normal ELE1 (RFG) protein is distributed [21]. Thus, different types of RET/PTC chimeric proteins, which have a similar RET tyrosine kinase portion but different N-terminal domains, may be distributed in various cytoplasmic compartments, allowing them to interact with different substrates. This may provide an explanation for some variations in biological properties recently found between different types of *RET*/PTC chimeric genes.

RET/PTC is tumorigenic in thyroid follicular cells. *RET*/PTC1 rearrangement has been originally isolated by virtue of its ability to transform NIH 3T3 cells [22], and in cooperation with *RAS*, it is capable of transforming PC Cl3 rat thyroid epithelial cells [23]. More recently, *RET*/PTC has been shown to induce PTCs in transgenic mice. This was demonstrated in animals with thyroid-specific expression of *RET*/PTC1 under the control of the rat or bovine thyroglobulin promoter and of *RET*/PTC3 under the control of bovine thyroglobulin promoter [24]. Thyroid tumors, developed in these transgenic mice, demonstrated architectural and cytologic features of human papillary carcinomas and were well differentiated. The progression from poorly differentiated to undifferentiated phenotypes was achieved by crossing *RET*/PTC1 mice with p53 -/- mice [25].

RET/PTC may be responsible for the characteristic microscopic features of papillary carcinoma cells. Thus, primary cultures of human thyroid follicular cells transfected with *RET*/PTC1 retroviral construct have been shown to acquire nuclear features typical of papillary carcinoma including open chromatin, irregularity of nuclear contours, and occasional nuclear grooves and pseudoinclusions [26]. This effect was not noticed in cells transfected with only the retroviral construct, suggesting that this is a direct effect of *RET*/PTC expression.

2.4. *Prevalence in thyroid tumors*

RET/PTC rearrangements occur only in tumors of the thyroid gland and are generally believed to be restricted to the papillary type of thyroid carcinoma [27,28]. Recently, it has also been identified in hyalinizing trabecular adenomas of the thyroid, the tumor that in all likelihood represents a peculiar variant of papillary carcinoma [29,30]. The presence of *RET*/PTC in follicular adenomas, hyperplastic thyroid nodules, and Hashimoto's thyroiditis, suggested in some reports, has not been confirmed in other studies and remains controversial (reviewed in [31]).

The prevalence of *RET*/PTC in papillary carcinomas varies significantly in different studies and geographic regions. In the United States, the five largest series of adult papillary carcinomas showed the frequency ranging from 11 to 43%, with the cumulative incidence of 35% [27–28,32–35]. A comparable rate of 30–40% has been noted in series from Canada [36] and Italy [27,37,38]. In other regions, a wide variation in frequency of *RET*/PTC has been reported, ranging from 3% in Saudi Arabia [39] to 85% in Australia [40]. Apart from the real geographic variability, which clearly exists, some differences are likely due to the variation in screening techniques, since different studies from the same regions revealed a highly variable prevalence of *RET*/PTC, such as 3% [41] and 36% [42] in Japan or 8% [43] and 85% [40] in Australia.

In the general population, *RET*/PTC1 represents the most common type, comprising up to 60–70% of all rearrangements, whereas *RET*/PTC3 accounts for 20–30% of positive cases and *RET*/PTC2 for less than 10% [28,34,35,38]. The novel types of *RET*/PTC are rare and typically associated with radiation exposure. *RET*/*ELKS* represents the only novel type of *RET*/PTC found in a papillary carcinoma with no history of radiation [16].

2.5. *Association with age and radiation exposure*

A higher prevalence of *RET*/PTC has been observed in papillary thyroid carcinomas from children and young adults [37,44–46]. Thus, in a series of 92 papillary carcinomas from Italy, 67% of tumors from patients aged 4–19 years harbored *RET*/PTC, in contrast to 32% in patients aged 31–80 years [37]. In the United States, a prevalence of 45–71% was noted in papillary carcinomas from children and young adults [44,46]. In all studies that reported a higher frequency of *RET*/PTC in younger patients, *RET*/PTC1 remained the major type of rearrangement.

Over the last several years it has been clearly documented that the prevalence of *RET*/PTC is higher in papillary carcinomas from patients with a history of radiation exposure, including those subjected to either accidental or therapeutic external irradiation. Thus, in children affected by the Chernobyl nuclear accident, 67–87% of papillary carcinomas removed 5–8 years after the exposure and 49–65% of tumors removed 7–11 years after the accident harbored *RET*/PTC [44,47–50]. Interestingly, in tumors developed less than 10 years after the accident, *RET*/PTC3 appeared to be the most common type, whereas tumors developed after the longer latency had predominantly *RET*/PTC1 [49,50]. In patients subjected to therapeutic external irradiation for benign or malignant conditions, the prevalence of *RET*/PTC was also higher than in the general population, being reported at 52–84% [51,52]. Exposure to ionizing radiation not only resulted in a higher prevalence in *RET*/PTC, but also promoted the fusion of *RET* to the unusual rearrangement partners, since six out of seven novel *RET*/PTC types were detected in tumors associated with radiation exposure. The novel types have been reported in up to 4% of post-Chernobyl papillary carcinomas [12,14,15,53,54] and in one papillary carcinoma from a patient with a history of external therapeutic irradiation [13].

The occurrence of *RET*/PTC has also been observed after high-dose *in vitro* irradiation of human undifferentiated thyroid carcinoma cells [55] and fetal human thyroid tissues transplanted into SCID mice [56,57]. In both studies, the rearrangements were detected by RT–PCR as early as 2 days after the exposure. In irradiated fetal thyroid cells, both *RET*/PTC1 and *RET*/PTC3 rearrangements were found 2–7 days after exposure, while only *RET*/PTC1 persisted and was detectable 2 months later [57]. The effective dose of radiation in these studies was high (50 Gy), and the cells irradiated by Ito and colleagues were already highly transformed and hence more susceptible to develop secondary genetic defects. Nevertheless, these observations suggest that radiation exposure may be directly associated with the generation of *RET*/PTC rearrangements in thyroid cells.

2.6. *Genotype-phenotype correlation*

It is likely that different types of *RET*/PTC are associated with distinct phenotypes of papillary carcinoma. In the general population, *RET*/PTC1 tends to be more common in microcarcinomas (<1 cm in size) and tumors with classical papillary architecture [28,58,59], whereas *RET*/PTC3 shows association with the more aggressive tall cell variant [60]. In tumors from children exposed to radiation after the Chernobyl accident, *RET*/PTC3 had a strong correlation with the solid variant of papillary carcinoma and *RET*/PTC1 with classical papillary carcinoma [44,50,61].

Interestingly, a similar correlation has been observed in transgenic mice. Thus, thyroid-specific expression of *RET*/PTC1 led to the development of thyroid tumors with micropapillary or mixed architecture and slow and non-metastatic growth [62–64]. In contrast, *RET*/PTC3 mice developed thyroid tumors with a solid histological phenotype and locally aggressive and metastatic behavior [24]. However, some caution should be used in direct comparison of these results because of the potential variability in the strains of mice, promoter constructs, and levels of chimeric gene expression between these animal models.

Recently, the potential mechanism responsible for such phenotypic difference has been proposed. Thus, it has been shown that, in PC Cl3 rat thyroid cells transfected with these chimeric genes, the *RET*/PTC3 transfected cells had a significantly higher proliferative activity, as determined by a fraction of cells in S and G2/M phases of the cell cycle [60]. Moreover, with the similar levels of expression and tyrosine phosphorylation, the MAPK activation, which is a common endpoint of receptor tyrosine kinase mitogenic signaling, appeared to be approximately threefold higher in the *RET*/PTC3 compared with *RET*/PTC1-transfected cells. This indicates that the increased proliferative activity found in cells harboring *RET*/PTC3 is likely due to a significantly higher level of MAPK phosphorylation.

2.7. *Characterization of breakpoint sites and possible mechanisms of* RET/PTC *rearrangement*

The mechanisms of *RET*/PTC generation in thyroid cells are not well understood. The higher prevalence of the rearrangement, especially of its *RET*/PTC3 type, in tumors associated with radiation exposure suggests the role of radiation-induced DNA damage in its generation. However, most papillary carcinomas with *RET*/PTC are not associated with such a history, indicating that other initiating factors do exist. Nevertheless, the availability of a large population of radiation-associated tumors with *RET*/PTC has provided an important resource to generate some insights into the mechanisms of *RET*/PTC formation.

The analysis of genomic sequences of the breakpoint sites revealed no long-sequence homology between the regions of genes involved in *RET*/PTC1 [65] and *RET*/PTC3 [66,67], indicating that these rearrangements are the result of illegitimate rather than homologous recombination.

An unexpected finding surfaced when breakpoint sites within the *RET* and *ELE1* genes were mapped and compared among 12 post-Chernobyl tumors with

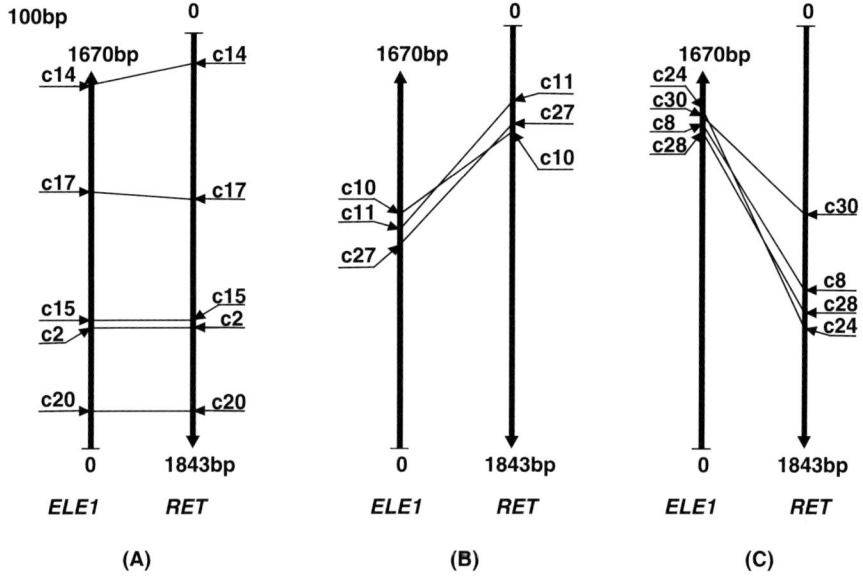

Fig. 2. Alignment of breakpoints involved in *RET*/PTC3 in post-Chernobyl tumors demonstrates three patterns of correspondence between the position of breakpoint sites in each tumor (A, B, C). Modified from Nikiforov et al. [67]. With permission.

RET/PTC3. It appeared that in each tumor, the relative position of a breakpoint in the *RET* gene corresponded to the location of a breakpoint in the *ELE1* gene [67]. Specifically, when the genes were aligned in opposite orientations, the breakpoints were located just across from each other in five (42%) tumors (Fig. 2A), while in the other tumors they could be aligned by sliding one gene with respect to another (Figs. 2B and C). A similar pattern can be observed if the breakpoints in the additional 22 post-Chernobyl tumors with *RET*/PTC3, mapped in a different study [68], are analyzed in the same way. In this series, eight (40%) tumors had the breakpoints located across from each other. Such a predilection for breakpoint sites in one gene to correspond to breakpoint sites located within the certain region of the other gene suggests the presence of a stable spatial relationship between these two chromosomal loci within the nucleus.

If the interaction between these loci exists, it should involve folding of chromosome 10, where both *RET* and *ELE1* genes reside separated by a linear distance of ~8 Mbp. This is conceivable since one of the levels of DNA packaging involves chromatin arrangement into loops of different size attached to a chromosomal backbone [69]. Thus, although two chromosomal loci are located at a considerable linear distance from each other, they may be closely spaced in the interphase nucleus because of their location at specific areas of chromosomal loop(s) (e.g., points a and e or f and g on Fig. 3). Similarly, folding of chromosome 10 may result in the approximation of *ELE1* and *RET* (*RET*/PTC3 partners) as well as *H4* and *RET* (*RET*/PTC1 partners) in the nuclei of thyroid cells.

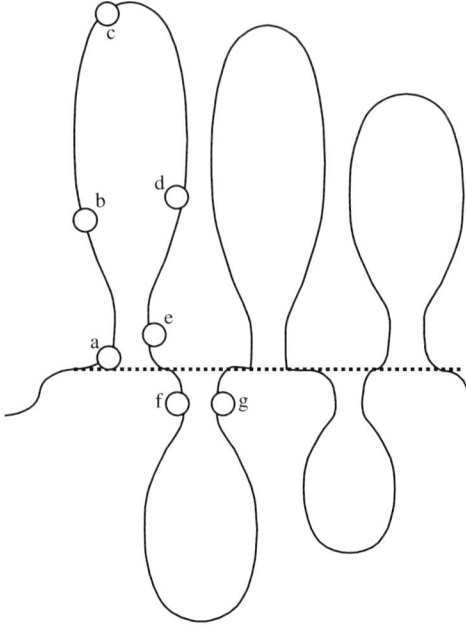

Fig. 3. A model of giant chromosomal loops attached to a flexible backbone provided by the nuclear matrix/ scaffold (dotted line). Modified from Yokota et al. [69]. Copyright Rockefeller University Press.

Indeed, we have recently demonstrated that chromosomal regions containing the *RET* and *H4* genes are juxtaposed to each other in the interphase nuclei of normal thyroid follicular cells [70]. Utilizing fluorescence *in situ* hybridization (FISH), we found that in 35% of primary cultured cells, at least one pair of *RET* and *H4* were juxtaposed. This contrasts with 6% juxtaposition observed in the control experiment between the *RET* and D10S539 loci, the latter located on chromosome 10q between *RET* and *H4* and is not known to participate in the rearrangement. In addition, two-dimensional interphase distances between *RET-H4* and *RET*-D10S539 were compared with a theoretical Rayleigh model that describes a distribution of distances between two points of linear polymers that fold in a random manner. Previous studies have shown that interphase distances between random chromosomal loci which are greater than 10 Mb apart, conform to the Rayleigh distribution [69,71]. Indeed, this was true for *RET*-D10S539 distances, indicating their random positioning in the nuclei of thyroid cells. However, *RET* and *H4* distances showed strong deviation from the Rayleigh model, primarily due to the loci that is either juxtaposed or closer than expected, indicating that *RET* and *H4* are non-randomly located with respect to each other (Fig. 4). These data suggest that the occurrence of *RET*/ PTC rearrangements in thyroid cells may be in part due to the structural organization of chromosome 10 resulting in non-random interaction and spatial approximation of potentially recombinogenic DNA loci in the nuclei of normal human thyroid cells.

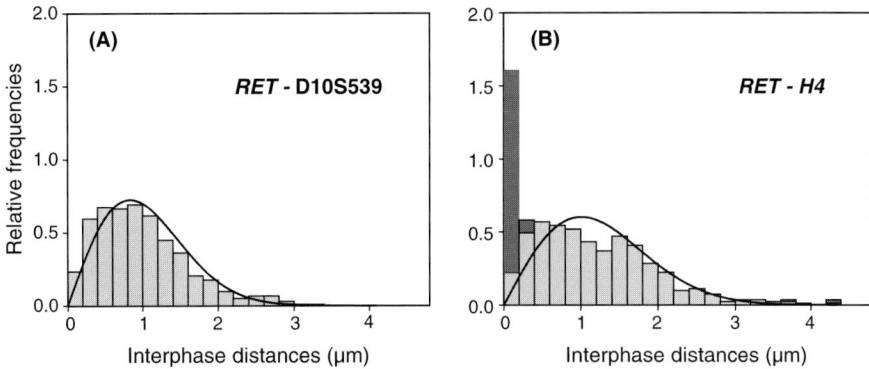

Fig. 4. Distribution of interphase distances between *RET* and D10S539 (A) and *RET* and *H4* (B) in thyroid cells as compared with the theoretical Rayleigh distribution (solid line). Dark bars indicate the *RET-H4* distances that were in excess over the number expected based on the Rayleigh distribution. Reprinted with permission from Nikiforova et al. [70]. Copyright 2000 American Association for the Advanced of Science.

It remains unclear, however, whether *RET*/PTC is a direct consequence of dsDNA breaks induced by ionizing radiation or other DNA-damaging agents, or it is formed indirectly after DNA damage is repaired. The mapping of breakpoint sites in the *RET* and *ELE1* genes in post-Chernobyl tumors with *RET*/PTC3 was expected to provide some answers. Thus, if the rearrangement occurred later as a result of activation or disruption of the recombination machinery, the breakpoints should be located within recombinase signal sequences at both participating loci, have similarity in nucleotide composition, or cluster at certain specific hypersensitive DNA regions. On the contrary, it has been clearly demonstrated that the breakpoints within and surrounding *ELE1* intron 5 and *RET* intron 11 were distributed randomly, with no breakpoints occurring at exactly the same base or within an identical sequence in any of the 41 tumors studied in three different series [66–68]. The breakpoints exhibited no particular nucleotide sequence or composition. In one study, no evidence of consistency in AT-rich regions, fragile sites, recombination-specific signal elements, or other target DNA sites (i.e., χ-like motifs, heptamer/nonamer signal sequences) implicated in illegitimate recombination in mammalian cells was found [6,7]. These data favor direct induction of *RET*/PTC as a result of random double-strand DNA breaks, rather than disruption of the recombination machinery. However, another study suggested an alternative mechanism and found at least one topoisomerase I site exactly at or in close proximity to all breakpoints, suggesting the role of DNA breaks induced by this enzyme in the generation of *RET*/PTC3 [68]. Irrespective of the exact initiation event, spatial contiguity of *RET*/PTC partners is likely to provide a structural basis for the generation of the rearrangement by facilitating simultaneous damage of adjacent DNA molecules or recombination between DNA loci located close to each other in the nuclear volume.

3. *PAX8–PPARγ* Rearrangement

Recently, a *PAX8–PPARγ* fusion has been identified in follicular thyroid carcinomas with cytogenetically detectable translocation t(2;3)(q13;p25) [72]. This finding declared the occurrence of chromosomal rearrangements in the second most common type of thyroid cancer and provided an additional evidence of distinct molecular pathways involved in the development of papillary and follicular carcinomas, both of which originate from thyroid follicular cells.

3.1. *Structure*

PAX8–PPARγ rearrangement involves the fusion between the *PAX8* and *PPARγ* genes. *PAX8* is located on chromosome 2q13 and encodes a paired domain transcription factor whose function is important in thyroid development and follicular cell differentiation [73,74]. Through its paired domain, PAX8 protein binds to the promoters of the thyroglobulin, thyroperoxidase, and sodium/iodide symporter genes and regulates their thyroid-specific expression [75,76]. Another partner of the rearrangement is the peroxisome proliferator-activated receptor *PPARγ*. PPARs are nuclear hormone receptors that, along with the receptors for thyroid hormones, retinoic acid, vitamin D, and the orphan receptors, require heterodimerization with the retinoid X receptor (RXR) for target gene activation [77]. Three related PPAR genes have been identified: *PPARα*, *PPARβ*, and *PPARγ*. *PPARγ* has been mapped to 3p25, and exists in three transcripts, PPARγ1–3, which share six common coding exons and differ at their 5′-ends as a consequence of alternate splicing [77,78]. Both *PPARγ*1 and *PPARγ*2 are highly expressed in human adipose tissue and at low level in skeletal muscles, and *PPARγ*1 has also been found in liver, heart, and some other tissues [77].

In follicular carcinomas with *PAX8–PPARγ* fusion, several transcripts are coexpressed, formed by the in-frame fusion of four *PAX8* variants (exons 1 to 7, 1 to 8, 1 to 9, or 1 to 7 plus 9) to *PPARγ* exons 1–6 [72] (Fig. 5). The different variants of the *PAX8* portion most likely result from alternate splicing involving exons 8 and 9, as shown for wild-type *PAX8* [79]. In our experience, the most commonly expressed transcripts in follicular thyroid carcinomas harboring the rearrangement are those containing exons 1 to 9 and 1 to 7 plus 9 of *PAX8*. Irrespective of the *PAX8* variant, the PAX8–PPARγ protein contains the paired and partial homeobox domains of PAX8 fused with the DNA binding, ligand binding, and RXR dimerization and transactivation domains of *PPARγ* (Fig. 6).

3.2. *Prevalence in thyroid tumors*

In the original study, *PAX8–PPARγ* fusion was identified in five of the eight (63%) follicular carcinomas, but not in follicular adenomas (0/20), papillary carcinomas (0/10) or multinodular goiter (0/10) [72]. Recently, we have extended the original study and analyzed the prevalence of *PAX8–PPARγ* in a series of 118 benign and malignant thyroid tumors [34,35]. Using RT–PCR, the fusion was detected in 8/15

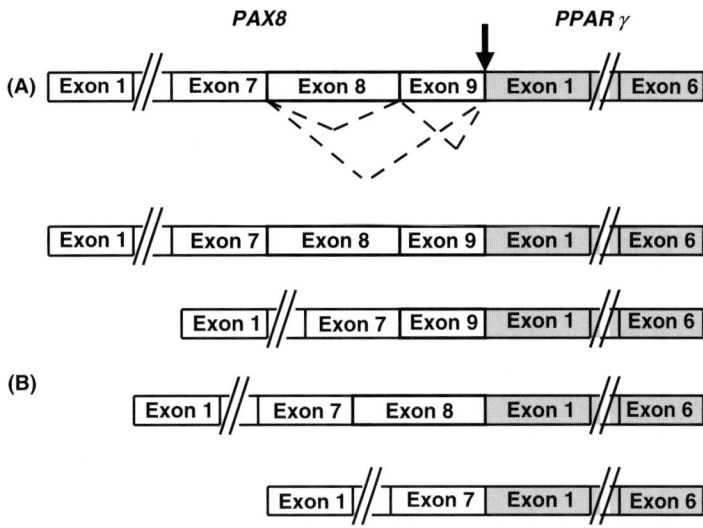

Fig. 5. Schematic representation of *PAX8–PPARγ* fusion gene (A) and different variants of the chimeric transcripts detectable in follicular thyroid tumors (B). Arrow indicates the fusion point and dashed lines the alternative splicing of the *PAX8* gene.

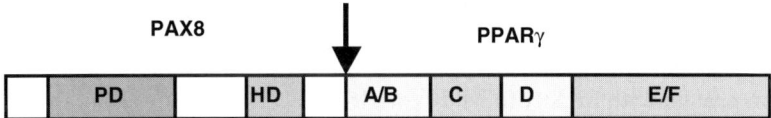

Fig. 6. Structure of PAX8–PPARγ fusion protein. It contains PAX8 paired (PD) and partial homeobox (HD) domains responsible for DNA binding, lacks PAX8 transactivation domain, and contains all PPARγ nuclear receptor domains (A–F). Arrow indicates the fusion point. Reprinted with permission from Kroll et al. [72]. Copyright 2000 American Association for the Advanced of Science.

(53%) follicular carcinomas and 2/25 (8%) follicular adenomas, but not in 35 papillary carcinomas, 12 Hurthle cell carcinomas, 12 Hurthle cell adenomas, 2 anaplastic carcinomas, 1 poorly differentiated carcinoma, or 16 hyperplastic nodules. Thus, *PAX8–PPARγ* appears to be restricted to follicular thyroid tumors, but, in addition to carcinomas, it was also found in two tumors meeting current diagnostic criteria for follicular adenomas. Both of these tumors demonstrated hypercellular trabecular growth pattern with minimal colloid formation (features of neoplastic process), but showed no invasion. It is conceivable that they are follicular carcinomas biologically programmed for invasive growth but removed at a preinvasive stage. By immunohistochemistry, diffuse nuclear immunoreactivity with *PPARγ* antibody was observed in all follicular tumors with *PAX8–PPARγ* rearrangement detectable by RT–PCR. All other types of malignant and benign thyroid tumors and normal thyroid cells demonstrated either no or very weak immunoreactivity with this anti-body, which recognizes both the rearranged and wild-type *PPARγ* protein.

Among follicular carcinomas, the prevalence of *PAX8–PPARγ* was 42% (5/12) in tumors from the general population and 100% (3/3) in tumors from patients with a history of radiation exposure [34,35]. Although only few radiation-associated follicular carcinomas were studied, a higher prevalence of *PAX8–PPARγ* in this group is intriguing. Papillary carcinoma is by far the most common type of thyroid tumors associated with radiation exposure, and, as discussed earlier, *RET*/PTC re-arrangements are highly prevalent in these populations. Follicular thyroid carcino-mas are less common in individuals subjected to irradiation, although an increased risk has been clearly documented [80]. In light of this finding, it is tempting to speculate that radiation exposure may also promote the development of follicular thyroid tumors through the generation of *PAX8–PPARγ* rearrangement.

3.3. *Biological function of* PAX8–PPARγ *and possible mechanisms of transformation*

A high prevalence of *PAX8–PPARγ* rearrangements suggests an important role of this genetic abnormality in the development of follicular thyroid cancer. However, the mechanism of *PAX8–PPARγ*-induced transformation is not yet clear. Typically, chromosomal rearrangements lead to the activation of an oncogene; this does not seem to be the case here. Thus, in U2OS cells transfected with *PAX8–PPARγ*, the fusion protein was found ineffective in inducing transactivation of several *PPARγ* response elements (PPREs) after stimulation with troglitazone [72]. Moreover, when coexpressed in the same cell with wild-type *PPARγ*, the PAX8–*PPARγ* protein com-pletely abrogated wild-type *PPARγ* activity, indicating a dominant-negative effect of the fusion protein with respect to wild-type *PPARγ* [72]. This suggested the possibility of a dominant-negative mechanism of *PAX8–PPARγ* action. Indeed, it has been shown that *PPARγ* ligands can inhibit growth and promote differentiation of certain cancer cell lines [77]. Therefore, it is conceivable that abrogation of normal *PPARγ* function is important in the development of different types of cancer, including thy-roid tumors. The potential problem with this mechanism, however, is that wild-type *PPARγ* is only weakly expressed in normal thyroid tissue and *PPARγ* protein is either undetectable or present in low amounts in thyroid follicular cells. This argues against the abrogation of normal *PPARγ* function as a key component of the molecular pathways toward follicular thyroid cancer. Another possibility is that PAX8–*PPARγ* deregulates PAX8 pathways in thyroid cell, and PAX8 function is known to be critical for thyroid cell differentiation. Finally, it is conceivable that PAX8–*PPARγ* promotes tumorigenesis through another and still unknown mechanism.

4. Concluding remarks

Thyroid cancer is an epithelial neoplasm that is characterized by chromosomal re-arrangements as a common genetic abnormality. This is unusual since large-scale rearrangements are typically found in lymphomas/leukemias and certain types of sarcomas, but not in epithelial tumors. One feature shared by thyroid cancer and other rearrangement-prone neoplasms is that all of them have ionizing radiation listed as a well-established etiologic factor. In thyroid tumors, *RET*/PTC and *PAX8–PPARγ* rearrangements are most common, and the frequency of both is significantly higher in tumors associated with radiation exposure. This points toward radiation as a possible factor directly involved in the induction of tumorigenic chromosomal rearrangements in human cells. However, overall, most thyroid tumors harboring these genetic aberrations arise in patients with no apparent history of irradiation. This raises the possibility of either unnoticed radiation exposure in many of those individuals or the existence of other factors acting in a similar way to promote the rearrangement. Another aspect of the puzzle is to understand why, despite a random distribution of radiation-induced DNA damage, some common cancer-associated chromosomal rearrangements are very specific. It is likely that the spatial proximity of different genes in the nucleus is part of the answer and needs further exploration. Finally, it remains unclear whether rearrangement occur directly by mis-rejoining of radiation-induced DNA breaks or in the indirect way. All these questions are crucial for the understanding of the mechanisms of chromosomal rearrangements in human cells and its association with radiation exposure, and should be addressed in the near future. In this respect, thyroid cancer represents a unique model of radiation carcinogenesis and is likely to be very helpful in these studies.

Acknowledgments

This work was supported by NIH grant R01 CA88041.

References

[1] M. Takahashi, J. Ritz, G.M. Cooper, Activation of a novel human transforming gene, ret, by DNA rearrangement, Cell 42 (1985) 581–588.

[2] M. Takahashi, Structure and expression of the ret transforming gene, IARC Sci. Publ. 92 (1988) 189–197.

[3] M.S. Airaksinen, A. Titievsky, M. Saarma, GDNF family neurotrophic factor signaling: four masters, one servant?, Mol. Cell. Neurosci. 13 (1999) 313–325.

[4] D.P. Smith, C. Eng, B.A. Ponder, Mutations of the RET proto-oncogene in the multiple endocrine neoplasia type 2 syndromes and Hirschsprung disease, J. Cell. Sci. Suppl. 18 (1994) 43–49.

[5] M. Grieco, M. Santoro, M.T. Berlingieri, R.M. Melillo, R. Donghi, I. Bongarzone, M.A. Pierotti, G. Della Porta, A. Fusco, G. Vecchio, PTC is a novel rearranged form of the ret proto-oncogene and is frequently detected *in vivo* in human thyroid papillary carcinomas, Cell 60 (1990) 557–563.

[6] I. Bongarzone, M.G. Butti, S. Coronelli, M.G. Borrello, M. Santoro, P. Mondellini, S. Pilotti, A. Fusco, G. Della Porta, M.A. Pierotti, Frequent activation of ret protooncogene by fusion with a new activating gene in papillary thyroid carcinomas, Cancer Res. 54 (1994) 2979–2985.

[7] M. Santoro, N.A. Dathan, M.T. Berlingieri, I. Bongarzone, C. Paulin, M. Grieco, M.A. Pierotti, G. Vecchio, A. Fusco, Molecular characterization of RET/PTC3; a novel rearranged version of the RETproto-oncogene in a human thyroid papillary carcinoma, Oncogene 9 (1994) 509 516.

[8] M.A. Pierotti, M. Santoro, R.B. Jenkins, G. Sozzi, I. Bongarzone, M. Grieco, N. Monzini, M. Miozzo, M.A. Herrmann, A. Fusco, et al., Characterization of an inversion on the long arm of

chromosome 10 juxtaposing D10S170 and RET and creating the oncogenic sequence RET/PTC, Proc. Natl. Acad. Sci. U S A 89 (1992) 1616–1620.

[9] F. Minoletti, M.G. Butti, S. Coronelli, M. Miozzo, G. Sozzi, S. Pilotti, A. Tunnacliffe, M.A. Pierotti, I. Bongarzone, The two genes generating RET/PTC3 are localized in chromosomal band 10q11.2, Genes Chromosomes Cancer 11 (1994) 51–57.

[10] I. Bongarzone, N. Monzini, M.G. Borrello, C. Carcano, G. Ferraresi, E. Arighi, P. Mondellini, G. Della Porta, M.A. Pierotti, Molecular characterization of a thyroid tumor-specific transforming sequence formed by the fusion of ret tyrosine kinase and the regulatory subunit RI alpha of cyclic AMP-dependent protein kinase A, Mol. Cell. Biol. 13 (1993) 358–366.

[11] S. Klugbauer, E.P. Demidchik, E. Lengfelder, H.M. Rabes, Detection of a novel type of RET rearrangement (PTC5) in thyroid carcinomas after Chernobyl and analysis of the involved RET-fused gene RFG5, Cancer Res. 58 (1998) 198–203.

[12] S. Klugbauer, H.M. Rabes, The transcription coactivator HTIF1 and a related protein are fused to the RET receptor tyrosine kinase in childhood papillary thyroid carcinomas, Oncogene 18 (1999) 4388–4393.

[13] R. Corvi, N. Berger, R. Balczon, G. Romeo, RET/PCM-1: a novel fusion gene in papillary thyroid carcinoma, Oncogene 19 (2000) 4236–4242.

[14] S. Klugbauer, A. Jauch, E. Lengfelder, E. Demidchik, H.M. Rabes, A novel type of RET rearrangement (PTC8) in childhood papillary thyroid carcinomas and characterization of the involved gene (RFG8), Cancer Res. 60 (2000) 7028–7032.

[15] K. Salassidis, J. Bruch, H. Zitzelsberger, E. Lengfelder, A.M. Kellerer, M. Bauchinger, Translocation t(10;14)(q11.2:q22.1) fusing the kinetin to the RET gene creates a novel rearranged form (PTC8) of the RET proto-oncogene in radiation-induced childhood papillary thyroid carcinoma, Cancer Res. 60 (2000) 2786–2789.

[16] T. Nakata, Y. Kitamura, K. Shimizu, S. Tanaka, M. Fujimori, S. Yokoyama, K. Ito, M. Emi, Fusion of a novel gene, ELKS, to RET due to translocation t(10;12)(q11;p13) in a papillary thyroid carcinoma, Genes Chromosomes Cancer 25 (1999) 97–103.

[17] Q. Tong, S. Xing, S.M. Jhiang, Leucine zipper-mediated dimerization is essential for the PTC1 oncogenic activity, J. Biol. Chem. 272 (1997) 9043–9047.

[18] S.M. Jhiang, The RET proto-oncogene in human cancers, Oncogene 19 (2000) 5590–5597.

[19] D. Salvatore, M.V. Barone, G. Salvatore, R.M. Melillo, G. Chiappetta, A. Mineo, G. Fenzi, G. Vecchio, A. Fusco, M. Santoro, Tyrosines 1015 and 1062 are *in vivo* autophosphorylation sites in ret and ret-derived oncoproteins, J. Clin. Endocrinol. Metab. 85 (2000) 3898–3907.

[20] M.A. Pierotti, I. Bongarzone, M.G. Borello, A. Greco, S. Pilotti, G. Sozzi, Cytogenetics and molecular genetics of carcinomas arising from thyroid epithelial follicular cells, Genes Chromosomes Cancer 16 (1996) 1–14.

[21] C. Monaco, R. Visconti, M.V. Barone, G.M. Pierantoni, M.T. Berlingieri, C. De Lorenzo, A. Mineo, G. Vecchio, A. Fusco, M. Santoro, The RFG oligomerization domain mediates kinase activation and re-localization of the RET/PTC3 oncoprotein to the plasma membrane, Oncogene 20 (2001) 599–608.

[22] A. Fusco, M. Grieco, M. Santoro, M.T. Berlingieri, S. Pilotti, M.A. Pierotti, G. Della Porta, G. Vecchio, A new oncogene in human thyroid papillary carcinomas and their lymph-nodal metastases, Nature 328 (1987) 170–172.

[23] M. Santoro, R.M. Melillo, M. Grieco, M.T. Berlingieri, G. Vecchio, A. Fusco, The TRK and RET tyrosine kinase oncogenes cooperate with ras in the neoplastic transformation of a rat thyroid epithelial cell line, Cell Growth Differ. 4 (1993) 77–84.

[24] D.J. Powell, J. Russell Jr., K. Nibu, G. Li, E. Rhee, M. Liao, M. Goldstein, W.M. Keane, M. Santoro, A. Fusco, J.L. Rothstein, The RET/PTC3 oncogene: metastatic solid-type papillary carcinomas in murine thyroids, Cancer Res. 58 (1998) 5523–5528.

[25] K.M. La Perle, S.M. Jhiang, C.C. Capen, Loss of p53 promotes anaplasia and local invasion in ret/PTC1-induced thyroid carcinomas, Am. J. Pathol. 157 (2000) 671–677.

[26] A.H. Fischer, J.A. Bond, P. Taysavang, O.E. Battles, D. Wynford-Thomas, Papillary thyroid carcinoma oncogene (RET/PTC) alters the nuclear envelope and chromatin structure, Am. J. Pathol. 153 (1998) 1443–1450.

[27] M. Santoro, F. Carlomagno, I.D. Hay, M.A. Herrmann, M. Grieco, R. Melillo, M.A. Pierotti, I. Bongarzone, G. Della Porta, N. Berger, et al., Ret oncogene activation in human thyroid neoplasms is restricted to the papillary cancer subtype, J. Clin. Invest. 89 (1992) 1517–1522.

[28] G. Tallini, M. Santoro, M. Helie, F. Carlomagno, G. Salvatore, G. Chiappetta, M.L. Carcangiu, A. Fusco, RET/PTC oncogene activation defines a subset of papillary thyroid carcinomas lacking evidence of progression to poorly differentiated or undifferentiated tumor phenotypes, Clin. Cancer Res. 4 (1998) 287–294.

[29] C.C. Cheung, S.L. Boerner, C.M. MacMillan, L. Ramyar, S.L. Asa, Hyalinizing trabecular tumor of the thyroid: a variant of papillary carcinoma proved by molecular genetics, Am. J. Surg. Pathol. 24 (2000) 1622–1626.

[30] M. Papotti, M. Volante, A. Giuliano, A. Fassina, A. Fusco, G. Bussolati, M. Santoro, G. Chiappetta, RET/PTC activation in hyalinizing trabecular tumors of the thyroid, Am. J. Surg. Pathol. 24 (2000) 1615–1621.

[31] Y.E. Nikiforov, RET/PTC rearrangement in thyroid tumors, Endocr. Pathol. 13 (2002) 3–16.

[32] S.M. Jhiang, D.R. Caruso, E. Gilmore, Y. Ishizaka, T. Tahira, M. Nagao, I.M. Chiu, E.L. Mazzaferri, Detection of the PTC/retTPC oncogene in human thyroid cancers, Oncogene 7 (1992) 1331–1337.

[33] A.K. Lam, K.T. Montone, K.A. Nolan, V.A. Livolsi, Ret oncogene activation in papillary thyroid carcinoma: prevalence and implication on the histological parameters, Hum. Pathol. 29 (1998) 565–568.

[34] M.N. Nikiforova, P.W. Biddinger, C.M. Caudill, Y.E. Nikiforov, Prevalence of RET/PTC rearrangements in Hashimoto's thyroiditis and papillary thyroid carcinomas, Int. J. Surg. Pathol. 10 (2002) 15–22.

[35] M.N. Nikiforova, P.W. Biddinger, C.M. Caudill, T.G. Kroll, Y.E. Nikiforov, PAX8–PPARg rearrangement in thyroid tumors: RT-PCR and immunohistochemical analyses, Am. J. Surg. Pathol., 26 (2002) 1016–1023.

[36] S.L. Sugg, S. Ezzat, L. Zheng, J.L. Freeman, I.B. Rosen, S.L. Asa, Oncogene profile of papillary thyroid carcinoma, Surgery 125 (1999) 46–52.

[37] I. Bongarzone, L. Fugazzola, P. Vigneri, L. Mariani, P. Mondellini, F. Pacini, F. Basolo, A. Pinchera, S. Pilotti, M.A. Pierotti, Age-related activation of the tyrosine kinase receptor protooncogenes RET and NTRK1 in papillary thyroid carcinoma, J. Clin. Endocrinol. Metab. 81 (1996) 2006–2009.

[38] I. Bongarzone, P. Vigneri, L. Mariani, P. Collini, S. Pilotti, M.A. Pierotti, RET/NTRK1 rearrangements in thyroid gland tumors of the papillary carcinoma family: correlation with clinicopathological features, Clin. Cancer Res. 4 (1998) 223–228.

[39] M. Zou, Y. Shi, N.R. Farid, Low rate of ret proto-oncogene activation (PTC/retTPC) in papillary thyroid carcinomas from Saudi Arabia, Cancer 73 (1994) 176–180.

[40] E.L. Chua, W.M. Wu, K.T. Tran, S.W. McCarthy, C.S. Lauer, D. Dubourdieu, N. Packham, C.J. O'Brien, J.R. Turtle, Q. Dong, Prevalence and distribution of ret/ptc 1, 2, and 3 in papillary thyroid carcinoma in New Caledonia and Australia, J. Clin. Endocrinol. Metab. 85 (2000) 2733–2739.

[41] W. Wajjwalku, S. Nakamura, Y. Hasegawa, K. Miyazaki, Y. Satoh, H. Funahashi, M. Matsuyama, M. Takahashi, Low frequency of rearrangements of the ret and trk proto-oncogenes in Japanese thyroid papillary carcinomas, Jpn. J. Cancer Res. 83 (1992) 671–675.

[42] T. Motomura, Y.E. Nikiforov, H. Namba, K. Ashizawa, S. Nagataki, S. Yamashita, J.A. Fagin, ret rearrangements in Japanese pediatric and adult papillary thyroid cancers, Thyroid 8 (1998) 485–489.

[43] D.L. Learoyd, M. Messina, J. Zedenius, A.I. Guinea, L.W. Delbridge, B.G. Robinson, RET/PTC and RET tyrosine kinase expression in adult papillary thyroid carcinomas, J. Clin. Endocrinol. Metab. 83 (1998) 3631–3635.

[44] Y.E. Nikiforov, J.M. Rowland, K.E. Bove, H. Monforte-Munoz, J.A. Fagin, Distinct pattern of ret oncogene rearrangements in morphological variants of radiation-induced and sporadic thyroid papillary carcinomas in children, Cancer Res. 57 (1997) 1690–1694.

[45] P. Soares, E. Fonseca, D. Wynford-Thomas, M. Sobrinho-Simoes, Sporadic ret-rearranged papillary carcinoma of the thyroid: a subset of slow growing, less aggressive thyroid neoplasms?, J. Pathol. 185 (1998) 71–78.

[46] C.L. Fenton, Y. Lukes, D. Nicholson, C.A. Dinauer, G.L. Francis, R.M. Tuttle, The ret/PTC mutations are common in sporadic papillary thyroid carcinoma of children and young adults, J. Clin. Endocrinol. Metab. 85 (2000) 1170–1175.

[47] L. Fugazzola, S. Pilotti, A. Pinchera, T.V. Vorontsova, P. Mondellini, I. Bongarzone, A. Greco, L. Astakhova, M.G. Butti, E.P. Demidchik, Oncogenic rearrangements of the RET proto-oncogene in papillary thyroid carcinomas from children exposed to the Chernobyl nuclear accident, Cancer Res. 55 (1995) 5617–5620.

[48] S. Klugbauer, E. Lengfelder, E.P. Demidchik, H.M. Rabes, High prevalence of RET rearrangement in thyroid tumors of children from Belarus after the Chernobyl reactor accident, Oncogene 11 (1995) 2459–2467.

[49] J. Smida, K. Salassidis, L. Hieber, H. Zitzelsberger, A.M. Kellerer, E.P. Demidchik, T. Negele, F. Spelsberg, E. Lengfelder, M. Werner, M. Bauchinger, Distinct frequency of ret rearrangements in papillary thyroid carcinomas of children and adults from Belarus, Int. J. Cancer 80 (1999) 32–38.

[50] H.M. Rabes, E.P. Demidchik, J.D. Sidorow, E. Lengfelder, C. Beimfohr, D. Hoelzel, S. Klugbauer, Pattern of radiation-induced RET and NTRK1 rearrangements in 191 post-chernobyl papillary thyroid carcinomas: biological, phenotypic, and clinical implications, Clin. Cancer Res. 6 (2000) 1093–1103.

[51] A. Bounacer, R. Wicker, B. Caillou, A.F. Cailleux, A. Sarasin, M. Schlumberger, H.G. Suarez, High prevalence of activating ret proto-oncogene rearrangements, in thyroid tumors from patients who had received external radiation, Oncogene 15 (1997) 1263–1273.

[52] R. Elisei, C. Romei, T. Vorontsova, B. Cosci, V. Veremeychik, E. Kuchinskaya, F. Basolo, E.P. Demidchik, P. Miccoli, A. Pinchera, F. Pacini, RET/PTC rearrangements in thyroid nodules: studies in irradiated and not irradiated, malignant and benign thyroid lesions in children and adults, J. Clin. Endocrinol. Metab. 86 (2001) 3211–3216.

[53] S. Klugbauer, E.P. Demidchik, E. Lengfelder, H.M. Rabes, Molecular analysis of new subtypes of ELE/RET rearrangements, their reciprocal transcripts and breakpoints in papillary thyroid carcinomas of children after Chernobyl, Oncogene 16 (1998) 671–675.

[54] H.M. Rabes, Gene rearrangements in radiation-induced thyroid carcinogenesis, Med. Pediatr. Oncol. 36 (2001) 574–582.

[55] T. Ito, T. Seyama, K.S. Iwamoto, T. Hayashi, T. Mizuno, N. Tsuyama, K. Dohi, N. Nakamura, M. Akiyama, *In vitro* irradiation is able to cause RET oncogene rearrangement, Cancer Res. 53 (1993) 2940–2943.

[56] T. Mizuno, S. Kyoizumi, T. Suzuki, K.S. Iwamoto, T. Seyama, Continued expression of a tissue specific activated oncogene in the early steps of radiation-induced human thyroid carcinogenesis, Oncogene 15 (1997) 1455–1460.

[57] T. Mizuno, K.S. Iwamoto, S. Kyoizumi, H. Nagamura, T. Shinohara, K. Koyama, T. Seyama, K. Hamatani, Preferential induction of RET/PTC1 rearrangement by X-ray irradiation, Oncogene 19 (2000) 438–443.

[58] G. Viglietto, G. Chiappetta, F.J. Martinez-Tello, F.H. Fukunaga, G. Tallini, D. Rigopoulou, R. Visconti, A. Mastro, M. Santoro, A. Fusco, RET/PTC oncogene activation is an early event in thyroid carcinogenesis, Oncogene 11 (1995) 1207–1210.

[59] S.L. Sugg, S. Ezzat, I.B. Rosen, J.L. Freeman, S.L. Asa, Distinct multiple RET/PTC gene rearrangements in multifocal papillary thyroid neoplasia, J. Clin. Endocrinol. Metab. 83 (1998) 4116–4122.

[60] F. Basolo, R. Giannini, C. Monaco, R.M. Melillo, F. Carlomagno, M. Pancrazi, G. Salvatore, G. Chiappetta, F. Pacini, R. Elisei, P. Miccoli, A. Pinchera, A. Fusco, M. Santoro, Potent mitogenicity of the RET/PTC3 oncogene correlates with its prevalence in tall-cell variant of papillary thyroid carcinoma, Am. J. Pathol. 160 (2002) 247–254.

[61] G.A. Thomas, H. Bunnell, H.A. Cook, E.D. Williams, A. Nerovnya, E.D. Cherstvoy, N.D. Tronko, T.I. Bogdanova, G. Chiappetta, G. Viglietto, F. Pentimalli, G. Salvatore, A. Fusco, M. Santoro, G. Vecchio, High prevalence of RET/PTC rearrangements in Ukrainian and Belarussian post-Chernobyl thyroid papillary carcinomas: a strong correlation between RET/PTC3 and the solid-follicular variant, J. Clin. Endocrinol. Metab. 84 (1999) 4232–4238.

[62] S.M. Jhiang, J.E. Sagartz, Q. Tong, J. Parker-Thornburg, C.C. Capen, J.Y. Cho, S. Xing, C. Ledent, Targeted expression of the ret/PTC1 oncogene induces papillary thyroid carcinomas, Endocrinology 137 (1996) 375–378.

[63] M. Santoro, G. Chiappetta, A. Cerrato, D. Salvatore, L. Zhang, G. Manzo, A. Picone, G. Portella, G. Santelli, G. Vecchio, A. Fusco, Development of thyroid papillary carcinomas secondary to tissue-specific expression of the RET/PTC1 oncogene in transgenic mice, Oncogene 12 (1996) 1821–1826.

[64] J.E. Sagartz, S.M. Jhiang, Q. Tong, C.C. Capen, Thyroid-stimulating hormone promotes growth of thyroid carcinomas in transgenic mice with targeted expression of the ret/PTC1 oncogene, Lab. Invest. 76 (1997) 307–318.

[65] P.A. Smanik, T.L. Furminger, E.L. Mazzaferri, S.M. Jhiang, Breakpoint characterization of the ret/PTC oncogene in human papillary thyroid carcinoma, Hum. Mol. Genet. 4 (1995) 2313–2318.

[66] I. Bongarzone, M.G. Butti, L. Fugazzola, F. Pacini, A. Pinchera, T.V. Vorontsova, E.P. Demidchik, M.A. Pierotti, Comparison of the breakpoint regions of ELE1 and RET genes involved in the generation of RET/PTC3 oncogene in sporadic and in radiation-associated papillary thyroid carcinomas, Genomics 42 (1997) 252–259.

[67] Y.E. Nikiforov, A. Koshoffer, M. Nikiforova, J. Stringer, J.A. Fagin, Chromosomal breakpoint positions suggest a direct role for radiation in inducing illegitimate recombination between the ELE1 and RET genes in radiation-induced thyroid carcinomas, Oncogene 18 (1999) 6330–6334.

[68] S. Klugbauer, P. Pfeiffer, H. Gassenhuber, C. Beimfohr, H.M. Rabes, RET rearrangements in radiation-induced papillary thyroid carcinomas: high prevalence of topoisomerase I sites at breakpoints and microhomology-mediated end joining in ELE1 and RET chimeric genes, Genomics 73 (2001) 149–160.

[69] H. Yokota, G. van den Engh, J.E. Hearst, R.K. Sachs, B.J. Trask, Evidence for the organization of chromatin in megabase pair-sized loops arranged along a random walk path in the human G0/G1 interphase nucleus, J. Cell Biol. 130 (1995) 1239–1249.

[70] M.N. Nikiforova, J.R. Stringer, R. Blough, M. Medvedovic, J.A. Fagin, Y.E. Nikiforov, Proximity of chromosomal loci that participate in radiation-induced rearrangements in human cells, Science 290 (2000) 138–141.

[71] G. van den Engh, R. Sachs, B.J. Trask, Estimating genomic distance from DNA sequence location in cell nuclei by a random walk model, Science 257 (1992) 1410–1412.

[72] T.G. Kroll, P. Sarraf, L. Pecciarini, C.J. Chen, E. Mueller, B.M. Spiegelman, J.A. Fletcher, PAX8–PPARgamma1 fusion oncogene in human thyroid carcinoma, Science 289 (2000) 1357–1360.

[73] A. Poleev, H. Fickenscher, S. Mundlos, A. Winterpacht, B. Zabel, A. Fidler, P. Gruss, D. Plachov, PAX8 a human paired box gene: isolation and expression in developing thyroid kidney, and Wilms' tumors, Development 116 (1992) 611–623.

[74] A. Mansouri, K. Chowdhury, P. Gruss, Follicular cells of the thyroid gland require Pax8 gene function, Nat. Genet. 19 (1998) 87–90.

[75] M. Zannini, H. Francis-Lang, D. Plachov, R. Di Lauro, Pax-8, a paired domain-containing protein, binds to a sequence overlapping the recognition site of a homeodomain and activates transcription from two thyroid-specific promoters, Mol. Cell Biol. 12 (1992) 4230–4241.

[76] M. Ohno, M. Zannini, O. Levy, N. Carrasco, R. di Lauro, The paired-domain transcription factor Pax8 binds to the upstream enhancer of the rat sodium/iodide symporter gene and participates in both thyroid-specific and cyclic-AMP-dependent transcription, Mol. Cell. Biol. 19 (1999) 2051–2060.

[77] B. Desvergne, W. Wahli, Peroxisome proliferator-activated receptors: nuclear control of metabolism, Endocr. Rev. 20 (1999) 649–688.

[78] M.E. Greene, B. Blumberg, O.W. McBride, H.F. Yi, K. Kronquist, K. Kwan, L. Hsieh, G. Greene, S.D. Nimer, Isolation of the human peroxisome proliferator activated receptor gamma cDNA: expression in hematopoietic cells and chromosomal mapping, Gene Expr. 4 (1995) 281–299.

[79] A. Poleev, F. Wendler, H. Fickenscher, M.S. Zannini, K. Yaginuma, C. Abbott, D. Plachov, Distinct functional properties of three human paired-box-protein, PAX8, isoforms generated by alternative splicing in thyroid, kidney and Wilms' tumors, Eur. J. Biochem. 228 (1995) 899–911.

[80] R.E. Shore, Issues and epidemiological evidence regarding radiation-induced thyroid cancer, Radiat. Res. 131 (1992) 98–111.

Chapter 2

Molecular markers of thyroid nodules

Nikolaos Stathathos[1], Matthew D. Ringel[1,2]

[1]Section of Endocrinology, Washington Hospital Center/MedStar Research Institute and Division of
Endocrinology and Metabolism, Georgetown University School of Medicine, Washington, DC 20010, USA;
[2]Division of Endocrinology, Oncology, and Human Cancer Genetics, The Ohio State University and Arthur
G. James Cancer Center, Columbus, OH 43210, USA

1. Introduction

Thyroid nodules are extremely common in the general population with prevalence
rates approaching 50–60% of adults under the age of 60 years. Although most nodules are benign, approximately 5% are malignant; thus, accurate preoperative characterization of thyroid nodules is critical for the best management of patients. Since
its initial description, fine needle aspiration (FNA) has become the diagnostic procedure of choice in the evaluation of thyroid nodules. For small, solid nodules, FNA
can accurately characterize the majority of benign nodules and papillary cancers.
However, cytological features are not helpful in distinguishing benign from malignant
follicular neoplasms, and cystic lesions that can occasionally represent papillary cancers may be difficult to interpret due to scant cellularity. Finally, cytopathology is
quite subjective, even in the most experienced hands. For these reasons, a major area
of research in thyroidology has been to identify new methods that may be applied to
FNA samples to aid in the preoperative characterization of thyroid nodules.

With the advent of molecular diagnostics, in which small amounts of clinical
samples can be analyzed by molecular analysis, the possibility of improving FNA-
based characterization of thyroid nodules is now possible. In the following review,
we will study the best-studied and most promising molecular markers (Table 1) for
thyroid FNA.

1.1. Telomerase

Telomeres are specialized structures at the ends of chromosomes that play an important
role in chromosome protection, positioning and replication [1]. In vertebrate chromosomes, telomeres consist of tandem repeats of the sequence TTAGGG. Chromosomes
lose about 50–200 nucleotides of telomeric sequence per cell division, because of an
inability of DNA polymerase to replicate the ends of linear DNA. This mechanism has

ADVANCES IN MOLECULAR AND CELLULAR ENDOCRINOLOGY
VOLUME 4   ISSN 1569-2566/DOI 10.1016/S1569-2566(04)04002-5

Table 1
Molecular markers

Potential diagnostic markers for thyroid nodules

1. Telomerase	11. GLUT-1
2. Galectin-3	12. CA 19-9, CD 15, HMBE-1[a]
3. Thyroid peroxidase (TPO)	13. CD 30
4. Oncofetal fibronectin	14. CD 57
5. ret/PTC oncogene	15. CD 97
6. Pax8/PPAR· oncogene	16. Leu-7, EMA, EGF[a]
7. Nm23	17. Cyclooxygenase 2
8. High-mobility group I (Y) protein	
9. Ceruloplasmin	
10. Cytokeratin 19	

Note: This represents only a partial list of all the potential markers investigated for the detection of various malignancies, but includes the ones best studied for thyroid tumors.
[a]Markers grouped were studied together.

been described as the 'biological clock' for cells because once they are shortened below a critical length, cell growth stops and apoptosis is induced. This process may also represent a defense mechanism against the development of malignancy.

Telomerase, an enzyme that extends telomeric structures, thereby slowing this 'biological clock' mechanism, was recently cloned and found to be a ribonucleic acid–protein complex containing a catalytic component, the human telomerase reverse transcriptase (hTERT) [2]. Telomerase expression and activity have been identified in immortalized human cell lines and cells from human malignant tissues but not in most normal human tissues. When telomerase activity was investigated by a PCR-based assay telomeric repeat amplification Protocol (TRAP) in various benign and malignant human tissues, expression was primarily noted not only in malignant tissues but also in other cells, such as germinal cells of the ovary and testis [1]. Based on these results, the potential value of using telomerase to distinguish the benign from malignant tissues has been the focus of intensive investigations for several types of human malignancies including thyroid cancers.

In a study of 30 papillary thyroid cancers, three benign nodules and 10 normal surgical thyroid specimens, Saji et al. [3] reported that 67% of the malignant tissues, compared with 0% of the benign nodules, had telomerase activity by TRAP assay. Of interest was the fact that 64% of the papillary thyroid cancers that had a non-diagnostic preoperative FNA were positive for telomerase activity. Haugen et al. [4] and Onoda et al. [5] also obtained similar results when they investigated similar surgical thyroid specimens.

The ability of telomerase to differentiate follicular cancer from follicular adenoma has also been reported. Umbricht et al. [6] studied frozen tissue samples from patients undergoing thyroidectomy for follicular neoplasm. TRAP assays were performed on 44 thyroid tissue specimens classified as follicular neoplasms by intraoperative FNA and 22 normal thyroid tissue samples. The authors report a sensitivity of 100% and a specificity of 76% using the final postoperative pathology as the gold-standard diagnostic technique. Potential complicating factors for this technique are the false-positive results due to the telomerase activity of lymphocytes often present in thyroid tissues (benign or malignant) and false-negative results due to PCR inhibitors in the tissues. An interesting statistical correlation ($p = 0.001$) was noted between the tumor size and telomerase activity. It is possible that the presence of telomerase activity in histologically 'benign' specimens may represent an early step in the development of an invasive tumor, prior to microscopically detectable invasion (capsular or vascular invasion, the most common finding that classifies a follicular tumor as malignant).

De Deken et al. [7] demonstrated a decrease in telomere length as well as increased variability in the telomere size in benign nodules as compared with normal thyroid tissues. This finding suggests that the cells of these benign nodules may have progressed through a greater number of mitotic divisions and therefore may be closer to their limit for further growth. The absence of telomerase activity in these nodules is probably consistent with their benign nature.

More recently, the human telomerase reverse transcriptase cDNA was cloned allowing for RT–PCR of its mRNA product. This created an opportunity to design a more user-friendly telomerase assay than the laborious TRAP assay. Saji et al. [8] studied 19 malignant and 18 benign thyroid tumors for the evidence of hTERT gene expression. hTERT mRNA was detected in 15 (79%) of the malignant tumors compared with 5 (28%) of the benign ones. All five benign lesions that were positive had a lymphocytic infiltration, a known source of telomerase activity that can cause false-positive results. HTERT mRNA was not detected in any of the normal thyroid specimens. The same authors also showed that this assay could be applied to FNA specimens [9].

FNA specimens were also investigated for telomerase activity by TRAP assay. Sebesta et al. [10] failed to show any additional usefulness of measuring telomerase activity in a small study of FNA samples. It is possible that RT–PCR of the hTERT is a more sensitive technique in the case of limited cellular material, as is commonly the case for FNA specimens.

The frequency of telomerase positivity by any method varies significantly between different studies. For example, some report that as many as 67% of papillary thyroid cancers are positive [3], while others indicate a much lower percentage of about 20% [11]. The small number of cases in many of these studies makes interpretation quite difficult. A similar conflict seems to exist for the ability of this test to predict aggressiveness of the thyroid tumors, with some studies indicating correlation between telomerase activity and tumor progression [5,12] while others do not [3]. It is clear that larger, more extensive studies are needed before telomerase can be considered an effective diagnostic tool.

1.2. *Galectin-3*

Galectin-3 is a member of the lectin family and is involved in regulating the function of specific protein targets by interacting with attached galactose-containing glycoproteins. As a group, galectins have been implicated in cell growth and differentiation, intercellular recognition and adhesion as well as malignant transformation. Galectin-3 has been directly correlated with neoplastic transformation and metastatic capacity in fibrosarcoma and melanoma cells. *In vitro* studies have indicated that expression of galectin proteins is elevated in thyroid cancer cell lines [13]. This has led to their investigation as molecular markers used to distinguish between benign and malignant thyroid tissues.

In a study of 41 surgical thyroid specimens, Xu et al. [14] performed western-blot analysis for galectin-1 and galectin-3 and found elevated levels of both proteins in thyroid cancer tissues compared with normal thyroid tissue. Similarly, immunohistochemistry demonstrated that normal thyroid tissue did not express galectin-1 or galectin-3, but the surrounding stromal cells stained for galectin, probably accounting for the weak bands seen in normal thyroid tissues on Western blots. In contrast to the benign specimens, all papillary and follicular thyroid carcinomas expressed high levels of galectin-1 and galectin-3. This strong positivity was maintained in one specimen from a regional lymph node metastasis of a primary papillary thyroid carcinoma.

In a similar study of 41 malignant and 35 benign thyroid tissue specimens [15], galectin-3 was found to be expressed in 18 of 18 papillary cancers (primary and metastatic lesions), 4 of 8 follicular cancers, 2 of 3 poorly differentiated cancers, 5 of 5 anaplastic cancers, 3 of 6 medullary and 1 of 1 Hurthle cell cancers. By contrast, none of the benign tissues, including normal tissue, hyperplastic nodules, nodular goiters and follicular adenomas expressed galectin-3. The only exception was noted in inflammatory areas of the benign tissues. This is consistent with early reports indicating that galectin-3 is a product of inflammatory cells such as macrophages and has some role in inflammatory processes [16]. As with other markers, differences were noted in the intensity and distribution of galectin-3 expression in the malignant tissues, but in contrast to other markers studied, galectin-3 seemed to be much more specific. Northern-blot analysis of galectin-3 mRNA was performed on a limited number of cases that suggested a correlation between mRNA and protein levels [15]. Galectin-3 mRNA was overexpressed in the papillary cancers studied while it was undetectable in benign tumors.

Galectin-3 immunocytochemistry has been investigated in FNA specimens from both benign and malignant thyroid tissues. In a retrospective study, Orlandi et al. [17] evaluated specimens from 64 patients who had undergone thyroidectomy. The preoperative diagnosis based on routine FNA cytology was malignant in 15 cases, indeterminate in 37 and benign in 12. The final histologic diagnosis included 18 papillary and 17 follicular cancers, as well as 29 follicular adenomas. All papillary thyroid cancers demonstrated strong expression of galectin-3 in both FNA and surgical specimens. For the follicular cancers, all were positive from the surgical specimens (although at varying degrees of intensity), but 3 FNA specimens were negative. These were noted to have the weakest galectin-3 expression in their corresponding surgical specimens. Three of twenty-nine benign follicular adenomas expressed galectin-3. These were noted to have some cellular features of malignancy, such as an increasing nucleus, cytoplasm ratio, hypercellularity and increased mitoses, but there was no invasion of the surrounding tissues, blood vessels and lymph channels. As a result, they were classified as benign follicular adenomas.

In a more recent study [18], antibodies against human, not mammalian, galectin-3 were used on 13 benign and 62 malignant thyroid surgical specimens. There was a clear predominance in reactivity for the papillary thyroid cancer (33 of 45), but some benign lesions were also positive (1 of 3 adenomas and 2 of 5 Hurthle cell adenomas). Also, some of the malignancies, including some of the papillary cancers (especially the tall variant), were negative.

Based on the above results, galectin-3 immunocytochemistry seems to be one of the best markers currently available for thyroid malignancies and may be useful in routine analysis of FNA samples. A large, multicenter trial evaluated the utility of galectin-3 as a marker for thyroid cancer (Bartolazzi A, Lancet 357, 1644, 2001). A retrospective component of this study revealed 96% sensitivity and 97% specificity on surgical specimens and a prospective study of 226 FNAB specimens showed a 100% sensitivity and 94% specificity for this molecular marker. While these data are encouraging, more prospective studies on FNAB cytology from indeterminate nodules are needed to recommend galectin-3 for routine use.

1.3. *Thyroid peroxidase*

Thyroid peroxidase (TPO) is a thyroid-specific enzyme that catalyzes iodide oxidation, thyroglobulin iodination and iodothyronine coupling. Reduced activity or expression of TPO impairs thyroid follicular cell function by reducing iodide trapping and impairing thyroid hormone synthesis. Moreover, TPO has also been shown to suppress thyroid cell proliferation and its loss has been associated with thyroid carcinogenesis. Thus, immunohistochemical staining for TPO expression of both FNA samples and surgical specimens has been investigated

In a retrospective study of 150 FNA samples from surgical specimens [19], more than 80% of cells from 113 of 125 benign lesions stained positive for TPO, while in all cases of thyroid malignancies, less than 80% of cells were positive, giving this test a sensitivity of 100% and a specificity of 90% using 80% staining as a cutoff.

In a large prospective study of 124 FNAs [20], immunohistochemical staining for TPO correctly identified all cases of cancer (as diagnosed by conventional FNA cytology and postoperative tissue examinations). The study used the same cutoff of 80% for the percentage of TPO-stained cells to distinguish between the benign and malignant tissues, as well as the same monoclonal antibody against TPO (MoAb47). Only one of the benign lesions (a follicular adenoma) was incorrectly identified as malignant by these immunohistochemical criteria as well as preoperative routine FNA cytology. The investigators concluded that TPO immunohistochemistry of FNA samples using the 80% cutoff values has a sensitivity of 100% and a specificity of 99%.

Because germline mutations resulting in a loss of TPO function have been identified as a cause of congenital hypothyroidism, loss of this heterozygocity has been implicated as a potential cause for the development of hypoactive thyroid nodules and thyroid cancer. In a study of 40 hypoactive thyroid nodules [21], loss of heterozygocity near the locus of the TPO gene was noted on six of the specimens. It is therefore probable that other mechanisms account for the reduced TPO levels in thyroid cancers.

1.4. *Oncofetal fibronectin*

Fibronectins are high-molecular-weight adhesive glycoproteins present in the extracellular matrix and in body fluids. Oncofetal fibronectin is characterized by the presence of the oncofetal domain (IIICS domain), which is absent in normal fibronectin. The usefulness of this molecule as a marker has been investigated in several malignancies such as cancers of the breast, colon and stomach. More recently, it has also been studied in thyroid tumors.

Several investigators have evaluated the utility of the oncofetal fibronectin mRNA as a marker. In a study of 19 malignant and 33 benign surgical thyroid specimens, Higashiyama et al. [22] found significantly elevated levels in papillary and anaplastic cancers as compared with benign tissues. Some follicular carcinomas had low and some high expressions making their distinction from benign follicular adenomas more difficult by this method. The same group next used *in situ* hybridization to detect oncofetal fibronectin mRNA and reported similar results [23].

Takano et al. [24] examined 72 surgical thyroid specimens (23 normal thyroid tissues, 14 adenomatous goiters, 13 follicular adenomas, 3 follicular carcinomas, 18 papillary carcinomas and 1 anaplastic tumor) for expression of oncofetal fibronectin. FNA specimens were obtained from these tissues immediately after surgical resection and RT–PCR was performed using the cells left in the syringe after the samples were placed on slides for cytologic examination. About 94.6% of the specimens diagnosed as papillary or anaplastic carcinomas by cytology also expressed oncofetal fibronectin compared with only 3.7% (4 of 109) of benign specimens. In contrast to papillary cancers, none of the 6 follicular tumors expressed oncofetal fibronectin. From all these patients, 50 underwent surgery and results of the RT–PCR could be compared with the gold standard of surgical histopathology. Based on the results of the surgical histologic examinations, the RT–PCR detecting oncofetal fibronectin mRNA was 96.9% sensitive and 100% specific, as all but one cancer sample in this study was papillary. Finally, the same investigators also demonstrated expression of oncofetal fibronectin in thyroid fibroblasts, suggesting a potential cause for false-positive amplification of this transcript from clinical samples [25]. These results suggest that measurement of oncofetal fibronectin expression may be useful as an adjunctive test for identifying papillary thyroid carcinoma, but its use for follicular tumors is limited. Thus, in most cases, determination of oncofetal fibronectin is not likely to alter clinical managements for patients with thyroid nodules.

1.5. *Ret/PTC*

Ret/PTC oncogenes have been identified in a significant percentage of papillary thyroid cancers and are thought to play an important role in the carcinogenesis of these tumors, especially in tumors associated with radiation exposure. This led to their investigation as molecular markers for the distinction between benign and malignant thyroid tissues, but so far conflicting results have been reported.

In a study of 73 cases of thyroid specimens [26], from which both FNA and surgically obtained tissue are available, the presence of the oncogenes ret/PTC1-5 was examined. Ret/PTC-4 and -5 were not detected in any specimens. Of the 39 benign tissues (including 11 follicular adenomas, 25 nodular hyperplasias and 3 Hashimoto's thyroiditis), no FNA or surgical specimens tested positive for the oncogenes by RT–PCR. In contrast, of the 33 papillary thyroid cancers, 17 FNA samples and 21 surgical specimens expressed Ret/PTC-1, -2 or -3. In comparison, based on FNA cytology, 12 of the 33 papillary cancers were correctly diagnosed, while 6 were 'insufficient' and 15 were 'indeterminate' specimens. Although detection of the ret/PTC oncogenes failed to detect all the cases of papillary cancer based on the FNA samples, their use correctly identified several cases classified as indeterminate by cytology, thereby reducing the number of false-negative results.

These results were not verified, however, by another study where 154 patients were studied prospectively [27]. This group of patients was referred to surgery for FNA-characterized benign nodules (65 cases) or papillary thyroid cancer ($n = 89$). Ret/PTC-1 and ret/PTC-3, the most common Ret/PTC oncogenes, were investigated by RT–PCR in this study. They were detected in both benign and malignant nodules. Of interest is the fact that they were detected in nodules of patients who were exposed to radiation, as well as of patients with no history of any radiation exposure, although patients exposed to post-Chernobyl fall-out seemed to have a higher frequency of ret/PTC-3.

Ret protein expression in surgical samples has also been evaluated immunohistochemically [28]. Its overexpression was heterogenous and was demonstrated in regions of cellular atypia in both malignant and benign lesions. These results indicate that the efficacy of preoperative testing for the presence of the ret/PTC oncogenes in cytologic specimens may be limited by a heterogenous expression pattern. More studies are needed to clarify a role for Ret/PTC rearrangement or Ret overexpression in the diagnosis of thyroid nodules.

1.6. *Pax8-PPAR·*

Pax8 is a transcription factor that plays a crucial role in thyroid cell differentiation and thyroid gland morphogenesis. *In vitro* studies have indicated that loss of Pax8 expression results in reduced expression of thyroid-specific genes such as thyroglobulin, thyroid peroxidase (TPO), the sodium-iodide symporter (NIS) and the thyroid-stimulating hormone receptor. Its re-expression in de-differentiated thyroid cancer cell lines induces the synthesis of these molecules [29].

A recent report [30] identified the presence of a fusion oncogene involving Pax8 in some follicular thyroid cancers, but not in benign thyroid tissues or other thyroid malignancies such as papillary thyroid cancer. This chimeric protein results from a chromosomal translocation t(2;3)(q13;p25), causing a fusion gene to develop between Pax8 and the peroxisome proliferator-activated receptor gamma (PPAR·). In this study, 5 of 8 thyroid follicular cancers were positive for this translocation while all of the 20 follicular adenomas, 10 papillary thyroid carcinomas and 10 benign multinodular hyperplasic nodules did not express the rearranged gene.

Unfortunately, other studies [31] have failed to confirm the specificity of this finding and, in particular, have identified the PAX8-PPAR· fusion in benign follicular adenomas, although not as frequently as follicular carcinomas. It is unclear at this point whether the presence of the Pax8-PPAR· product in follicular adenomas predicts a higher likelihood of progression to follicular carcinoma. It is also important to note that there are some important differences in the methods of detection (RT–PCR vs. immunohistochemistry) employed by the different investigators that may be significant in determining their clinical utility.

1.7. *Nm23*

Nm23 gene is a tumor suppressor gene; re-expression of nm23 decreases metastatic potential of malignant cells (studied in human breast cancer and murine melanoma cell lines [32,33] *in vitro*. Reduced expression of Nm23 mRNA has been described in breast carcinoma and this associates with an increased tendency for lymph node metastasis [34]. The mechanism of nm23 participation in metastatic spread is unclear. The proposed biochemical properties include nucleoside diphosphate kinase (NDPK) activity, activation of G proteins and effects on microtubule polymerization.

Because of these data, Nm23 has also been investigated in thyroid tissues. Farley et al. [35] evaluated 34 thyroid tumors (4 follicular adenomas, 19 papillary carcinomas, 6 follicular carcinomas and 5 medullary carcinomas) for levels of Nm23 mRNA. Although higher levels of expression of Nm23 were detected in follicular and medullary cancers, significant overlap between benign and malignant tissues was noted. There was also no consistent difference between nm23 mRNA levels in metastatic and non-metastatic tumor tissues.

Similarly, in another study of 101 specimens [36], immunocytochemical staining with antibodies against Nm23 failed to distinguish between the benign and malignant lesions. However, a predilection for nuclear staining in normal tissues (93%) and its loss in malignant ones (29%) was identified. The biological significance of this finding has not yet been reported.

1.8. *High-mobility group I(Y) protein-HMGI(Y)*

The high-mobility group I proteins are a group of nuclear proteins involved in the regulation of chromatin structure and function. HMGI(Y) is a member of this family that has been found to be highly expressed during embryogenesis [37] as well as in malignant tumors [38,39] but is relatively absent in normal adult tissues.

In order to evaluate the utility of this molecule as a marker of thyroid malignancy, Chiappetta et al. [40] investigated 358 thyroid tissue samples by immunohistochemistry. HMGI(Y) was detected in 18 of 19 follicular carcinomas, 92 of 96 papillary tumors and 11 of 11 anaplastic cancers. In contrast, HMGI(Y) was detected only in 1 of 20 hyperplastic nodules, 44 of 200 benign follicular adenomas and 0 of 12 normal thyroid tissue samples. They also measured HMGI(Y) mRNA levels by RT–PCR in 12 FNA specimens. HMGI(Y) was detectable in 4 of 4 malignant tumors while the 8 benign FNA samples (6 follicular adenomas and 2 normal thyroid tissue) were negative. The authors conclude that HMGI(Y) may be a potentially useful diagnostic tool for thyroid cancer and its use warranted further investigation. These preliminary results have not yet been confirmed, but suggest a potential usefulness of HMGI(Y) in the preoperative characterization of thyroid nodules.

1.9. *Ceruloplasmin*

Ceruloplasmin is a serum glycoprotein involved in the transport of copper. However, because of its amino acid homology to lactoferrin, a molecular marker for several tumor types [41,42], ceruloplasmin has also been investigated for this purpose.

Tuccart and Barresi [43] evaluated 56 surgical thyroid specimens for the presence of ceruloplasmin by immunohistochemistry. None of the 15 follicular adenomas expressed ceruloplasmin, 2 of 2 Hurthle cell tumors, all 21 follicular, and all 6 papillary carcinomas were positive. All of the medullary thyroid cancers were negative for ceruloplasmin, as was the normal thyroid tissue surrounding the thyroid cancers. The functional role of ceruloplasmin in thyroid tumors as well as its full potential as a marker for distinguishing between benign and malignant thyroid tissues in FNA samples need to be further clarified.

1.10. *Cytokeratin 19*

Cytokeratins are integral structural proteins of benign and malignant epithelial cells. Several types of keratins have been described and their potential role as molecular markers in various malignancies has been investigated for different thyroid tumors. Immunocytochemical expression for prekeratin was detected in papillary thyroid cancer but not normal thyroid tissues, follicular adenomas and follicular thyroid carcinomas [44]. These results, however, were not confirmed using a more specific keratin monoclonal antibody. The intensity and distribution of cytokeratin staining is also debated in the literature, probably related to differences in antibodies, methods and the particular thyroid samples.

With the development of antibodies to specific types of cytokeratins a more comprehensive evaluation was undertaken. Schelfhout et al. [45] used monoclonal antibodies against cytokeratin 8, 18 and 19 to evaluate cytokeratin expression in thyroid tissues. Of these, only cytokeratin-19 antibody demonstrated preferential staining for papillary thyroid cancer; 12 of 12 papillary cancers all expressed cytokeratin 19, while follicular cancers, follicular adenomas, colloid nodules and normal thyroid tissue were negative or had only weak staining. The authors concluded that staining with antibodies against cytokeratin-19 is a useful diagnostic tool for papillary thyroid cancer.

The above results could not be confirmed though by later studies. In a study of 35 surgical thyroid specimens cytokeratin-19 expression was evaluated [46]. Although papillary cancers tended to display more intense staining, the presence or absence of positivity to these antibodies could not reliably distinguish between the different tissue types.

1.11. *GLUT 1*

In general, malignant cells have an increased rate of glucose utilization to compensate for a deficient capacity for oxidative metabolism or to allow for accelerated cellular growth. This frequently requires upregulation of the necessary membrane transport mechanisms for glucose transport into these cells. Of the different glucose transporters that have been described, Glut-1 has been found to be highly expressed in various cancers. In thyroid cancer, Glut-1 expression was investigated as a tumor marker in 38 benign and 28 malignant surgical thyroid specimens by immunohistochemistry [47]. No expression was seen in any of the benign tissues; however, 9 of 17 papillary cancer specimens, 2 of 6 follicular and 2 of 2 anaplastic tumors expressed Glut-1. These results suggest that Glut-1 could be a potentially useful marker. Also, in agreement with these results are reports of [18F]-2-fluoro-deoxyglucose PET scan positivity of more anaplastic thyroid tumors, with the loss of I^{131} uptake [48], suggesting a potential role and prognostic significance for Glut-1 expression in these tumors.

1.12. *CA 19-9, CD15 and HMBE-1*

CA 19-9 and CD15 (Leu-M1) are two antigens that have been previously identified as markers of various malignancies, such as pancreatic and gastrointestinal tumors for CA 19-9 [49] and Hodgkin's disease for CD-15 [50].

CA19-9 and CD15 were both identified in both benign thyroid tumors and in papillary carcinomas using immunohistochemistry [51]. By contrast, HMBE-1 was detected in 21 of 21 papillary cancer samples and in 9 of 31 benign lesions including 4 of 18 follicular adenomas and 5 of 10 benign goiters. Unfortunately, follicular carcinomas were not evaluated in this study. Based on these results, these markers are potentially useful for the evaluation of cytologic specimens, which were difficult to interpret from FNAs of thyroid glands.

1.13. *CD30*

The CD30 antigen (also called antigen Ki-1) is a cytokine receptor that belongs to the tumor necrosis factor (TNF)/nerve growth factor (NGF) receptor superfamily [52]. Under normal conditions, CD30 is expressed in activated B and T lymphocytes. In malignant cells, it was first described in Hodgkin's disease [53] as well as other lymphomas (such as Burkitt's lymphoma).

The presence and distribution of both CD30 and the CD30 ligand were investigated using immunohistochemistry in a study of 131 surgical thyroid specimens and 6 normal thyroid glands (at autopsy) [54]. Normal thyroid tissue did not express CD30 or the CD30 ligand. Normal thyroid tissue adjacent to benign nodular or follicular cancer thyroid tissue did not express either molecule, while tissue adjacent to papillary and medullary cancer (possibly by a paracrine mechanism) expressed

CD30 ligand. A 20% of follicular adenomas showed coexpression of CD30 and CD30L, while 7% of the follicular, 33% of the anaplastic, 76% of the papillary and 67% of the medullary cancers expressed both proteins. Medullary and papillary cancers along with oncocytic adenomas were the only tissues to have nuclear expression. The significance of this difference is uncertain. The overlap in expression between benign and malignant thyroid tissues may ultimately limit the use of this marker in identifying thyroid cancer.

1.14. *CD97*

CD97 is a glycoprotein that belongs to a subclass of transmembrane leukocyte cell surface molecules. Although CD97 was originally described on leukocytes, its expression was later identified in other tissues including thyroid tissues [55]. Immunohistochemical analysis revealed that expression of CD97 was mostly found in poorly differentiated thyroid cancers (11 of 12). Expression of CD97 also correlated with tumor stage, being absent or weakly reactive in T1 tumors and strongly expressed in T4 tumors. These data suggest potential functional relevance of CD97 in thyroid cancer, but do not indicate that CD97 will be able to distinguish benign from malignant thyroid tumors.

1.15. *Epithelial membrane antigen, Leu-7 (CD57), epidermal growth factor receptor*

Epithelial membrane antigen (EMA) is a glycoprotein, which is known to be expressed by malignant cells of epithelial origin [56], Leu-7 is an antigen expressed by lymphocytes and natural killer cells and has also been identified in a variety of epithelial and non-epithelial tumors [57], and epidermal growth factor receptor (EGF-R) is a known prognostic indicator in colon and breast cancers [58,59]. In a study of 40 thyroid nodules with both a benign and malignant histology, Cheifetz et al. [60] evaluated the utility of these markers in distinguishing malignant from benign thyroid tumors in 40 nodules by immunohistochemistry of surgical specimens. For EMA, 16 of 22 malignant (73%) and 5 of 18 benign (28%) tumors were positive, a difference that was statistically significant and resulted in a sensitivity of 75% and a specificity of 90%. Leu-7 expression was detected in 20 of 22 malignant tumors and 6 of 18 benign tumors, also representing a statistically significant difference. In contrast, EGF-R expression was not different between benign and malignant lesions.

The utility of Leu-7 expression as a marker of thyroid malignancy was further investigated in a study of 83 malignant and 77 benign surgical specimens [61]: 95% of the malignant and 21% of the benign lesions were positive. The authors also reported that staining of the benign tissues was weaker compared with the malignant tumors. An overall tumor sensitivity of 97.5% and a specificity of 82% were estimated. As with other markers, differences in the intensity and distribution of the staining were also noted between benign and malignant tissues, thus the analysis is quite subjective. Also, these markers have not yet been reported for FNA samples.

1.16. *Cyclooxygenase-2*

The two distinct isoforms of cyclooxygenase enzymes have been described to date, cyclooxygenase 1 and 2. Cyclooxygenase type 2 (Cox-2) is a highly inducible enzyme that is involved in carcinogenesis. It has been shown to be upregulated in many malignancies including colon [62], gastric [63], pancreatic [64] and lung [65] cancers. Cox-2 gene and protein expression were investigated in a study of 14 benign and 14 malignant surgical thyroid specimens by quantitative RT–PCR and immunohistochemistry [66]. Elevated levels of COX-2 mRNA were noted in malignant thyroid tissues as compared with adjacent normal thyroid tissue and in malignant nodules compared with benign nodules. Immunohistochemical staining and western-blot demonstration were also positive. Of interest in this study was the fact that COX-2 expression was identified in FNA samples (by RT–PCR) as well as surgical specimens. These data suggest that COX-2 is upregulated in thyroid malignancies and this could be used as a potential marker for differentiating benign from malignant tissue preoperatively.

Table 2
Summarized results

Marker	Method	Sensitivity (%)	Specificity (%)	Reference
Telomerase	TRAP	37–100[a]	36–92[a]	[6,10,11]
	HTERT	66–79[a]	62–72[b]	[8]
Galectin-3	Immunohistochemistry	70–91[b]	77–100[b]	[13–16]
TPO	Immunohistochemistry	100	90–99	[17,18]
Oncofetal fibronectin	RT–PRC	84–94	96–100	[20,22]
	In situ hybridization	53	100	[21]
Ret/PTC	RT–PCR	51	100	[23]
Pax8/PPAR ·	RT–PCR[c]	56–62	87–100	[27,28]
	Immunohistochemistry[c]	78	69	[28]
HMGI(Y)	Immunohistochemistry	96	80	[34]
Ceruloplasmin	Immunohistochemistry[d]	100	88	[35]
GLUT-1	Immunohistochemistry	46	97	[39]
CA19-9	Immunohistochemistry	38	97	[43]
CD15	Immunohistochemistry	71	94	[43]
HMBE-1	Immunohistochemistry	100	76	[43]
CD30	Immunohistochemistry	44	73	[46]
CD57	Immunohistochemistry	91	67	[52]
EMA	Immunohistochemistry	73	72	[52]
EGF-R	Immunohistochemistry	25	76	[52]

[a]Combined for tissue and FNA specimens.
[b]Cumulative for all types of thyroid cancer.
[c]For follicular thyroid cancer.
[d]Medullary tumors excluded.

2. Conclusion

A large and exciting volume of evidence is accumulating about the usefulness of molecular markers in the diagnosis of various human malignancies (refer to Table 2 below for summarized results). Immunohistochemical analysis of FNA samples for galectin-3 and thyroid peroxidase may soon be used in routine clinical practice, as they appear to be useful adjunctive tests and utilize standard pathology laboratory methods. Other tests that utilize molecular biology are under active investigation by many groups. The combination of analysis of protein and mRNA expression with routine cytology from FNA specimens could greatly improve the sensitivity and accuracy of this diagnostic tool, ultimately limiting the number of patients undergoing unnecessary thyroid surgery for benign thyroid nodules.

References

[1] N.W. Kim, M.A. Piatyszek, K.R. Prowse, et al., Specific association of human telomerase activity with immortal cells and cancer, Science 266 (1994) 2011–2015.

[2] J. Feng, W.D. Funk, S.S. Wang, et al., The RNA component of human telomerase, Science 269 (1995) 1236–1241.

[3] M. Saji, W.H. Westra, H. Chen, et al., Telomerase activity in the differential diagnosis of papillary carcinoma of the thyroid, Surgery 122 (1997) 1137–1140.

[4] B.R. Haugen, S. Nawaz, N. Markham, et al., Telomerase activity in benign and malignant thyroid tumors, Thyroid 7 (1997) 337–342.

[5] N. Onoda, T. Ishikawa, K. Yoshikawa, et al., Telomerase activity in thyroid tumors, Oncol. Rep. 5 (1998) 1447–1450.

[6] C.B. Umbricht, M. Saji, W.H. Westra, R. Udelsman, M.A. Zeiger, S. Sukumar, Telomerase activity: a marker to distinguish follicular thyroid adenoma from carcinoma, Cancer Res. 57 (1997) 2144–2147.

[7] X. De Deken, C. Vilain, J. Van Sande, J.E. Dumont, F. Miot, Decrease of telomere length in thyroid adenomas without telomerase activity, J. Clin. Endocrinol. Metab. 83 (1998) 4368–4372.

[8] M. Saji, S. Xydas, W.H. Westra, et al., Human telomerase reverse transcriptase (hTERT) gene expression in thyroid neoplasms, Clin. Cancer Res. 5 (1999) 1483–1489.

[9] M.T. Siddiqui, K.L. Greene, D.P. Clark, et al., Human telomerase reverse transcriptase expression in diff-quik-stained FNA samples from thyroid nodules, Diagn. Mol. Pathol. 10 (2001) 123–129.

[10] J. Sebesta, T. Brown, W. Williard, et al., Does telomerase activity add to the value of fine needle aspirations in evaluating thyroid nodules?, Am. J. Surg. 181 (2001) 420–422.

[11] P. Brousset, N. Chaouche, F. Leprat, et al., Telomerase activity in human thyroid carcinomas originating from the follicular cells, J. Clin. Endocrinol. Metab. 82 (1997) 4214–4216.

[12] A.J. Cheng, J.D. Lin, T. Chang, T.C. Wang, Telomerase activity in benign and malignant human thyroid tissues, Br. J. Cancer. 77 (1998) 2177–2180.

[13] L. Chiariotti, M.T. Berlingieri, P. De Rosa, et al., Increased expression of the negative growth factor, galactoside-binding protein, gene in transformed thyroid cells and in human thyroid carcinomas, Oncogene 7 (1992) 2507–2511.

[14] X.C. Xu, A.K. el-Naggar, R. Lotan, Differential expression of galectin-1 and galectin-3 in thyroid tumors, Potential diagnostic implications, Am. J. Pathol. 147 (1995) 815–822.

[15] P.L. Fernandez, M.J. Merino, M. Gomez, et al., Galectin-3 and laminin expression in neoplastic and non-neoplastic thyroid tissue, J. Pathol. 181 (1997) 80–86.

[16] H.J. Woo, L.M. Shaw, J.M. Messier, A.M. Mercurio, The major non-integrin laminin binding protein of macrophages is identical to carbohydrate binding protein 35 (Mac-2), J. Biol. Chem. 265 (1990) 7097–7099.

[17] F. Orlandi, E. Saggiorato, G. Pivano, et al., Galectin-3 is a presurgical marker of human thyroid carcinoma, Cancer Res. 58 (1998) 3015–3020.

[18] M.E. Herrmann, V.A. LiVolsi, T.L. Pasha, S.A. Roberts, E.M. Wojcik, Z.W. Baloch, Immunohistochemical expression of galectin-3 in benign and malignant thyroid lesions, Arch. Pathol. Lab. Med. 126 (2002) 710–713.

[19] C. De Micco, P. Zoro, S. Garcia, et al., Thyroid peroxidase immunodetection as a tool to assist diagnosis of thyroid nodules on fine-needle aspiration biopsy, Eur. J. Endocrinol. 131 (1994) 474–479.

[20] L. Christensen, M. Blichert-Toft, M. Brandt, et al., Thyroperoxidase (TPO) immunostaining of the solitary cold thyroid nodule, Clin. Endocrinol. (Oxf.) 53 (2000) 161–169.

[21] K. Krohn, R. Paschke, Loss of heterozygocity at the thyroid peroxidase gene locus in solitary cold thyroid nodules, Thyroid 11 (2001) 741–747.

[22] T. Higashiyama, T. Takano, F. Matsuzuka, et al., Measurement of the expression of oncofetal fibronectin mRNA in thyroid carcinomas by competitive reverse transcription-polymerase chain reaction, Thyroid 9 (1999) 235–240.

[23] T. Takano, F. Matsuzuka, A. Miyauchi, et al., Restricted expression of oncofetal fibronectin mRNA in thyroid papillary and anaplastic carcinoma: an in situ hybridization study, Br. J. Cancer 78 (1998) 221–224.

[24] T. Takano, A. Miyauchi, T. Yokozawa, et al., Accurate and objective preoperative diagnosis of thyroid papillary carcinomas by reverse transcription-PCR detection of oncofetal fibronectin messenger RNA in fine-needle aspiration biopsies, Cancer Res. 58 (1998) 4913–4917.

[25] T. Takano, A. Miyauchi, F. Matsuzuka, K. Kuma, N. Amino, Expression of oncofetal fibronectin messenger ribonucleic acid in fibroblasts in the thyroid: a possible cause of false positive results in molecular-based diagnosis of thyroid carcinomas, J. Clin. Endocrinol. Metab. 85 (2000) 765–768.

[26] C.C. Cheung, B. Carydis, S. Ezzat, Y.C. Bedard, S.L. Asa, Analysis of ret/PTC gene rearrangements refines the fine needle aspiration diagnosis of thyroid cancer, J. Clin. Endocrinol. Metab. 86 (2001) 2187–2190.

[27] R. Elisei, C. Romei, T. Vorontsova, et al., RET/PTC rearrangements in thyroid nodules: studies in irradiated and not irradiated, malignant and benign thyroid lesions in children and adults, J. Clin. Endocrinol. Metab. 86 (2001) 3211–3216.

[28] A. Fusco, G. Chiappetta, P. Hui, et al., Assessment of RET/PTC oncogene activation and clonality in thyroid nodules with incomplete morphological evidence of papillary carcinoma: a search for the early precursors of papillary cancer, Am. J. Pathol. 160 (2002) 2157–2167.

[29] M. Pasca di Magliano, R. Di Lauro, M. Zannini, Pax8 has a key role in thyroid cell differentiation, Proc. Natl. Acad. Sci. USA 97 (2001) 13144–13149.

[30] T.G. Kroll, P. Sarraf, L. Pecciarini, et al., PAX8-PPARgamma1 fusion oncogene in human thyroid carcinoma [corrected], Science 289 (2000) 1357–1360.

[31] A.R. Marques, C. Espadinha, A.L. Catarino, et al., Expression of PAX8-PPARgamma1 rearrangements in both follicular thyroid carcinomas and adenomas, J. Clin. Endocrinol. Metab. 87 (2002) 3947–3952.

[32] A. Leone, U. Flatow, K. VanHoutte, P.S. Steeg, Transfection of human nm23-H1 into the human MDA-MB-435 breast carcinoma cell line: effects on tumor metastatic potential, colonization and enzymatic activity, Oncogene 8 (1993) 2325–2333.

[33] A. Leone, U. Flatow, C.R. King, et al., Reduced tumor incidence, metastatic potential, and cytokine responsiveness of nm23-transfected melanoma cells, Cell 65 (1991) 25–35.

[34] G. Bevilacqua, M.E. Sobel, L.A. Liotta, P.S. Steeg, Association of low nm23 RNA levels in human primary infiltrating ductal breast carcinomas with lymph node involvement and other histopathological indicators of high metastatic potential, Cancer Res. 49 (1989) 5185–5190.

[35] D.R. Farley, N.L. Eberhardt, C.S. Grant, et al., Expression of a potential metastasis suppressor gene (nm23) in thyroid neoplasms, World J. Surg. 17 (1993) 615–620 (discussion 620-1).

[36] P. Bertheau, A. De La Rosa, P.S. Steeg, M.J. Merino, NM23 protein in neoplastic and nonneoplastic thyroid tissues, Am. J. Pathol. 145 (1994) 26–32.

[37] G. Chiappetta, V. Avantaggiato, R. Visconti, et al., High level expression of the HMGI (Y) gene during embryonic development, Oncogene 13 (1996) 2439–2446.

[38] Y. Tamimi, H.G. van der Poel, M.M. Denyn, et al., Increased expression of high mobility group protein I(Y) in high grade prostatic cancer determined by in situ hybridization, Cancer Res. 53 (1993) 5512–5516.

[39] M. Fedele, A. Bandiera, G. Chiappetta, et al., Human colorectal carcinomas express high levels of high mobility group HMGI(Y) proteins, Cancer Res. 56 (1996) 1896–1901.

[40] G. Chiappetta, G. Tallini, M.C. De Biasio, et al., Detection of high mobility group I HMGI(Y) protein in the diagnosis of thyroid tumors: HMGI(Y) expression represents a potential diagnostic indicator of carcinoma, Cancer Res. 58 (1998) 4193–4198.

[41] J. Caselitz, T. Jaup, G. Seifert, Lactoferrin and lysozyme in carcinomas of the parotid gland. A comparative immunocytochemical study with the occurrence in normal and inflamed tissue, Virchows Arch. A Pathol. Anat. Histol. 394 (1981) 61–73.

[42] G. Tuccari, G. Barresi, Immunohistochemical demonstration of lactoferrin in follicular adenomas and thyroid carcinomas, Virchows Arch. A Pathol. Anat. Histopathol. 406 (1985) 67–74.

[43] G. Tuccari, G. Barresi, Immunohistochemical demonstration of ceruloplasmin in follicular adenomas and thyroid carcinomas, Histopathology 11 (1987) 723–731.

[44] W. Permanetter, W.B. Nathrath, U. Lohrs, Immunohistochemical analysis of thyroglobulin and keratin in benign and malignant thyroid tumours, Virchows Arch. A Pathol. Anat. Histopathol. 398 (1982) 221–228.

[45] L.J. Schelfhout, G.N. Van Muijen, G.J. Fleuren, Expression of keratin 19 distinguishes papillary thyroid carcinoma from follicular carcinomas and follicular thyroid adenoma, Am. J. Clin. Pathol. 92 (1989) 654–658.

[46] S. Sahoo, S.A. Hoda, J. Rosai, R.A. DeLellis, Cytokeratin 19 immunoreactivity in the diagnosis of papillary thyroid carcinoma: a note of caution, Am. J. Clin. Pathol. 116 (2001) 696–702.

[47] R.S. Haber, K.R. Weiser, A. Pritsker, I. Reder, D.E. Burstein, GLUT1 glucose transporter expression in benign and malignant thyroid nodules, Thyroid 7 (1997) 363–367.

[48] R. Robbins, W. Drucker, L. Hann, R.M. Tuttle, Advances in the detection of residual thyroid carcinoma, Adv. Intern. Med. 46 (2001) 277–294.

[49] H. Koprowski, M. Herlyn, Z. Steplewski, H.F. Sears, Specific antigen in serum of patients with colon carcinoma, Science 212 (1981) 53–55.

[50] S.M. Hsu, E.S Jaffe, Leu M1 and peanut agglutinin stain the neoplastic cells of Hodgkin's disease, Am. J. Clin. Pathol. 82 (1984) 29–32.

[51] K.H. van Hoeven, A.J. Kovatich, M. Miettinen, Immunocytochemical evaluation of HBME-1, CA 19-9, and CD-15 (Leu-M1) in fine-needle aspirates of thyroid nodules, Diagn Cytopathol. 18 (1998) 93–97.

[52] C.A. Smith, H.J. Gruss, T. Davis, et al., CD30 antigen a marker for Hodgkin's lymphoma, is a receptor whose ligand defines an emerging family of cytokines with homology to TNF, Cell 73 (1993) 1349–1360.

[53] U. Schwab, H. Stein, J. Gerdes, et al., Production of a monoclonal antibody specific for Hodgkin and Sternberg-Reed cells of Hodgkin's disease and a subset of normal lymphoid cells, Nature 299 (1982) 65–67.

[54] M. Trovato, D. Villari, R.M. Ruggeri, et al., Expression of CD30 ligand and CD30 receptor in normal thyroid and benign and malignant thyroid nodules, Thyroid 11 (2001) 621–628.

[55] G. Aust, W. Eichler, S. Laue, et al., CD97: a dedifferentiation marker in human thyroid carcinomas, Cancer Res. 57 (1997) 1798–1806.

[56] G.S. Pinkus, P.J. Kurtin, Epithelial membrane antigen — a diagnostic discriminant in surgical pathology: immunohistochemical profile in epithelial, mesenchymal, and hematopoietic neoplasms using paraffin sections and monoclonal antibodies, Hum. Pathol. 16 (1985) 929–940.

[57] L. Si, T.L. Whiteside, Tissue distribution of human NK cells studied with anti-Leu-7 monoclonal antibody, J. Immunol. 130 (1983) 2149–2155.

[58] A.W. Hemming, N.L. Davis, A. Kluftinger, et al., Prognostic markers of colorectal cancer: an evaluation of DNA content, epidermal growth factor receptor, and Ki-67, J. Surg. Oncol. 51 (1992) 147–152.

[59] M. Toi, T. Nakamura, H. Mukaida, et al., Relationship between epidermal growth factor receptor status and various prognostic factors in human breast cancer, Cancer 65 (1990) 1980–1984.

[60] R.E. Cheifetz, N.L. Davis, B.W. Robinson, K.W. Berean, J.C. LeRiche, Differentiation of thyroid neoplasms by evaluating epithelial membrane antigen, Leu-7 antigen, epidermal growth factor receptor, and DNA content, Am. J. Surg. 167 (1994) 531–534.

[61] A. Khan, S.P. Baker, N.A. Patwardhan, J.M. Pullman, CD57 (Leu-7) expression is helpful in diagnosis of the follicular variant of papillary thyroid carcinoma, Virchows Arch. 432 (1998) 427–432.

[62] C.E. Eberhart, R.J. Coffey, A. Radhika, F.M. Giardiello, S. Ferrenbach, R.N. DuBois, Up-regulation of cyclooxygenase 2 gene expression in human colorectal adenomas and adenocarcinomas, Gastroenterology 107 (1994) 1183–1188.

[63] A. Ristimaki, N. Honkanen, H. Jankala, P. Sipponen, M. Harkonen, Expression of cyclooxygenase-2 in human gastric carcinoma, Cancer Res. 57 (1997) 1276–1280.

[64] O.N. Tucker, A.J. Dannenberg, E.K. Yang, et al., Cyclooxygenase-2 expression is up-regulated in human pancreatic cancer, Cancer Res. 59 (1999) 987–990.

[65] T. Hida, Y. Yatabe, H. Achiwa, et al., Increased expression of cyclooxygenase 2 occurs frequently in human lung cancers, specifically in adenocarcinomas, Cancer Res. 58 (1998) 3761–3764.

[66] M.C. Specht, O.N. Tucker, M. Hocever, D. Gonzalez, L. Teng, T.J. Fahey 3rd., Cyclooxygenase-2 expression in thyroid nodules, J. Clin. Endocrinol. Metab. 87 (2002) 358–363.

Chapter 3

Ultrasound in the diagnosis and management of thyroid cancer

H. Jack Baskin

Florida Thyroid Clinic, 2921 N. Orange Avenue, Orlando, FL 32804

Thyroid ultrasound has been used to determine thyroid size, to detect anatomic variations in the thyroid, to identify extrathyroidal masses, and to screen for endemic goiter. However, it is in the diagnosis and management of thyroid cancer that thyroid ultrasound has proven to be most valuable.

Although high resolution, real-time ultrasound has been available since the early 1980s, it did not make a significant impact on the diagnosis and management of thyroid cancer until the mid-1990s. Initially, an ultrasound of the thyroid entailed referring the patient to a radiology department where the ultrasound was performed by a sonographer, who took spot films that were interpreted by the radiologist for the clinician. This delay in diagnosis and increase in cost of going to another specialist deterred the application of ultrasound to the study of thyroid cancer. Furthermore, the separation of the real-time procedure from the clinician resulted in loss of information and hampered the appreciation of subtle changes that have proven valuable in treating patients diagnosed with or suspected of having thyroid cancer.

Advances in ultrasound engineering and electronic technology in the 1990s make modern ultrasound more user-friendly. This coincides with a marked reduction in equipment cost, which allows clinicians who treat thyroid patients to have an access to a machine dedicated to thyroid ultrasound. The performance of real-time ultrasound by the examining physician, who has taken a history, performed a physical examination, and anticipated what may be seen on ultrasound imaging prevents loss of information and allows the ultrasound findings to be integrated with the patients' clinical palpation findings. The recent introduction of small linear phased-array transducers greatly facilitates ultrasound-guided fine-needle aspiration (FNA) biopsy that decreases the number of inadequate biopsies. The increased convenience and the decreased cost of thyroid ultrasound by not having to refer the patient out to another level of specialty care make thyroid ultrasound an essential part of the examination of a patient who has or is suspected to have thyroid cancer.

ADVANCES IN MOLECULAR AND CELLULAR ENDOCRINOLOGY   © 2005 Elsevier B.V.
VOLUME 4   ISSN 1569-2566/DOI 10.1016/S1569-2566(04)04003-7   All rights reserved.

1. Ultrasound analysis of thyroid nodules

Ultrasound is the most sensitive test for detecting a thyroid nodule or an early thyroid cancer. It can detect lesions as small as 2–3 mm in size before they are large enough to be palpated on physical examination or imaged by an isotope scan, computer tomography, or magnetic resonance imaging [1]. It was by using ultrasound that physicians were effectively able to screen thousands of children exposed to radiation in the USSR and Eastern Europe following the Chernobyl nuclear accident, where the incidence of thyroid cancer increased 100-fold within 4 years. The early ultrasound detection of cancer, followed by thyroidectomy, in these young children was responsible for saving many lives. In this country ultrasound screening is used mainly in examining the thyroid of people exposed to radiation during childhood and in families with hereditary cancer – even when the physical examination is normal. Unlike an isotope scan, ultrasound can be performed during pregnancy, in patients taking levothyroxine, and in incidences in which exogenous iodine contamination precludes performance of a radioiodine scan.

The primary concern when a patient presents with a thyroid nodule is whether the nodule is benign or malignant and needs surgery. FNA biopsy is the standard diagnostic test for evaluating possible malignancy in a thyroid nodule, but it has limitations. It cannot differentiate between follicular adenoma and follicular carcinoma, and up to 20% of FNA biopsies yield inadequate material for diagnosis [2]. Ultrasound extends the clinician's diagnostic acumen by allowing visualization of the architectural characteristics of thyroid nodules that have predictive value in deciding if a nodule is benign or malignant. Ultrasound also allows observation of changes in thyroid nodules over time, which often helps in making the decision regarding surgery. Obviously, a nodule that is decreasing in size is unlikely to be malignant or require surgical intervention, but a nodule that is increasing in size while on thyroid stimulating hormone (TSH) suppression needs re-evaluation. In a study of patients referred to a thyroid nodule clinic because of an abnormal thyroid physical examination, ultrasound altered the clinical management in 109 of 173 (63%) patients [3]. The results of ultrasound complement results from FNA biopsy, and it is the combination of the two procedures that provides the clinician with the optimal amount of information.

Various ultrasound characteristics of thyroid nodules have proven to have predictive diagnostic value in determining which nodules are malignant and which are not. Among these characteristics of thyroid nodules are echogenecity, smoothness of the border around the nodule, presence and type of calcifications, vascularity, and the finding of enlarged adjacent lymph nodes. Other characteristics such as nodule size, presence of fluid or cysts, and number of nodules seen have been less helpful in detecting malignancy.

1.1. *Echogenecity*

The echo density or *echogenecity* refers to the echo pattern of the nodule in comparison to the surrounding thyroid tissue, and it correlates to the actual tissue density. Nodules that appear darker on the screen are referred to as *hypoechoic* and are less dense (Fig. 1); nodules that appear lighter are called *hyperechoic* and are more dense (Fig. 2). Rarely, a nodule will have the same density (*isoechoic*) as the surrounding thyroid tissue and may be difficult to delineate unless there is a halo around the nodule. Modern ultrasound equipment has 256 shades of gray; therefore, most nodules can be categorized as either hypoechoic or hyperechoic. Nodules that are hyperechoic (more dense than the surrounding thyroid tissue) are unlikely to be malignant. Although exceptions do occur, most large published series report a very low rate of malignancy in these dense nodules. Solbiati et al. [4] reported only three hyperechoic nodules out of 139 malignant nodules.

Although most malignant thyroid nodules are hypoechoic, over 90% of *all* thyroid nodules are hypoechoic indicating that the tissue is less dense than normal thyroid tissue. Finding that a nodule is hypoechoic does not mean that it is cancerous. Ultrasound of a thyroid with Hashimoto thyroiditis frequently reveals many hypo-echoic areas that will vary in size and location over time. When these are not palpable, they are referred to as *pseudonodules* and represent areas of inflammation that often disappear on subsequent ultrasound.

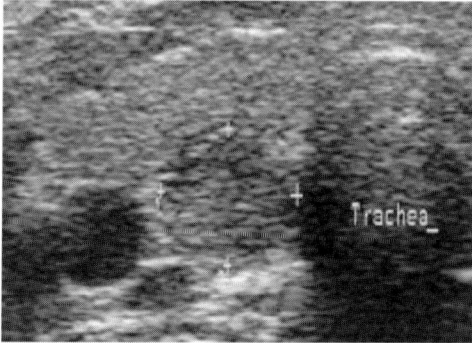

Fig. 1. This hypoechoic nodule in the right lobe is less dense than the surrounding thyroid tissue.

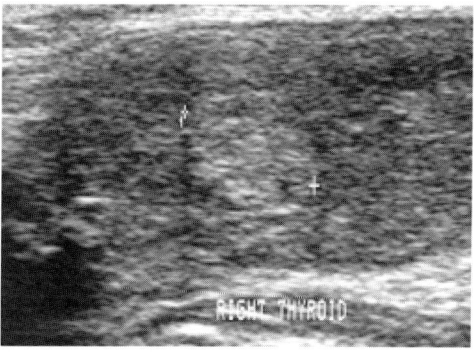

Fig. 2. This hyperechoic nodule is denser than the surrounding tissue; such nodules are seldom malignant.

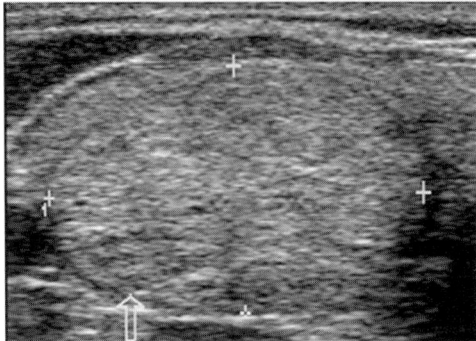

Fig. 3. The thin sonolucent rim around this isoechoic nodule (arrow) provides a smooth border or margin that clearly delineates the nodule.

1.2. *Margins*

The border or margin of a nodule on ultrasound represents the interface of nodule tissue with the surrounding thyroid. This border tends to be smooth and well defined in benign nodules as opposed to malignant nodules. Frequently, there will be a *halo* or a smooth sonolucent rim around the nodule (Fig. 3). The cause for the halo is an enigma since it does not correlate with an anatomical capsule. It may represent compressed blood vessels, inflammation, or just a sound wave characteristic that occurs when sound waves pass from one tissue to another. Haloes are much more common around benign nodules although they occasionally are seen with papillary carcinoma [5].

A halo is sometimes the only way to discern an isoechoic nodule where the tissue density of the nodule is the same as the thyroid. The width of a halo is variable and can affect the measurement of a nodule if it is included in the measurement. When following the size of a nodule, it is important to be consistent in including or not including the width of the halo in the measurement. This avoids the misconception that a nodule is shrinking or enlarging when actually it is not.

When one examines a malignant nodule closely using ultrasound, invasive growth of the tumor into the surrounding structures may be seen. If the edge of a nodule is not smooth but has an obscure or irregular border, it may indicate malignancy. Sometimes invasion of the surrounding structures such as the strap muscles or trachea can be visualized with ultrasound and confirms the diagnosis of malignancy.

1.3. *Calcifications*

The presence of calcifications within and around thyroid nodules is common and may have considerable significance. Because calcifications are quite dense, they reflect sound waves, causing bright images on the ultrasound screen. If the calcifications are large, the area distal to the calcification will be dark due to blockage of the sound waves (*acoustic shadowing*). This type of calcification takes time to deposit and is indicative that a nodule is slow growing or stable, and thus not likely to be malignant. The calcifications may be one or more amorphous deposits within the nodule or be deposited as rings of calcification around the periphery of the nodule where they are referred to as 'eggshell' calcifications (Fig. 4). All of these types of calcification have one thing in common – they are large enough to block sound waves and cause acoustic shadowing distally. Occasionally a bright spot is seen in a nodule that resembles a calcification, but instead of shadowing, a blurred brightness is seen distally. This is referred to as a 'comet tail' caused by a colloid crystal in a benign colloid nodule (Fig. 5).

Another type of calcification has a different clinical significance. Tiny punctate flecks of calcium scattered within the nodule are called *microcalcifications*, and they

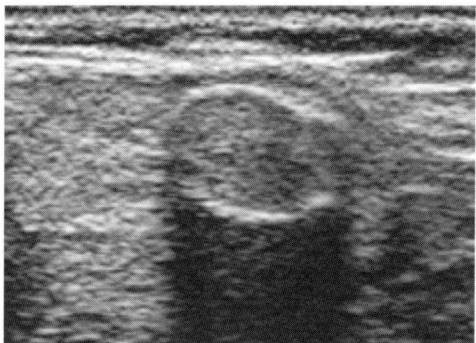

Fig. 4. The rim of calcium (eggshell calcifications) around this nodule causes acoustic shadowing distal to the nodule.

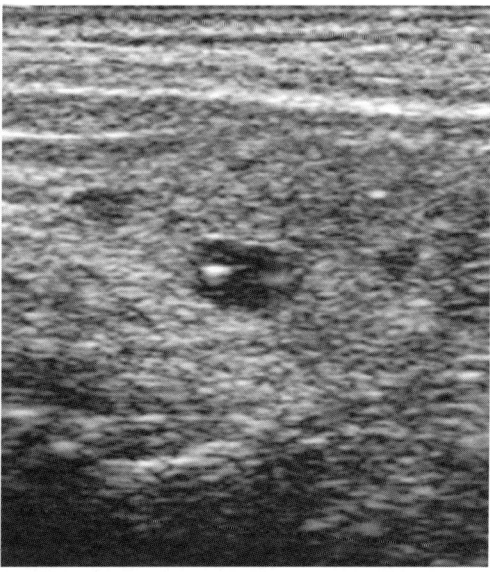

Fig. 5. The bright spot in the center of this small nodule has a distal 'comet tail' and is commonly referred to as a 'cat's eye'- a sign of a benign colloid nodule.

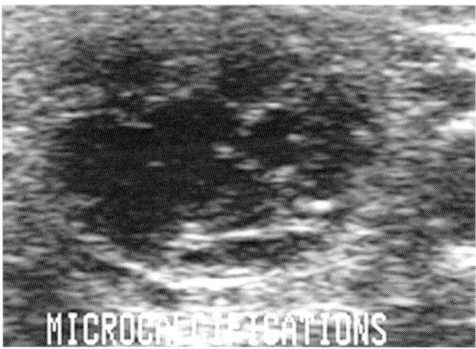

Fig. 6. These punctate flecks of calcium are called microcalcifications and are much more apparent on real-time ultrasound. They should raise the suspicion for malignancy.

are too small to cause shadowing. They are frequently difficult to see on spot images but appear as bright pinpoints of light on real-time ultrasound resembling twinkling stars in a dark sky (Fig. 6). Microcalcifications probably represent calcified psammoma bodies and have a high correlation with papillary carcinoma [6,7]. Because these fine calcifications may only be seen by the person performing the real-time ultrasound, it is critical that the person be a clinician.

1.4. *Vascularity*

Power Doppler detects the power of the shifted Doppler signal or the peaked systolic flow. While it does not determine the direction of blood flow it is sensitive to small amplitude flow typical in the tissues of the neck. Thyroid nodules that are malignant are more likely to have intranodular blood flow, whereas benign nodules show more blood flow in the perinodular area.

1.5. *Cervical lymphadenopathy*

Ultrasound of a thyroid nodule also includes ultrasound of the surrounding area of the neck to look for enlarged cervical lymph nodes. The finding of unsuspected enlarged lymph nodes in the neck of a patient with a thyroid nodule increases the risk of malignancy [8]. Metastatic lymph nodes may occur in the corotid sheath and along the internal jugular vein as well as in the lateral neck. They frequently show cystic degeneration or microcalcifications. While lymph node enlargement is not an absolute sign that a nodule is cancerous, it increases the likelihood significantly and provides a way for a quick diagnosis by allowing an FNA of the lymph node.

1.6. *Other nodule characteristics*

Other ultrasound characteristics have been less helpful than originally hoped in differentiating malignant from benign nodules. It was once thought that the presence of a cystic nodule decreased the chance of malignancy. However, modern ultrasound has revealed that a simple cyst in the thyroid is extremely rare and that virtually all cystic nodules have a solid component [9]. Only if a cyst can be fully evacuated and the nodule eliminated can one be certain that a cyst is benign. This is rarely possible. Many papillary carcinomas develop central necrosis that results in cyst formation (cystic degeneration) (Fig. 7); therefore, the presence of a cyst does not rule out malignancy.

When ultrasonography of a fluid-filled cyst is done, the posterior wall of the cyst and area distal to the cyst is bright or *enhanced* (Fig. 8). Some solid nodules are so hypoechoic that they may initially appear to be cysts, but careful study of the nodule reveals the absence of *enhancement* behind the nodule indicating that the nodule is solid and not liquid (Fig. 9). When ultrasound reveals that a nodule is cystic, it alerts the clinician that fluid is present so that a larger needle can be used to drain the fluid before biopsy of the solid component.

Although size of a nodule is important, once a nodule is known to be present, size does not correlate with whether a nodule is benign or malignant. In fact, ultrasound is often helpful in locating a small non-palpable primary cancer when a patient presents with a lymph node that contains thyroid metastasis. The discovery

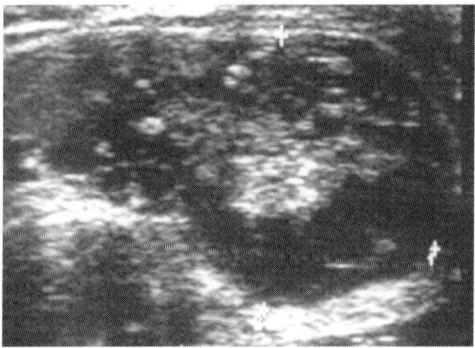

Fig. 7. This complex nodule proved to be a cystic papillary carcinoma. FNA without ultrasound guidance may have prevented biopsy of the solid component of the nodule and resulted in a false-negative test.

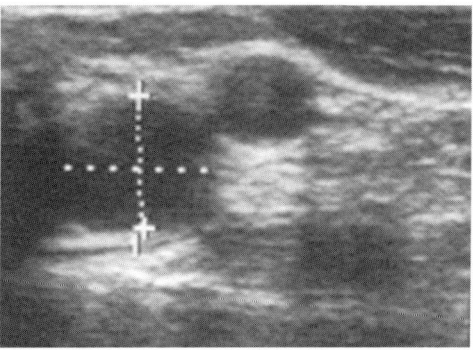

Fig. 8. The small nodule can be identified as a cyst by the bright area of enhancement below the nodule. Note the carotid artery also shows distal enhancement since it is fluid filled.

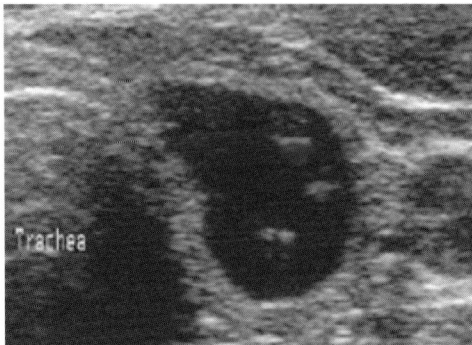

Fig. 9. This very hypoechoic nodule initially appeared cystic with debris in the fluid; however the absence of enhancement distally means the nodule is solid.

of a small non-palpable nodule cannot be ignored because several studies have shown that the incidence of malignancy in these non-palpable nodules is the same as in palpable nodules [10–13].

Micronodules (nodules 0.5–1 cm) are common in the population, hence the question arises when to perform ultrasound-guided FNA (UG FNA). Nodules this size seldom presents a threat to life and are so numerous that routine biopsy of all such nodules is neither practical nor cost effective. Clearly some judgment is required in deciding which micronodules require FNA. Patients who received external radiation during childhood and those with a family history of thyroid cancer (medullary or papillary) should have their micronodules biopsied. The occurrence of a nodule >0.5 cm in a patient who had only a hemithyroidectomy for thyroid cancer also requires an UG FNA. Many also recommend an UG FNA for hypoechoic micronodules accompanied by one or more of the following: blurred margins, microcalcifications, intranodular vascularity, or nodules that appear taller than wide in transverse view. Most other nodules 1 cm or less in size can safely be observed over a period of time using ultrasound, and FNA can be avoided if there is no increase in size. Ultrasound provides a much more objective measure of a nodule's dimensions and volume than that provided by a physical examination. While size is not important, *the change in the size* of a nodule over time is often significant and can be helpful in determining treatment.

For years it was assumed that a multinodular goiter presents a low risk of malignancy [14,15]. This might have been correct when the diagnosis of multinodular goiter was made by physical examination. Ultrasound has redefined the term multinodular goiter because many small and previously unfelt nodules are discovered when ultrasound is used to evaluate what was thought to be a solitary thyroid nodule. Recent studies have shown that malignancy is just as common in multinodular goiter as in uninodular goiter [16]. Ultrasound is used in deciding which of the nodule(s) are dominant and require FNA, but does not eliminate the need for biopsy.

The decision to do an ultrasound before a FNA biopsy has been controversial. Many felt that it was unnecessary because it delayed the biopsy and increased the cost by having to refer the patient to another specialist [17]. Now that endocrinologists perform the ultrasound at the initial examination, the time and cost considerations are minimized and many advantages of a pre-biopsy ultrasound have become obvious. It allows an objective baseline measurement of the size of a nodule. Since most nodules do not require surgery but are followed medically, ultrasound provides an accurate method to determine if a nodule is changing its size over a period of time. It permits the clinician to see the physical characteristics mentioned above that determine how aggressively a nodule is treated. For example, a hypoechoic nodule having an irregular border and microcalcifications is much more likely to require surgery than a hyperechoic nodule with a halo. Similarly, the finding of enlarged cervical lymph nodes may redirect the FNA biopsy. Pre-biopsy ultrasound also allows appropriate selection of needle length and size, using small (25–27 G) needles for solid nodules and larger needles for cyst aspiration. It also helps in detecting which nodule(s) require biopsy in multinodular goiter. Finally, it can determine if there is a need for an ultrasound-guided FNA.

2. Ultrasound-guided FNA

Although many thyroid nodules are superficial and large enough to be biopsied using only palpation, the widespread availability of 'bedside' ultrasound now makes it possible for the physician to perform FNA using ultrasound guidance. This technique facilitates the biopsy of material from the periphery of the nodule for the best cytological analysis and avoids biopsy of the surrounding normal thyroid tissue, which may yield a false-negative diagnosis. Various studies have demonstrated a marked decrease in inadequate specimens from 15–20% down to 3–4% when FNA is performed using ultrasound [18,19]. There are also studies that show improvement in specificity and sensitivity when nodules are biopsied under ultrasound guidance [20–25]. Ultrasound-guidance allows biopsy of nodules that were not previously amenable to FNA biopsy [26]. UG FNA is essential for small nodules that are less than 1.5 cm and for non-palpable nodules such as those located posteriorly in the thyroid or in the upper mediastinum. Even large nodules may not be palpable in the large muscular individual or the elderly patient with kyphosis, especially when placed in the supine position. UG FNA permits proper placement of the needle in these patients. Indeed, UG FNA allows tissue sampling of virtually all nodules 1 cm or greater in size.

As many as one-half of thyroid nodules >2 cm in size have a cystic component and biopsy of this fluid yields inadequate follicular cells for diagnosis. Therefore, it is critical that needle placement into the solid component of the nodule be assured. UG FNA accomplishes this easily. Alternatively, ultrasound may be used to place the needle tip in the liquid portion of the nodule for drainage prior to the FNA biopsy. UG FNA also prevents accidental puncture of the corotid artery, internal jugular vein, or trachea. There is a general agreement that a repeat biopsy performed because of inadequate material should always be done using ultrasound guidance. The overall decrease in inadequate specimens and the improvement in diagnostic accuracy have resulted in making UG FNA the standard method in performing FNA in many thyroid clinics.

3. Ultrasound in the post-operative surveillance of thyroid cancer

The use of ultrasound in the diagnosis of thyroid cancer is equally important in managing patients who have been treated for thyroid cancer. Because of its propensity to occur at any age, even in the very young, and to recur many years later, thyroid cancer must be monitored for the lifetime of the patient. Surveillance of these patients in a cost-effective manner has been a challenge. Until the 1990s, the only diagnostic tool available was a ^{131}I whole body scan (WBS) done after withdrawing the patient from their thyroid hormone replacement. The sensitivity of a WBS in the early detection of residual, recurrent, or metastatic thyroid cancer is poor [27]. This is apparent from the many patients who have increased thyroglobulin (Tg), but negative diagnostic scans who are treated with ^{131}I and have positive post-treatment scans [28–30]. Park et al. [31] have also shown that the doses of ^{131}I used for WBS can stun the uptake of iodine in metastatic lesions and interfere with the subsequent treatment dose of [131]I. The expense, poor sensitivity, and risk of stunning with WBS make it an unsatisfactory test with which to follow patients with thyroid cancer. In the last decade, several new probes have been developed that aid the early detection of recurrent thyroid cancer. These include: (1) sensitive, reliable, reproducible Tg assays that biochemically detect the earliest sign of cancer recurrence; (2) development of recombinant human TSH (rhTSH) that allows scanning and Tg stimulation without thyroid hormone withdrawal; and (3) ultrasound of the post-operative neck to identify early lymph node recurrence. Using these new tools, especially Tg after rhTSH stimulation and neck ultrasound combined with UG FNA of suspicious lymph nodes, has greatly improved cancer surveillance in these patients.

Physical examination of the neck of a patient who has undergone a thyroidectomy for thyroid cancer is seldom helpful in the *early* detection of a recurrence. The scar tissue following surgery and the propensity of metastatic lymph nodes to lie deep in the neck or beneath the sternocleidomastoid muscle combine to make palpation of the neck difficult. Even lymph nodes, several centimeters in diameter, are often not palpable. High-resolution ultrasound has solved this problem by proving to be a very sensitive method to find and locate early recurrent cancer and lymph node metastasis. Simeone et al. [14] reported 25 cases of recurrent cancer found by ultrasound in which only eight could be detected by palpation. Gorman et al. [32] reported nine patients found to have recurrent medullary cancer by ultrasound; only three could be detected by palpation. Sutton et al. [33] reported 29 cases of recurrent cancer found by UG FNA; only eight had a palpable mass. Using ultrasound, Antonelli et al. [34] found 12 patients with recurrence that even had a negative WBS. Since most thyroid cancer metastasizes to the neck, it is rare for thyroid cancer to spread elsewhere without neck lymph node involvement. Therefore, neck ultrasound has proven very helpful in locating early recurrent disease when serum Tg is elevated. It is also valuable in following patients with positive Tg antibodies.

While performing ultrasound of the neck of a patient who has undergone a thyroidectomy, one sees that the carotid artery and jugular vein have migrated medially close to the trachea and the thyroid bed has been filled with a varying amount of hyperechoic connective tissue that appears white (dense) on ultrasound (Fig. 10).

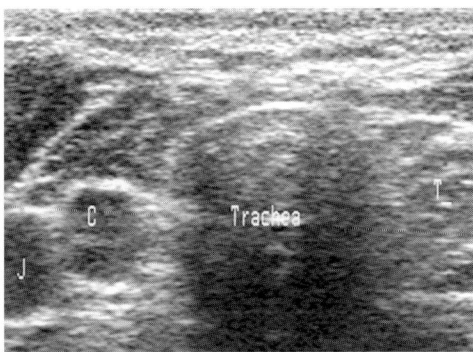

Fig. 10. This patient had a right hemithyroidectomy with a normal lobe on the left. The right common corotid artery and internal jugular vein have shifted medially and lie next to the trachea. A small amount of white connective tissue is in the thyroid bed.

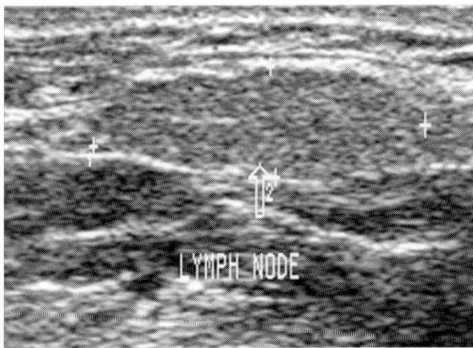

Fig. 11. This normal lymph node is flat in shape with a partial hilar line.

This serves well in demarcating a recurrence of cancer or a metastatic lymph node, which will appear dark or hypoechoic. The commonest areas for detecting cancer are the thyroid bed and the jugular chain of lymph nodes, but metastatic lymph nodes may occur anywhere in the neck. In performing ultrasound, the thyroid bed is examined first. Next, the entire length of the jugular vein from the head of the clavicle up to the mandible is searched, paying close attention to the area between the carotid artery and the jugular vein. Finally, the lateral neck is examined.

One finds that normal lymph nodes in the neck are common, especially in the upper neck near the pharynx. These are usually less than 0.5 cm in height and flattened in the transverse view of the neck with a width greater than twice their height. If they become inflamed or hyperplasic, they enlarge but generally maintain this flattened or oval shape and often show a white line of fat and blood vessels running through the center referred to as a *hilar line* (Fig. 11). Because lymph node hyperplasia is so common in the neck, only those lymph nodes greater than 0.5 cm (>0.8 cm in pharyngeal area) in height without a hilar line are usually biopsied. Those with a height <0.5 cm should have their location marked and be re-examined in 6 months. Metastatic lymph nodes generally have a more rounded appearance in the transverse view with a height/width ratio >0.5 [35]. Since all lymph nodes appear elongated in the longitudinal view, ultrasound surveillance for cancer is done in the transverse view.

In addition to a rounded shape and the absence of a hilar line, there are other ultrasound findings, which may also suggest that a lymph node is malignant. Since metastatic nodes commonly occur in proximity with the internal jugular vein or in the carotid sheath, jugular compression or deviation of the jugular vein away from the carotid artery strongly suggest malignancy. Microcalcifications (punctate flecks of calcium within the node) also suggest malignancy. Cystic necrosis within the lymph node, often recognized because of distal enhancement, is another sign of metastatic involvement with thyroid cancer, although it may also occur with tuberculosis. Power Doppler is also used in evaluating lymph nodes. Normal nodes have hilar vascularization, but malignant nodes have chaotic vascularization with recruitment of vessels into the cortex or the periphery of the node. Unlike malignant thyroid *nodules*, metastatic lymph nodes may have sharp borders until they become quite large. Normal and malignant lymph nodes are hypoechoic compared to thyroid; therefore, echogenecity may not be helpful in determining malignancy since papillary metastasis may be relatively hyperechoic. Matting of lymph nodes occurs with malignancy, but is also seen with inflammation or in patients who have had radiation.

The sonographic features of malignant lymph nodes are not always present and there is overlap in the ultrasound appearance of benign and malignant lymph nodes, therefore, biopsy of suspicious lesions is essential for a definitive diagnosis. Lymph nodes with a height >0.5 cm, and a height/width ratio >0.5, which do not have a hilar line must have an UG FNA (Fig. 12). UG FNA of a suspicious lymph node in the neck is carried out in the same manner as an UG FNA of a thyroid nodule with aspirate slides prepared and sent for cytology interpretation. In addition, the needle(s) should be washed with $1 \, cm^3$ normal saline and the washout sent for Tg assay [36]. Either a positive cytology report or the presence of Tg in the needle washout confirms that the lymph node is malignant [37]. Using either positive cytology or the presence of Tg as proof of recurrent cancer, Lee et al. [38] reported 100% sensitivity and specificity of UG FNA in detecting recurrent thyroid cancer.

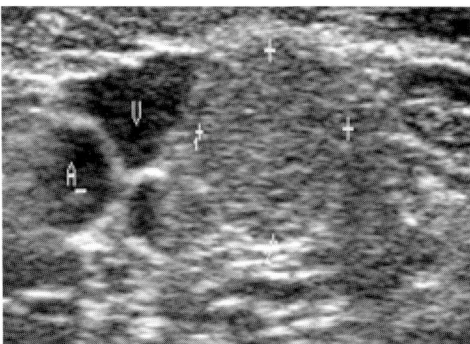

Fig. 12. This lymph node in the left neck contained papillary carcinoma. Its rounded appearance, location next to the neck vessels, and absence of a hilar line are typical of metastatic disease.

4. Summary

Real-time ultrasound of the neck coupled with UG FNA biopsy is a powerful new tool in diagnosing and managing patients with thyroid cancer. The ultrasound instrument is as helpful in examining the patient with thyroid cancer as the stethoscope is in examining the patient who has a heart murmur. As with the stethoscope, ultrasound must be incorporated into the physical examination and performed by the examining physician in order to reach its full potential.

References

[1] H. Baskin, Thyroid ultrasonography – a review, Endocrine Pract. 3 (1997) 153–157.

[2] H. Gharib, Thyroid Fine Needle Aspiration Biopsy, in: H. Baskin (Ed.), Thyroid Ultrasound and Ultrasound-Guided FNA Biopsy, Kluwer Academic Publishers, Boston, 2000, pp. 103–123.

[3] E. Marqusee, C.B. Benson, M.C. Frates, P.M. Doubilet, R. Larson, E.M. Cibas, S.J. Mandel, Usefulness of ultrasonography in the management of nodular thyroid disease, Ann. Int. Med. 133 (2000) 696–700.

[4] L. Solbiati, L. Volterrani, G. Rizzatto, M. Bazzocchi, P. Busilacchi, F. Candiani, F. Ferrari, G. Giuseppetti, G. Maresca, P. Mirk, L. Rubaltelli, F. Zappasodi, The thyroid gland with low uptake lesions: evaluation by ultrasound, Radiology 155 (1985) 187–191.

[5] R. Propper, L. Skolnick, B. Weinstein, A. Dekker, The nonspecificity of the halo sign, J. Clin. Ultrasound 8 (1980) 129–132.

[6] S. Takashima, H. Fukuda, N. Nomura, H. Kishimoto, T. Kim, T. Kobayashi, Thyroid nodules: re-evaluation with ultrasound, Clin. Ultrasound 23 (1995) 179–184.

[7] L. Solbiati, V. Cioffi, E. Ballarati, Ultrasonography of the neck, Radiol. Clin. North Am. 30 (1992) 941–954.

[8] M. Cignarelli, V. Triggiani, A. Ciampolillo, A. Ambrosi, F. Giorgino, V. Liso, R. Giorgino, The frequency of incidental diagnosis of extrathyroidal neoplastic diseases at the fine-needle aspiration biopsy of laterocervical lymph nodes in patients with thyroid nodules, Thyroid 11 (2001) 65–71.

[9] J. Simeone, G. Daniels, P. Mueller, F. Maloof, E. vanSonnenberg, D. Hall, R. O'Connell, J. Ferrucci, J. Wittenberg, High-resolution real-time sonography of the thyroid, Radiology 145 (1982) 431–435.

[10] T. Yokozawa, A. Miyauchi, K. Kuma, M. Sugawara, Accurate and simple method of diagnosing thyroid nodules by modified technique of ultrasound-guided fine needle aspiration biopsy, Thyroid 8 (1995) 141–145.

[11] P. Hagag, S. Strauss, M. Weiss, Role of ultrasound-guided fine-needle aspiration biopsy in evaluation of nonpalpable thyroid nodules, Thyroid 8 (1998) 989–995.

[12] L. Leenhardt, G. Hejblum, B. Franc, F.L. du Pasquier, T. Delbot, C. le Guillouzic, F. Menegaux, C. Guillausseau, C. Hoang, G. Turpin, A. Aurengo, Indications and limits of ultrasound-guided cytology in the management of nonpalpable thyroid nodules, J. Clin. Endocrinol. Metab. 84 (1999) 24–28.

[13] T. Yokozawa, S. Fukata, K. Kuma, F. Matsuzuka, A. Kobayashi, K. Harai, A. Miyauchi, M. Sugawara, Thyroid cancer detected by ultrasound-guided fine-needle aspiration biopsy, World J. Surg. 20 (1996) 848–853.

[14] J. Simeone, G. Daniels, D. Hall, K. McCarthy, D. Kopans, R. Butch, P. Mueller, D. Stark, J. Ferrucci, C. Wang, Sonography in the follow-up of 100 patients with thyroid carcinoma, AJR 148 (1987) 45–49.

[15] J. Katz, R. Kane, G. Reyes, M. Clarke, T. Hill, Thyroid nodules: sonographic–pathologic correlations, Radiology 151 (1984) 741–745.

[16] S.R. Tollin, G.M. Mery, N. Jelveh, E.F. Fallon, M. Mikhail, W. Blumenfeld, S. Perlmutter, The use of fine-needle aspiration biopsy under ultrasound guidance to assess the risk of malignancy in patients with a multinodular goiter, Thyroid 10 (2000) 235–241.

[17] A.J. Van Herle, P. Rich, B.E. Ljung, M.W. Ashcraft, D.H. Solomon, E.B. Keeler, The thyroid nodule, Ann. Int. Med. 96 (1982) 221–232.

[18] S. Takashima, H. Fukuda, T. Kobayashi, Thyroid nodules: clinical effect of ultrasound-guided fine-needle aspiration biopsy, Clin. Ultrasound 22 (1994) 535–542.

[19] D. Danese, S. Sciacchitano, A. Farsetti, M. Andreoli, A. Pontecorvi, Diagnostic accuracy of conventional sonography-guided fine-needle aspiration biopsy of thyroid nodules, Thyroid 8 (1998) 15–21.

[20] I. Rosen, A. Azadian, P. Walfish, S. Salem, E. Lansdown, Y. Bedard, Ultrasound-guided fine-needle aspiration biopsy in the management of thyroid disease, Am. J. Surg. 166 (1993) 346–349.

[21] B. Cochand-Priollet, P. Guillausseau, S. Chagnon, C. Hong, C. Guillausseau-Scholer, P. Chanson, H. Dahan, A. Warnet, P. Tran Ba Huy, P. Valleur, The diagnostic value of fine-needle aspiration biopsy under ultrasonography in nonfunctional nodules: a prospective study comparing cytologic and histologic findings, Am. J. Med. 97 (1994) 152–157.

[22] C. Carmeci, B. Jefrey, R. McDougall, K. Nowels, R. Weigel, Ultrasound-guided fine-needle aspiration biopsy of thyroid masses, Thyroid 8 (1998) 283–289.

[23] G.C.H. Yang, D. Liebeskind, A.V. Messina, Ultrasound-guided fine-needle aspiration of the thyroid assessed by ultrafast Papanicolaou stain: data from 1135 biopsies with a two-to-six year follow-up, Thyroid 11 (2001) 581–589.

[24] T. Hatada, K. Okada, H. Ishii, S. Ichii, J. Utsunomiya, Evaluation of ultrasound-guided fine-needle aspiration biopsy for thyroid nodules, Am. J. Surg. 175 (1998) 133–136.

[25] G. Boland, M. Lee, P. Mueller, W. Mayo-Smith, S. Dawson, J. Simeone, Efficacy of sonographically guided biopsy of thyroid masses and cervical lymph nodes, AJR 161 (1993) 1053–1056.

[26] K. Khurana, V. Richards, P. Chopra, R. Izquierdo, D. Rubens, C. Mesonero, The role of ultrasonography-guided fine-needle aspiration in the management of nonpalpable and palpable thyroid nodules, Thyroid 8 (1998) 511–515.

[27] H.J. Baskin, Recombinant human thyrotropin stimulation of thyroglobulin in the follow-up of patients with stage I or II differentiated thyroid carcinoma, Endocrine Pract. 6 (2000) 430–434.

[28] J. Pineda, T. Lee, K. Ain, et al., Iodine-131 therapy for thyroid cancer patients with elevated thyroglobulin and negative diagnostic scan, J. Clin. Endocrinol. Metab. 80 (1995) 1488–1492.

[29] M. Schumberger, O. Arcangioli, J. Piekarski, et al., Detection and treatment of lung metastases of differentiated thyroid carcinoma in patients with normal chest X-ray, J. Nucl. Med. 29 (1988) 1790–1794.

[30] F. Pacini, R. Lari, S. Mazzeo, et al., Diagnostic value of a single serum thyroglobulin determination on and off thyroid suppressive therapy in the follow-up of patients with differentiated thyroid cancer, Clin. Endocrinol. 23 (1985) 405–411.

[31] H. Park, O. Perkins, J. Edmondson, et al., Influence of diagnostic radioiodines on the uptake of ablative dose of iodine-131, Thyroid 4 (1994) 49–54.

[32] B. Gorman, J. Charboneau, E. James, C. Reading, L. Wold, C. Grant, H. Gharib, I. Hay, Medullary thyroid carcinoma: role of high-resolution US, Radiology 162 (1987) 147–150.

[33] R. Sutton, C. Reading, J. Charboneau, M. James, C. Grant, I. Hay, US-guided biopsy of neck masses in postoperative management of patients with thyroid cancer, Radiology 168 (1988) 769–772.

[34] A. Antonelli, P. Miccoli, M. Ferdeghini, G. Di Coscio, B. Alberti, P. Iacconi, V. Baldi, P. Fallahi, L. Baschieri, Role of neck ultrasonography in the follow-up of patients operated on for thyroid cancer, Thyroid 5 (1995) 25–28.

[35] P. Vassallo, K. Wernecke, N. Ross, P. Peters, Differentiation of benign from malignant superficial lymphadenopathy: the role of high-resolution US, Radiology 183 (1992) 215–220.

[36] A. Frasoldati, E. Toschi, M. Zini, M. Flora, A. Caroggio, C. Dotti, R. Valcavi, Role of thyroglobulin measurement in fine-needle aspiration biopsies of cervical lymph nodes in patients with differentiated thyroid cancer, Thyroid 9 (1999) 105–111.

[37] H. Baskin, Detection of recurrent thyroid carcinoma by thyroglobulin assessment in the needle washout after fine-needle aspiration of suspicious lymph nodes, Thyroid 11 (2004) 959–963.

[38] M. Lee, D. Ross, P. Mueller, G. Daniels, S. Dawson, J. Simeone, Fine-needle biopsy of cervical lymph nodes in patients with thyroid cancer: a prospective comparison of cytopathologic and tissue marker analysis, Radiology 187 (1993) 851–854.

Chapter 4

Controversies in the use of radioiodine for remnant ablation and therapy of thyroid carcinoma

Richard T. Kloos

Internal Medicine and Radiology, Divisions of Endocrinology, Diabetes and Metabolism & Nuclear Medicine, The Ohio State University, OH, USA

1. Introduction

Radioactive iodine (^{131}I) represents a cornerstone of therapy for papillary thyroid carcinoma (PTC) and follicular (FTC) thyroid carcinoma, collectively referred to here as 'differentiated' thyroid carcinoma (DTC), along with thyroidectomy and thyroid-stimulating hormone (TSH) suppression. However, each of these therapeutic modalities is fraught with controversy because there are no prospective, randomized clinical studies to provide definitive data to guide clinical decision-making. Clinical investigations are confounded by the low incidence of thyroid carcinoma, its prolonged course, and the relatively good outcome for the majority of patients. The numerous controversies of thyroid neoplasms are perhaps reflected by the fact that every year there are about as many papers published on the topic as there are patients who die from thyroid carcinoma in the United States. An example of a controversy with ^{131}I is the finding of Samaan et al. [1] that ^{131}I therapy was the most significant treatment factor to increase the disease-free interval and survival; yet others have found little or no benefit from ^{131}I [2–9]. This chapter explores some of the current radioiodine controversies.

2. ^{131}I Thyroid remnant ablation

2.1. *Rationale for thyroid remnant ablation*

Since it is uncommon to remove all thyroid tissue with thyroidectomy, ^{131}I uptake is almost always seen postoperatively in the thyroid bed and any thyroglossal duct

ADVANCES IN MOLECULAR AND CELLULAR ENDOCRINOLOGY
VOLUME 4   ISSN 1569-2566/DOI 10.1016/S1569-2566(04)04004-9

remnant. The use of therapeutic doses of ^{131}I in the setting of unknown residual malignancy is referred to as remnant 'ablation.' [131]I administered to treat residual or recurrent carcinoma is referred to as 'therapy.' Prospective, randomized studies of remnant ablation are lacking and data from large, non-randomized retrospective studies are conflicting. Thus, the efficacy of ^{131}I ablation remains a controversial topic in the literature [5,7,10,11]. In practice, however, the current majority opinion favors remnant ablation as reflected in three questionnaire studies and a consensus panel of experts. In 1987, at an international symposium, 160 specialists from 13 countries recommended total thyroidectomy and remnant ablation for most patients with DTC [12]. In 1989, the majority of 157 thyroid experts recommended total or near-total thyroidectomy followed by 60–115 mCi [131]I (1.62–3.11 MBq; (1 mCi = 37 MBq, 100 mCi = 3.7 GBq).) remnant ablation for a hypothetical patient with a solitary DTC tumor [13]. In 1996, most of the clinical members of the American Thyroid Association recommended near-total thyroidectomy and ^{131}I ablation for a hypothetical patient with PTC [14]. The majority did not alter their recommendations regardless of radiation exposure, extremes of age, or a neoplasm less than 1 cm, and multiple foci in the contralateral lobe or capsular invasion by the neoplasm. In 1999, the National Comprehensive Cancer Network® (NCCN®) convened a multidisciplinary panel of experts that established annually updated consensus practice guidelines for the management of thyroid nodules and thyroid cancers based on a process that integrated the evaluation of scientific results and expert opinion. Version 1.2000 of the guidelines, published in November 1999 [15], favors total thyroidectomy and remnant ablation for all DTC except unifocal tumors < 1 cm in diameter.

Wong et al. [16] performed decision analysis to examine the effects of thyroid remnant ablation on survival, recurrence, and ^{131}I-induced leukemia and sialadenitis. In all cases, the benefit of ablation outweighed the risks, and the absolute loss of life expectancy from thyroid carcinoma exceeded that from leukemia by 4–40 fold.

2.1.1. *Decreased cancer recurrence after* [131]I *ablation*

Rationale for remnant ablation, along with rebutting literature, is outlined in Table 1. Cancer recurrence is associated with both morbidity and disease-specific mortality. For example, Voutilainen et al. [17] reported that carcinoma-specific 5- and 15-year survival after lymph node recurrence for patients up to 45 years old was 100 and 90%, while for those older than 45 years it was only 61 and < 30%, respectively. In a stepwise Cox proportional hazards regression model, the development of lymph node recurrence after original treatment, age, distant metastases, and the presence of lymph node metastases at the time of the original surgery were all independent predictors of survival. Death resulted mainly, but not exclusively, from distant metastases. An example of the effect of remnant ablation toward decrease in cancer recurrence is seen when comparing the incidences of pulmonary metastases after the initial therapy of thyroidectomy plus 100 mCi ^{131}I ablation, thyroidectomy alone, partial thyroidectomy plus ^{131}I, and partial thyroidectomy alone which were 1.3, 3, 5, and 11%, respectively [18].

Table 1
Rationale of thyroid remnant ablation

Outcome[a]	Rationale
Decrease recurrence [1,5,11,18,20,125,182–186]	Ablation of normal tissue destined to become malignant [187]
	Ablation of microscopic residual malignancy in the remnant
	Ablation of microscopic residual malignancy outside the remnant [43]
	Ablation of residual malignancy outside the remnant obscured by uptake in a large remnant [25,48,188]
	Demonstrate unsuspected residual malignancy on post-therapy scan to alter disease stage and further management (as in Fig. 1) [11,27,189]
Decrease death [5,19,20]	As above for recurrence
Simplify follow-up [11,28,32,33]	Eliminate all 'thyroid bed' uptake and its confusion with central compartment lymph nodes [134]
	Eliminate normal tissue as a source of thyroglobulin (Tg) production to simplify care of those without disease, while promoting early identification of those with residual cancer
	Eliminate normal tissue serving as a nidus for continued anti-Tg antibody production
Psychological reassurance	Patient and/or physician's consolation from being proactive rather than risk regret
	Reassurance of an undetectable or low stimulated Tg with or without a negative whole body scan
[131]I side effects	Side effects are usually mild with uncommon severe side effects
Cost	Regulations permitting outpatient ablation has safely reduced cost

[a]References including supporting and rebutting literature.

DeGroot et al. [19] reported that remnant ablation decreased recurrence of tumors larger than 1 cm, including those predicted to have a good prognosis (class I or II disease).

Samaan et al. [1] performed a stepwise proportional hazards (Cox model) regression on 1599 patients and found that remnant ablation was the most significant single factor to increase the disease-free interval. This was true for low risk patients, while the slight advantage seen in high-risk patients was not statistically significant.

Among patients with tumors > 1.5 cm, Mazzaferri reported that both local cancer recurrence and distant recurrence were significantly lower following remnant ablation than with levothyroxine (LT4) alone or no medical therapy [10]. In the latest analysis of this series, 230 patients had undergone remnant ablation, 789 had been treated with only LT4 and 163 had received no medical therapy; their median follow-up, respectively, was 14.7, 20.8 and 21.2 years [20]. With LT4 therapy alone, the recurrence rate was fourfold ($P < 0.0001$) and the distant recurrence rate was fivefold ($P < 0.02$) the rates of those who received remnant ablation. Based on regression modeling on 1510 patients without distant metastases at the time of initial therapy, remnant ablation was an independent variable that reduced all cancer recurrences and distant recurrences.

Other investigators have not found similar beneficial effects on tumor recurrence [2–5], including patients with PTC $\leqslant 1$ cm with metastatic lymph nodes [6], or inter- mediate- or high risk patients [7].

2.1.2. *Decrease in cancer-specific death after* ^{131}I *ablation*
In addition to reducing DTC recurrence, some investigators have noted a decrease in incidence of death from DTC after remnant ablation. DeGroot et al. [19] reported that remnant ablation reduced the risk of death only in patients with more advanced disease (class III or IV).

Mazzaferri reported significantly lower cancer death rates for patients older than 40 years with tumors > 1.5 cm following remnant ablation as compared to those with LT4 alone or no medical therapy [10]. In the latest analysis of this series, there were fewer cancer deaths 40 years after thyroid remnant ablation than after the other treatment strategies (20% versus 2%, $P < 0.001$). Based on regression modeling on 1510 patients without distant metastases at the time of initial therapy, remnant ablation was an independent variable that reduced cancer death [20].

Other investigators have not found similar beneficial effects on cause-specific mortality [5–7].

2.1.3. *Simplified patient follow-up and early detection of disease*
In the past, tumor recurrence was defined by the clinical detection of tumor in a patient previously thought to be free of disease, based on the criteria that usually did not include serum thyroglobulin (Tg) values. In such studies, the average risk of tumor recurrence during long-term follow-up was about 15–35% [20–22]. About three-fourths of all recurrences and two-thirds of distant recurrences occur in the first 10 years after initial therapy [21–23]. Using modern methodologies and criteria, it is likely that most of the patients with 'recurrences' after thyroidectomy and remnant ablation would never have been deemed free of disease. The rate of disease recur- rence after achieving and undetectable serum Tg despite thyroid hormone with- drawal (THW) may be $< 1\%$ when followed for as long as an average of 12 years [24,25].

The major goal of follow-up is to promptly differentiate the patients who are free of disease from those who are not, because early detection and intervention might diminish morbidity and mortality. For example, limited extent of disease was an independent predictor of survival in a study of pulmonary and bone metastases [26]. Schlumberger et al. [27] reported that the chest X-ray was normal in patients with pulmonary metastases before and after institution of routine Tg determination in 13 and 43% of patients, respectively, suggesting that Tg measurement enabled earlier disease detection. Complete remission occurred in 64% of patients with lung or bone metastases and a normal X-ray (Fig. 1), as opposed to only 8% of those with an abnormal X-ray. Additionally, pulmonary metastases were detected in 18 patients by the post-therapy whole body scan (RxWBS), while they were undetected by the 2 mCi diagnostic whole body scan (DxWBS) [27]. Thus, patients (Fig. 1) are at a risk of delayed diagnosis of distant metastases when remnant ablation and post-therapy imaging are not practiced.

Ant 48 HR   Post   Ant   Post

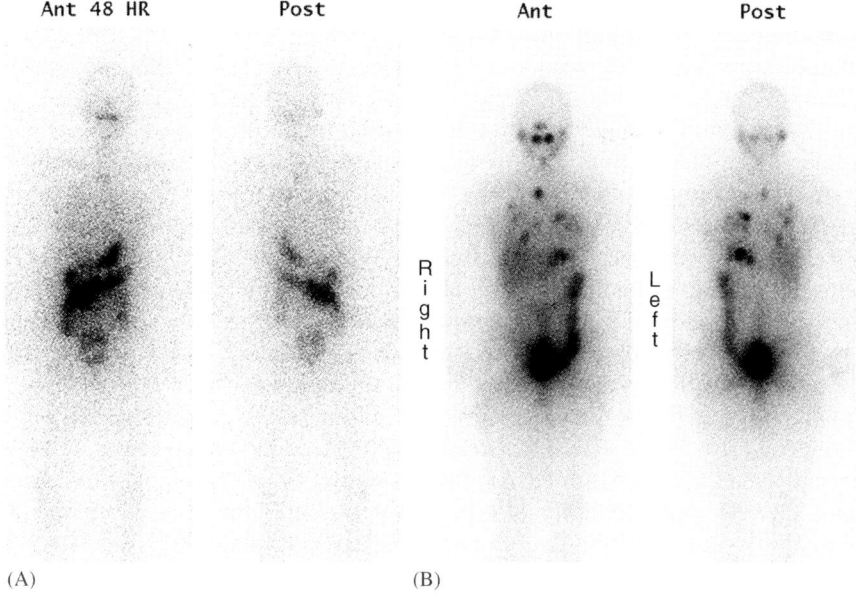

(A)   (B)

Fig. 1. Twenty-eight-year-old female, at age 27 years, underwent a total thyroidectomy that yielded a left 1.2 cm PTC, central neck and superior mediastinal dissections with 6 of 9 metastatic lymph nodes, and a left modified neck dissection with 3 of 24 metastatic lymph nodes. A peri-operative chest X-ray was normal and she was given 30 mCi ^{131}I- after a diagnostic scan revealed thyroid bed uptake with a TSH of 77 µIU mL^{-1}, qualitative serum Tg antibodies were positive, and serum was Tg 5.3 ng mL^{-1}. The post-therapy scan revealed diffuse and focal pulmonary uptake. A subsequent bone scan was normal and a chest CT demonstrated 'small' pulmonary nodules. The patient was referred to the Ohio State University Medical Center where she underwent hypothyroid lithium dosimetry where her 2 mCi 48 h diagnostic WBS (A) showed faint superior mediastinal uptake, her 48 h whole body retention was 13.1%, and her whole blood (beta plus gamma) dosimetry revealed 0.543 rad mCi^{-1}. Her serum TSH was 117.8 µIU mL^{-1}, serum TG antibodies were positive at 3.6 U mL^{-1} (normal <2.0 U mL^{-1}), and serum Tg was <0.5 ng mL^{-1}. She was prescribed 365 mCi of ^{131}I- and her 7-day post-therapy WBS (B) showed probable superior mediastinal uptake, and bilateral pulmonary metastases. Ten months later she underwent hypothyroid lithium 2 mCi ^{131}I- 48 h WBS that was normal (image not shown) with a serum TSH of 120.9 µIU mL^{-1}, negative Tg antibodies, and serum Tg <0.5 ng mL^{-1}.

Patient surveillance depends on measurement of serum Tg during both TSH suppression and stimulation, usually with an ^{131}I DxWBS. The sensitivities of all of these diagnostic tests have remarkably improved after remnant ablation. This is true to such a degree for available Tg assays that routine whole body imaging in patients thought to be free of disease (undetectable serum Tg during TSH suppression) is largely being replaced by THW- or rhTSH-stimulated serum Tg measurement alone [24,25,28]. Neither of these diagnostic maneuvers requires a low iodine diet and both eliminate the additional cost, inconvenience, and radiation exposure of ^{131}I imaging.

2.1.3.1. *Scan sensitivity after ^{131}I ablation.* It is well appreciated that substantial thyroid remnants can obscure the presence of local and distant metastases. Besides, there is little consensus on the importance, or definition, of small residual thyroid remnants that can be attained only after total thyroidectomy. In the setting of a low, stimulated serum Tg, some view small remnants as 'trivial' and clinically insignificant, and with no proven benefit to their ablation. Others feel that all remnants must be fully ablated, and some believe that the RxWBS must be negative before ablation is considered complete. Continuing with controversy, no consensus exists on the level of serum Tg that one can attribute to a visible thyroid remnant versus the level of serum Tg that is excessive and suggests the presence of disease in addition to the visualized remnant [29]. Finally, the distinction of remnant uptake in the thyroid bed or thyroglossal duct remnant versus uptake in malignant tissue is not always clear-cut. The boundaries where normal thyroid tissue may be seen include paramedical uptake between the suprasternal notch and thyroid cartilage and/or nearly midline uptake superior to the thyroid cartilage from a thyroglossal duct remnant. However, central compartment lymph nodes commonly contain metastases in papillary thyroid carcinoma and are found within the same boundaries. Thus, there seems to be more agreement that it is easier to interpret the clinical status of a patient with a frankly negative DxWBS than the status of a patient with visible thyroid bed uptake [30].

Given these controversies, patient care is often simplified by ^{131}I ablation that eliminates all thyroid bed uptake in the majority and leaves very small residual remnants in almost all of the rest, which are associated with very low or undetectable stimulated serum Tg levels in those free of disease [28].

2.1.3.2. *Serum Tg during TSH suppression.* Both normal thyroid epithelial cells and DTC produce serum Tg. It follows that Tg measurement is a much more sensitive and specific test for carcinoma when measured after near-total or total thyroidectomy and remnant ablation [31,32]. For example, in one series of patients considered free of disease after total or near-total thyroidectomy, the serum Tg levels during thyroid hormone therapy were $> 10 \, \text{ng} \, \text{mL}^{-1}$ in 1.8% and 9.1% in those treated with and without ^{131}I ablation, respectively [33]. In another series of patients treated with total thyroidectomy, who had remnant uptake of less than 2% and no ^{131}I ablation, the Tg level was detectable in 7% during thyroid hormone therapy and in 20% after THW [11]. In contrast, only 1% of patients free of disease after thyroidectomy and remnant ablation from a separate series had a serum Tg $> 0.5 \, \text{ng} \, \text{mL}^{-1}$ during TSH suppression [28]. In this series, the specificity of a detectable serum Tg during TSH suppression for residual or recurrent thyroid carcinoma was 99%; however, the sensitivity was still low at 36% because 7 of 11 patients with disease had serum Tg levels $\leqslant 0.5 \, \text{ng} \, \text{mL}^{-1}$ during TSH suppression.

2.1.3.3. *Accuracy of serum Tg during TSH stimulation.* The recurrence rate of DTC is high and recurrences occur over a span of decades [20]. Except for patients with residual normal thyroid tissue, it is likely that these 'recurrences' are actually cases of persistent disease that have progressed to the point of detection. The most concerning fact is that disease 'recurrence' is a predictor of an adverse outcome, including death [17]. The logical conclusion, therefore, is that the persistent disease that progresses is likely a predictor of an unfavorable outcome. The cutoff value of stimulated serum Tg that warns the clinician of possible persistent or recurrent disease has been declining and this decline is likely to continue. At the current cutoff levels, false-positive test results from residual normal tissue are common and diminish the utility of the test when the thyroid remnant is not ablated. The current sensitive Tg assays allow more reliable measurement of low serum Tg levels that allow for the early diagnosis of residual or recurrent DTC when the tumor bulk is low, and the therapy is more likely to be effective. High specificity of low-serum Tg cutoff levels for DTC can be reliably achieved only after ^{131}I ablation.

Tg measurement is more sensitive when thyroid hormone has been stopped or rhTSH is given to elevate the serum TSH as opposed to during TSH suppression [26,28,34–36], and under these conditions Tg is more sensitive than ^{131}I WBS [34,36].

After THW, a serum Tg above $5–10 \, \text{ng mL}^{-1}$ or after rhTSH stimulation, a Tg above $2 \, \text{ng mL}^{-1}$ is a sign of disease or a persistent thyroid remnant, with the former much more likely when the 2- to 4-mCi [131]I DxWBS is negative [15,28,35,37–39]. One recent study of thyroid cancer patients with no clinical evidence of disease and undetectable or very low serum Tg levels during thyroid hormone therapy evaluated the serum Tg in response to rhTSH [28]. Serum Tg remaining at $\leqslant 0.5 \, \text{ng mL}^{-1}$ in 64% of patients, increase to levels between 0.6 and $2 \, \text{ng mL}^{-1}$ in 18% and to levels $> 2 \, \text{ng mL}^{-1}$ in 19%. Ten percent of the patients, who all had rhTSH-stimulated serum Tg levels above $2 \, \text{ng mL}^{-1}$, were proven to have persistent tumor. A rhTSH-stimulated $\text{Tg} > 2 \, \text{ng mL}^{-1}$ had a sensitivity of 100%, a negative predictive value of 100%, and a false-positive rate of 9%. Over time, it is likely that more of these patients will be found to have disease (including false-positive patients), likely at a rate proportional to their rise in Tg after rhTSH. In fact, this has already begun to occur among the false-positive patients. This degree of accuracy and clinical utility with low-serum Tg cutoff values can be reliably achieved only after remnant ablation.

2.1.3.4. *Resolution of interfering antithyroglobulin antibodies.*   Serum anti-Tg antibodies are present in up to 20–25% of DTC patients at diagnosis and initial management, and are about twice as common in them as in the general population. These antibodies almost always compromise, if not invalidate, the serum Tg measurement [32,40]. In patients treated with thyroidectomy and ^{131}I, a stable or increase in anti-Tg antibody titer is indicative of active disease, whereas a decrease in antibody titer occurs in those who have become free of disease (Fig. 1) [31,32]. [131]I contributes to the elimination of these interfering antibodies by destroying residual antigen that would otherwise serve as a source for continued antibody stimulation. Following ^{131}I administration, there may be a transient increase in antibody titer (presumably due to antigen release from cell destruction) and then gradual antibody resolution (usually within a year) that largely simplifies patient care by restoring the reliability of serum Tg determination.

2.1.4. *Psychological comfort*
It is logical that the attitude of the physician influences the attitude of the patient. This effect may have influenced the observation that most patients view the risk to

benefit ratio of remnant ablation favorably only for the *possibility* of reduced disease recurrence, mortality, or improved accuracy of follow-up. Many patients are psychologically comforted, or even strengthened, by being proactive (and possibly without benefit on an individual basis) against cancer and its possibilities. To most, this 'aggressive' course of action appears favorable to risking regret.

2.2. *Candidate patients for remnant ablation*

2.2.1. *DTC surgery as it relates to remnant ablation*

For patients to be considered for ^{131}I remnant ablation (or residual thyroid cancer therapy), they should ideally have had a total or near-total thyroidectomy. Attempted total thyroid ablation (or treatment of residual cancer) after only lobectomy followed by ^{131}I therapy should be discouraged. This often results in incomplete destruction of the large normal remnant. Meanwhile, TSH stimulation is inadequate to drive ^{131}I into malignant cells with their characteristically reduced Na^+/I^- symporter (NIS) function, and overall the maneuver is associated with an appreciable rate of acute complications from radiation thyroiditis [41,42].

2.2.1.1. *Initial thyroid surgery.*   Most experts [15,37,43], but not all [44,45], recommend total or near-total thyroidectomy for all patients with DTC when the diagnosis of cancer is known preoperatively as it improves disease-free survival, even in children and adults with low-risk tumors [46–49]. This procedure removes multifocal and bilateral carcinoma, and provides the opportunity to ablate residual thyroid bed uptake with smaller doses of ^{131}I [41,49]. Pacini et al. [43] reported that 44% of patients undergoing completion thyroidectomy had tumor in the contralateral lobe with almost one-third demonstrating lymph node metastases. Bilateral disease was correlated with lymph node metastases at the initial surgical treatment and the time interval between initial surgery and the completion thyroidectomy, but not with initial tumor size, multifocality, or risk group classification. An additional 5% of the patients had no contralateral tumor, but did have lymph node metastases. When there is a local or distant tumor recurrence following lobectomy, cancer is found in more than 60% of the excised contralateral lobes [50].

Papillary thyroid cancers $\leqslant 1$ cm are multifocal in 20–46% of cases, associated with lymph node metastases in about a 15–35%, recurrent in about 3–11%, and cause death or distant metastases in about 1% [51–54]. Lobectomy is adequate surgery for papillary microcarcinoma discovered serendipitously on histological analysis postoperatively, provided the patient has no other risk factors such as significant exposure to radiation or a family history of DTC, and has a truly low-risk cancer: a tumor that is unifocal, confined to the thyroid, smaller than 1–1.5 cm, and without vascular invasion or histologic variation that predicts more aggressive behavior [21,51,53,55–59]. Similarly, lobectomy may be considered adequate for minimally invasive small (<4 cm) follicular carcinomas (without penetration through the tumor capsule or vascular invasion) confined to the thyroid and discovered postoperatively as they rarely recur or cause death. Follicular carcinomas with any vascular invasion or penetration through the tumor capsule should be treated with total thyroidectomy and ^{131}I ablation. In a study of follicular carcinomas that included small-to-medium vessel invasion, all tumor recurrences and death occurred in patients treated with less than a subtotal thyroidectomy, while total thyroidectomy treatment combined with ^{131}I ablation had a significantly better outcome ($P = 0.02$). Despite these findings, the authors concluded that therapy beyond lobectomy was unnecessary, given the groups overall excellent long-term prognosis and good patient outcome [60].

2.2.1.2. *Completion thyroidectomy.* When lobectomy with or without isthmusectomy has been performed, completion thyroidectomy should be considered for lesions with the potential to reoccur. There is no reason to preserve intrinsic thyroid function because thyroid hormone therapy is routinely used to achieve TSH suppression.

Completion thyroidectomy, by properly skilled surgeons, has a low complication rate [43] and is appropriate for thyroid carcinomas as outlined in Table 2. A study of Chernobyl children with thyroid cancer found that completion thyroidectomy allowed for the diagnosis and treatment of recurrent cancer and lung or lymph node metastases in 61% of patients, in whom residual carcinoma was not preoperatively recognized [48]. Machens et al. [61] performed 88 consecutive completion thyroidectomies for incidental DTC with negative surgical margins (cases of unifocal PTC

Table 2
Indications for total or near-total thyroidectomy for thyroid carcinoma [50,58,59,62,190–195]

Factors for consideration
- Patient and doctor decision
- Presence of hypothyroidism eliminates the rationale to spare thyroid tissue
- Presence of anti-thyroglobulin antibodies (eventual hypothyroidism risk if anti-microsomal antibodies are also present, and interference with serum Tg measurement)

Risk of adverse outcome from thyroid cancer
- Previous neck radiation therapy
- Active hyperthyroidism from Graves' disease or presence of thyroid-stimulating immunoglobulin (TSI)
- Papillary carcinoma >1–1.5 cm in diameter
- FTC with any penetration of tumor all the way through the tumor capsule or any vascular invasion (tumor penetration into but not through the tumor capsule is referred to as minimal invasion)
- FTC larger than 4 cm with minimal capsule invasion
- Multifocal carcinoma of any size

Factors suggesting higher risk of adverse outcome
- Familial differentiated thyroid carcinoma
- Aggressive thyroid cancer variants
- Carcinoma with a high histologic grade (nuclear atypia, necrosis or vascular invasion)
- Carcinoma that has metastasized
- Carcinoma with extrathyroidal extension
- Carcinoma with a positive surgical margin/incomplete resection

---

measuring $\leqslant 10$ mm were not re-operated) in conjunction with a systematic en bloc resection of the central compartment. Despite all patients having negative pre-operative clinical examinations and ultrasonography, 22% were found to harbor residual tumor including 11% with intrathyroidal tumor, 6% with extrathyroidal soft tissue infiltrates, and 10% with lymph node metastases. Scheumann et al. [62] reported that when patients underwent a subtotal thyroid resection and a decision was taken to re-operate for completion thyroidectomy, a delay of more than 6 months increased the relative risk of death by 4.31 times compared with patients re-operated within 6 months. Beierwaltes et al. [63] had previously suggested the importance of completion thyroidectomy within 6 months while Pacini et al. [43] did not see this effect.

2.2.2. Selection of patients for ^{131}I remnant ablation

Several staging and prognostic scoring systems have been devised that discriminate between low-risk patients who might require less aggressive therapy and higher risk patients who generally require more aggressive therapy to avoid morbidity and mortality from thyroid carcinoma [64–66]. While these systems are helpful and important, they fail to identify a group of patients who are not at a risk of disease recurrence or death [67]. For example, the TNM classification of the American Joint Commission on Cancer (AJCC) and International Union Against Cancer (UICC) is widely available and accepted for many malignancies, including thyroid carcinoma [68]. With this system, most tumors are classified as Stage I, thus *de facto* categorizing most patients with DTC as being at low risk [69]. However, patients with stage I TNM tumors had a 15% recurrence rate after a median of 11 years follow-up in one study [69], which indicates that aggressive therapy for this group is appropriate. In another study, Hundahl et al. [70] reported a relative 96 and 68% 10-year survival rates for patients categorized as low and high risk, respectively, according to the classification age-metastases-extent-size (AMES); however, almost two-thirds of the cancer deaths in this series occurred in the low-risk group because they outnumbered high-risk patients almost by a ratio 15:1.

Most staging systems use advancing patient age at diagnosis to predict survival, which is problematic. Although mortality increases as age advances, death rates may be high in children under the age of 10 years [71–73]. Further, relatively less importance is assigned to tumor recurrence and its associated morbidity in these staging systems, which is a problem because recurrence rates are high, especially in patients diagnosed with DTC during the first two decades [20]. Finally, the application of scoring systems to patients at institutions other than where the system was developed may not yield wholly reproducible results [74].

Accordingly, staging systems may offer less support for the notion of performing lobectomy followed by only thyroid hormone as opposed to total or near-total thyroidectomy and ^{131}I ablation for tumors at low risk of causing cancer mortality, because these tumors are often at substantial risk of recurrence. ^{131}I ablation (or therapy) is advised for the same group of patients for whom total or near-total thyroidectomy is recommended and is outlined in Table 2.

2.3. *Patient preparation for remnant ablation*

2.3.1. *Stable iodine depletion*
2.3.1.1. *Low-iodine diet.* A low-iodine diet is recommended whenever ^{131}I imaging or therapy is to occur [75]. A daily iodine diet of about 50 g for 1 week can raise thyroidal ^{131}I uptake and can double the Gy per 100 mCi of ^{131}I administered [76,77]. It is unknown if a longer period of iodine deprivation would be more beneficial. It is also unknown if the same result could be achieved with a shorter duration of iodine deprivation. In the study by Lakshmanan et al. [75], athyreotic patients deviating from the diet demonstrated clearance of excess iodine by the next day. This finding may not be applicable to patients with residual remnant tissue or carcinoma. One approach is to start the diet 2 weeks before ^{131}I therapy, as this gives patients the opportunity to raise questions and possibly make mistakes in the first week, so that the diet is more optimal in the second week. While it is possible that compliance with the diet could diminish over time and have a negative impact in the second week, Lakshmanan et al. [75] showed good compliance with the diet over a 4-week time period. A free low-iodine cookbook is available from the Thyroid Cancer Survivors' Association website [78].

While there is some question as to how soon the diet should be started before dosing with ^{131}I, greater uncertainty exists as to how long the diet should be maintained after ^{131}I therapy. Reasons to continue the low-iodine diet after ^{131}I administration include maximizing ^{131}I uptake in order to deliver its radiation effects to the target thyroidal tissue. In euthyroid iodine sufficient humans, thyroid uptake is maximal at 24–48 h [79]. In hyperthyroid subjects (e.g. thyroid autonomy) with small thyroid iodine pools that turn over rapidly (which may be more similar to thyroidectomized subjects with high TSH levels on low-iodine diets), peak thyroid uptake may occur before 24 h [80]. In a small sample group of patients, metastatic thyroid carcinoma lesions achieved their maximal uptake 1–3 days following ^{131}I therapy [81]. However, despite the static moment of 'peak' [131]I uptake, there is some dynamic element of ^{131}I recirculation such that the ^{131}I may be taken up and processed through the thyroid on more than one occasion, delivering therapeutic radiation with each passage [79].

A reason to terminate the low-iodine diet and initiate therapy with stable non-radioactive iodine is to try and 'trap' the ^{131}I in the target tissue after it has been organified via the Wolff–Chaikoff effect. Stable iodine loading is known to rapidly block release of thyroid hormone secretion. Stable iodide is proposed to directly inhibit intrathyroidal lysosomal activity and colloid resorption [82,83]. Theoretically, these latter effects may be used to prolong the retention of organified ^{131}I in target tissues and deliver greater radiation therapy, although this effect lasts no longer than 7 days in normal adults [79].

Despite these uncertainties, no study has investigated the optimal duration to continue the low-iodine diet after ^{131}I therapy or the use of stable iodine in this setting. Some experts advise stopping the diet 3–24 h after ^{131}I therapy [84]. Alternatively, one may stop the low-iodine diet in the morning 2 days after the therapy, knowing that an earlier discontinuation is possible, especially under unique circumstances.

2.3.1.2. *Stable iodine from CT, angiography, and ERCP contrast.* Physicians must be aware of the many dietary, dietary supplement, and medical sources of stable iodine that can reduce ^{131}I uptake into target tissues. Three common medical sources include iodinated contrast used for computed tomography (CT) imaging, coronary angiography, and endoscopic retrograde cholangio-pancreatography (ERCP).

Ionic and non-ionic CT contrast media contain an average of less than $10 \mu g \, mL^{-1}$ of free inorganic iodide and are typically administered in 150 mL intravenous doses [85]. This iodine load is 30 times the recommended daily allowance of the low-iodine diet [75]. The duration and intensity of impaired RAIU after currently utilized iodinated contrast agents is not well defined, and is expected to vary based on the volume of contrast administered, the content of free iodide, and other biological variables including renal function and volume of residual thyroid tissue or tumor. Nygaard et al. [86] found that the RAIU reduced by 53% 1 week after 100 mL of iohexol. One patient was reported to return to normal within a few weeks. In the absence of more explicit data and knowing that hypothyroidism is associated impaired iodine excretion, a minimum of 6 weeks duration from CT in contrast to ^{131}I administration is preferred, but every effort to allow for more than a 12-week interval is probably prudent. Impaired RAIU is not seen with MR gadolinium contrast [87].

Systemic iodine absorption from radiographic contrast agents used for ERCP is significant and can impair RAIU. Urinary iodine concentrations have been shown to return to normal after 2–3 weeks [88], while others have found elevated levels after 6 weeks [89].

Elevated urinary iodine levels are present at 6 [90] and 12 weeks [91] after coronary angiography with a return to normal levels at 24 weeks [90].

2.3.2. *TSH stimulation*

2.3.2.1. *Thyroid hormone withdrawal (THW).* The optimal magnitude of TSH elevation prior to ^{131}I therapy and the duration of TSH elevation after ^{131}I therapy to destroy target tissue are not well characterized. Historically, a target TSH level $>30 \mu IU \, mL^{-1}$ for ^{131}I imaging and therapy has been cited [84], based on only one study. In their study, Edmonds et al. [92] reported 2 patients with no significant ^{131}I uptake in their tumor despite modest TSH elevation ($\sim$10–30 mU L^{-1}), which demonstrated considerable uptake when the TSH was further elevated (probably 50–90 mU L^{-1}). Importantly, Torres et al. [93] suggested that TSH receptors become saturated at serum TSH concentrations between 51 and 82 mU L^{-1}.

The duration of THW required to achieve adequate TSH elevation has historically been cited as 4–6 weeks with some patients given liothyronine (LT3) until the final 3 weeks [94,95]. The duration of THW needed to adequately raise the TSH is likely dependent partly upon the amount of residual functioning thyroidal tissue, the degree and duration of any previous TSH suppression therapy, age, and other factors [92,96–99].

Edmonds et al. [92] found that 42% patients had TSH levels $>30 \mu IU \, mL^{-1}$ 2–3 weeks after total thyroidectomy despite incomplete tumor resection. In a subset of patient treated twice with ^{131}I and 4 weeks of LT4 withdrawal, the TSH exceeded 50 mU L^{-1} in 75% patients.

Schlumberger et al. [98] studied patients whose thyroid extract was replaced with LT3 for 3 weeks and then withdrawn. Sixteen days after LT3 withdrawal, 87% of patients had TSH levels $\geqslant 37$ mU L^{-1}. Maxon performed a similar study and found that 90% of patients had TSH levels of at least 30 mU L^{-1} 3 weeks after stopping LT3 [95].

Guimaraes and DeGroot [100] found that 5 of 7 patients with baseline TSH levels < 1 μU mL^{-1} had TSH levels above 25–30 mU L^{-1} after reducing the LT4 dose by 50% for 8–10 weeks, while 5 of 6 patients with baseline TSH levels > 1 μU mL^{-1} had similar TSH elevations after 5 weeks. Maxon [101] performed a modified LT4 reduction protocol with baseline TSH levels < 0.1 μU mL^{-1} in 71% and found that LT4 reductions to about 25% of baseline resulted in a TSH of > 25 μU mL^{-1} in all patients after a mean of 8 weeks. Patients felt better on the reduced LT4 protocol as compared with the standard LT4 + LT3 withdrawal.

TSH exerts stimulatory effects on all steps of iodine metabolism from the initial active transport of iodine into thyroid follicular cells to secretion of thyroid hormones into the blood. Thus, optimal destruction of the target tissue would appear to require a balance between TSH-stimulated uptake and organification of ^{131}I versus TSH-stimulated secretion of the organified products out of the target tissue. Thus, radiation of the target thyroidal tissue may be enhanced by rapid suppression of TSH following ^{131}I organification. However, as with the discontinuation of the low-iodine diet, there are no studies as to when and how thyroid hormone should be reinstituted. Some experts have reported restarting thyroid hormone 5 days after therapy [27]. However, this delay may not be needed as simple reinitiation of LT4 at the dose used for chronic maintenance results in prolonged elevation of TSH levels [102]. Several protocols designed to rapidly treat myxedema or more rapidly suppress TSH elevation have been reported using LT4 with or without LT3 [102]. The effect of these protocols on ^{131}I retention in target tissues is unknown.

2.3.2.2. *Recombinant human TSH (rhTSH).* Recently, recombinant human TSH (Thyrogen®) has been developed for diagnostic use in thyroid cancer patients while maintaining euthyroidism [28,35]. Thyrogen produces average peak TSH levels > 120 mU L^{-1} [103,104]. The 22 h half-life of rhTSH produces TSH levels of ~ 10 mU L^{-1} at 4 days following the last administration [105]. This rapid reduction of TSH may suppress ^{131}I turnover from the target thyroidal tissue. This potentially enhanced radiation retention in target tissue, coupled with the known, enhanced whole body clearance of iodine during euthyroidism [84,106], may differentially increase the radiation dose delivered to target tissues compared with non-target tissues. However, a randomized study of the dosimetry or outcome from rhTSH-mediated thyroid remnant ablation or therapy is necessary [106]. In 2001, Robbins and colleagues [196] reported their findings from 10 non-randomized patients who received 'remnant ablation' (2 patients had reported metastases on pre-ablation DxWBS) with 30–250 mCi (mean 110 mCi) 24 h after the second of two daily 0.9 mg rhTSH injections. All patients subsequently had a visually negative rhTSH-stimulated DxWBS 72 h after ~ 5 mCi ^{131}I between 5 and 13 months later, although 4 of the 10 had concurrent rhTSH-stimulated Tg levels $\geqslant 3.4$ ng mL^{-1} consistent with residual disease. While these results are consistent with effective remnant ablation, the presence of residual disease emphasizes the necessity of a randomized controlled study comparing rhTSH remnant ablation with THW before decisive conclusions can be drawn.

2.3.3. *Diagnostic whole body scan (DxWBS)*

2.3.3.1. *Utility.* There is a general, but not universal, agreement that a RxWBS should be obtained after ^{131}I therapy as it is more sensitive in detecting remnant and malignant tissue than is the DxWBS performed with a substantially lower ^{131}I dose [107–111]. For example, Fatourechi et al. found abnormal ^{131}I uptake undetected on the 3 mCi DxWBS in 13%, and this changed management strategy in 9% [109]. More controversial is the use of a DxWBS prior to ^{131}I therapy or ablation [112]. Logically, the DxWBS may be omitted when the results will not alter therapy [25,104,107]. Reasons to obtain the image include the chance to confirm the presence of iodine concentrating tissue to be ablated [108]. Physicians tend to base their decision on ^{131}I ablation based on the amount of residual remnant uptake, the stimulated serum Tg level, or both. While even the most experienced surgeons typically leave some residual thyroid tissue behind, occasionally there is no residual thyroid bed uptake combined with an undetectable serum Tg level. Most physicians would not administer ^{131}I ablative therapy in this setting [108]. Whether patients having small amounts of residual bed uptake ($<0.5\%$) with undetectable or low ($<5\,ng\,dL^{-1}$) serum Tg levels are benefited from remnant ablation is not yet established [24,25,108]. A DxWBS having no or less remnant uptake with disproportionately high serum Tg may identify patients with poor iodine avid metastatic disease or those contaminated by stable iodine. Conversely, the presence of an unexpected large thyroid remnant should prompt consideration of further surgery prior to ^{131}I ablation [113]. Detection of the presence or absence of metastatic lesions on the DxWBS may alter the activity of therapeutic ^{131}I to be administered [106,108]. Uncommonly, central nervous system metastases may be detected on the DxWBS and can prompt hospitalization and institution of glucocorticoid therapy if ^{131}I treatment were to be given.

2.3.3.2. *Stunning.* Administering $\geqslant 3$ mCi of ^{131}I may have a sufficiently harmful effect upon the tissue in which it concentrates to interfere with subsequent uptake of ^{131}I, an effect first described in 1951 [114–117]. Using $\leqslant 2$ mCi of ^{131}I or 500 µCi of ^{123}I may avoid stunning, but is less sensitive than larger ^{131}I doses in identifying remnants or metastases [116–119]. Using more ^{123}I may improve DxWBS images [104,120,121], but the cost is higher and production requires a cyclotron [108]. Delaying ^{131}I therapy may be responsible for the stunning effect [116–118], which was not visually apparent in 172 patients treated with ^{131}I within 72 h of receiving 5 mCi for a DxWBS [122]. Similarly, Morris et al. [107] found no difference in the rate of ablation if treatment was given without a DxWBS compared with the ablation rate when therapy was given within 2–5 days after a 3–5 mCi diagnostic dose. However, the possibility of quantitative stunning below the threshold of visible stunning has not been excluded in these studies [123,124].

2.4. ^{131}I dose for remnant ablation

There are no randomized studies of the ablation dose and long-term DTC outcome to help in guiding the clinician. Current clinical practice has been derived largely from empiric experience. For many years the standard ^{131}I dose for remnant ablation was between 75 and 150 mCi, but now many use lower doses of 30–50 mCi, at least for uncomplicated cases [21,125,126]. In one non-randomized series of 100 patients, 43 received 29–50 mCi (mean 45 mCi) and 57 received 51–200 mCi (mean 111 mCi), with both groups experiencing similar clinical recurrence rates (7 and 9%, respectively, $P = 0.7$) [10]. The effect of selection bias on the results of this study is not known.

In a prospective, randomized clinical study of various ^{131}I doses on remnant ablation (but not cancer outcome) from New Delhi, India [126], successful thyroid remnant ablation was achieved in 63 and 78%, respectively, given $\sim$30 and 51 mCi of ^{131}I, and the rate of successful ablations did not increase with even larger doses of ^{131}I. This optimal dose of $\sim$51 mCi was reported to deliver $\sim$30,000 rad (1 Gy = 100 rad) to the thyroid remnant. A study from the United States found that a mean ^{131}I dose of $\sim$87 mCi was necessary to deliver 30,000 rad to the remnant, which ablated in 86% of the cases [41].

Interest in low-dose ablation is derived from a desire to minimize radiation exposure (and presumably side effects), reduce radiopharmaceutical cost, and avoid the cost and inconvenience of patient hospitalization previously required by the Nuclear Regulatory Commission (NRC) until activity was < 30 mCi (or < 5 mrem h^{-1} at 1 m). However, 1997 NRC changes (Code of Federal Regulations, title 10, part 35.75) now permit the outpatient use of much larger ^{131}I doses throughout most of the United States [127]. Recent commentary on the previous 30 mCi limitation found it seriously flawed but quiescently accepted and lamented that it may have been responsible for the inappropriate therapy of thyroid cancer patients, unnecessary hospitalizations, and increased health care costs for nearly 50 years [128]. A recent study [129] of the current practice found that radiation exposure to household members of patients receiving outpatient ^{131}I therapy for thyroid carcinoma, which ranged from $\sim$75 to 150 mCi of ^{131}I were well below the limit (5.0 mSv) mandated by current regulations. For comparison, German patients are not discharged with > 75 MBq (2 mCi) and in Europe the annual public dose limit is 1 mSv [130].

Given these data, candidates for relatively low-dose remnant ablation (50–100 mCi) may be those who have undergone a total or near-total thyroidectomy or completion thyroidectomy and have visible uptake only in the thyroid bed or thyroglossal duct remnant, a measurable serum Tg that is proportionate to the neck RAIU [29], and are at relatively low risk of having residual tumor deposits (Table 2). Patients at high risk of having residual disease should be considered for higher (therapy dose magnitude) activity of ^{131}I.

Patients with large amounts of residual tissue in the neck, such as an entire lobe or tissue sufficient to prohibit frank hypothyroidism, should undergo completion thyroidectomy. High levels of circulating TSH, necessary to enhance tumor ^{131}I uptake and destruction, cannot be achieved in the presence of a large thyroid remnant [97].

Only under unusual circumstances should large thyroid remnants be treated with ^{131}I. In such compromised situations, consideration may be given to using a low-^{131}I dose (~30 mCi) to incompletely ablate the thyroid remnant intentionally. A subsequent attempt at remnant ablation would likely be associated with greater TSH stimulation and produce less local side effects. Patients with large thyroid remnants ablated with substantial ^{131}I doses often develop severe radiation thyroiditis (occasionally associated with thyrotoxicosis), sometimes with airway compromise, and often require large cumulative doses of ^{131}I to completely destroy the remnant [41,42].

2.5. *Definition of complete ablation and selection of patients for repeat ^{131}I ablation*

Remnant ablation should be performed at 6–12-month intervals until complete ablation has been accomplished. The criteria for this endpoint are, however, relatively arbitrary and may include visual or quantitative limits of residual uptake in the thyroid bed, stimulated serum Tg levels, or both [131,132]. Nonetheless, small amounts of residual normal tissue (such as <0.5% uptake at 24–72 h) are unlikely to be the source of serum Tg levels above 10 ng mL^{-1} [25,29,133].

Whether evaluated by THW or rhTSH, successful ablation may be defined as a negative DxWBS and a rhTSH-stimulated Tg <2 ng mL^{-1} or a THW Tg <5 ng mL^{-1} [28,35,103]. However, patients with similar Tg values who have little residual uptake (<0.5%) in the thyroid bed (paramedially between the suprasternal notch and thyroid cartilage) or in a thyroglossal duct remnant (near the midline above the thyroid cartilage) are probably not benefited from further ^{131}I ablation [25]. Moreover, most patients who are free of thyroid cancer and in whom normal thyroid tissue has been completely ablated have undetectable TSH-stimulated Tg levels within about a year after therapy, and have lower recurrence rates than patients with low but detectable Tg levels [25]. Recent experience with rhTSH-stimulated Tg levels has suggested that diagnostic ^{131}I scanning can usually be omitted in patients suspected to be free of disease with undetectable serum Tg levels during thyroid hormone therapy that reduces cost, inconvenience, and radiation exposure [28]. One approach to patients whose rhTSH-stimulated Tg level rises >2 ng mL^{-1} is careful neck ultrasonography by an experienced ultrasonographer inspecting the superior mediastinum, bilateral central, and bilateral lateral compartments. In this setting, suspicious or obviously malignant disease is often found and ultrasound-guided FNA is performed if needed. Cancer identified by ultrasonographic appearance or biopsy is resected by en block compartmental dissection rather than selective-node resection. When disease is not identified in the neck (or as an alternative to the above ultrasonographic approach to find resectable disease), patients may undergo THW imaging and/or THW-stimulated Tg evaluation, and probably ^{131}I therapy followed by a RxWBS. CT imaging of the chest without contrast may be done at this time to guide the dose of ^{131}I, or reserved for those patients with a negative post-therapy whole body scan despite an elevated serum Tg.

Patients with a negative DxWBS or uptake <0.5% and hypothyroid-stimulated Tg between 5 and 10 ng mL^{-1} should be viewed with strong suspicion for having residual carcinoma. Patients with a negative WBS or uptake <0.5% and hypothyroid-stimulated Tg levels above $10\,ng\,mL^{-1}$ are highly likely to harbor residual cancer [25,35].

Patients with significant visible remnant uptake (such as >0.5%) and detectable Tg levels during THW warrant further ablation, which can be easily done as an outpatient, usually (and ideally [122]) on the day of diagnostic imaging. Patients with significant visible rhTSH-stimulated uptake >0.5% and rhTSH-stimulated serum Tg level $>2\,ng\,mL^{-1}$ should also undergo repeat remnant ablation.

3. ^{131}I Therapy of differentiated thyroid carcinoma

Some have questioned the effectiveness of ^{131}I therapy against metastatic disease [8,9], while the majority find it beneficial for a large number of patients (Fig. 1) [15].

In 1973, Leeper [134] reported 46 patients with distant metastases who were studied dosimetrically, of which some were treated with ^{131}I therapy. About one-third of patients with FTC responded to ^{131}I therapy and the survival time of treated patients was significantly better than for untreated patients. Metastatic PTC in patients under the age of 40 years was quite responsive to ^{131}I therapy while similar disease in patients over the age of 40 was lethal and responded poorly to ^{131}I therapy that did not enhance survival.

Beierwaltes et al. [63] found that PTC metastasized outside the neck, in descending order, to the lung, mediastinum, and bone, while ^{131}I was most effective in treating the disease in descending order in the mediastinum, lung, and bone. Patients alive without the disease were more likely to have been treated within 3 months of their thyroidectomy and were more likely to have their disease treated with more than 150 mCi of ^{131}I. FTC metastatic to the mediastinum was also effectively treated, while most patients with FTC metastatic to bone died despite of ^{131}I therapy.

Bernier et al. [54] studied 109 patients with bone metastases and found, after multivariate analysis, that ^{131}I therapy had a significant impact on their survival.

In our experience with patients without distant metastases, ^{131}I therapy of residual disease was found to be an independent variable that favorably reduced the likelihood of recurrence, distant recurrence, and death from thyroid cancer [20].

Most experts agree that there is a hierarchy of therapeutic efficacy among the treatments for DTC. Surgery is preferred when the tumor is resectable. Tumor debulking of unresectable disease is generally encouraged, especially for cervical disease. If the tumor, or part of it, is not amenable to surgery, ^{131}I therapy is recommended for tumors that concentrate the radionuclide and external-beam radiotherapy for tumors that do not, although in some cases both may be used sequentially to treat tumors that concentrate ^{131}I. TSH suppression is added to the above strategy. High-dose ^{131}I therapy has little or no effect on the viability of the majority of fluorodeoxyglucose (FDG)-avid metastases, although a few show favorable responses [135].

Patients with unresectable T_4 category disease or distant metastases (M_1) from thyroid cancer are at a high risk of death from their tumor (especially those with high-volume FDG-PET positive lesions [136]). A recent general oncology study from

Australia provides an opportunity to consider interactions with high-risk patients. These investigators determined the amount of information given by consultant cancer specialists to patients with incurable cancer (not specific to thyroid cancer), and the patient's opportunity for participation in management decisions [137]. Three-quarters of the patients were informed that their disease was incurable, about half were informed about life expectancy, one-third were offered a management choice, and the patient's understanding of the information was checked in only 10%. Greater disclosure of information did not elevate patient's anxiety, while greater participation in the decision-making process did.

3.1. ^{131}I Dosing for tumor therapy

Despite the apparent effectiveness of ^{131}I therapy in many patients, the optimal therapeutic dose remains uncertain and controversial [138]. There are three approaches to ^{131}I therapy: empiric fixed doses, therapy determined by the upper-bound limit of blood and body dosimetry, and quantitative tumor dosimetry [127]. Dosimetric methods are often reserved for distant metastases, unusual cases such as when renal failure is present, or when therapy with rhTSH stimulation is deemed necessary. Comparison of the outcome between these methods from published series is difficult and unreliable; [138], they are confounded by investigators measuring different outcomes, changing equipment sensitivities such as radiology equipment or Tg assays, duration of follow-up differences, incomparable stages of disease, and inequalities of supportive care. No prospective randomized trial to address the optimal therapeutic approach has been published. Similarly, no randomized trial comparing THW therapy to rhTSH-mediated therapy has been reported, despite a growing non-randomized literature regarding this use [139–147] and associated complications that may include rapid swelling of metastatic lesions [145,148–150]. Arguments in favor of higher doses cite a positive relationship between the total ^{131}I uptake per tumor mass and outcome [95], while others have not confirmed this relationship [37,151].

In the absence of controlled trials, it is not surprising that many questions regarding ^{131}I therapy of metastatic thyroid carcinoma remain. Are there comparable empiric doses of ^{131}I that can be administered to patients after rhTSH stimulation as compared to THW? Is a single, large dose more effective than the same total dose administered over several smaller therapies, or do smaller therapies deliver sublethal injury and the chance for cellular repair? Does stunning from a small sublethal dose ever resolve, or is the residual tissue more likely to be non-iodine avid? Should mediastinal lymph nodes unresponsive to THW 150–200 mCi ^{131}I therapies be subjected to upper-bound limiting dosimetry and therapy with doses potentially greater than 300 mCi?

3.1.1. Empiric fixed doses
The most common method employed currently uses a fixed amount of ^{131}I activity, often based on tumor stage. This method is the easiest, has a long history of use, and

a reasonable rate and severity of side effects [138]. Generally, about 30–100 mCi are given to ablate thyroid remnants, 150–200 mCi for residual carcinoma in cervical nodes or neck tissues, and 200 mCi or more for distant metastases. Tumor ^{131}I uptake in amounts adequate for imaging with 4 mCi [131]I DxWBS is usually sufficient for ^{131}I therapy using these empiric doses [152]. Some routinely treat distant metastases with relatively low empiric doses of 100–150 mCi for adults [37]. Conversely, ^{131}I doses up to 300 mCi for distant metastases only infrequently result in serious complications when renal function is normal [153]. However, much smaller doses used under special circumstances, such as diffuse bone marrow metastases, may be associated with severe myelosuppression [154].

3.1.2. *Maximum safety limit of the ^{131}I dose established by dosimetry*

This method, which is technically easier than tumor dosimetry described below, does not require an estimate of tumor mass. An upper ^{131}I dose limit is established for the amount that can be given safely as a single dose, which is usually 200 rad to the whole blood [155]. This limit may be increased to 300 rad in unusual circumstances, which may exist in patients with rapidly growing or large tumor deposits; however, it is associated with a higher complication rate. In patients with diffuse pulmonary metastases, the dose is limited so that < 80 mCi of ^{131}I remains in the whole body after 48 h to avoid pulmonary fibrosis [134]. Without diffuse pulmonary metastases, the dose is limited so that less than 120–150 mCi remain in the whole body after 48 h [134,155,156]. Based on these calculations, therapy doses in excess of 300 mCi are common (Fig. 1). Benua et al. [155] reported that serious complications were related to exceeding these dosimetric limits or administering individual doses of more than 300 mCi of [131]I. Of their 14 cases of serious radiation complications, one case of bone marrow depression occurred with a treatment dose of 324 mCi when the total blood radiation dose was 170 rad and 81 mCi were retained at 48 h. Others have uncommonly reported complications of ^{131}I therapy despite the careful use of dosimetry [157].

3.1.3. *Quantitative tumor dosimetry*

The purpose of quantitative tumor dosimetry is to provide sufficient ^{131}I for effective therapy, while minimizing excess ^{131}I to avoid therapy complications. For example, about half of the patients treated with an empiric 150 mCi ^{131}I dose for metastatic disease are undertreated [158]. With quantitative tumor dosimetry, the ^{131}I dose is calculated to deliver 30,000 rad to the thyroid remnant or 8000 to 12,000 rad to nodal or discrete soft tissue metastases [127]. Diffuse pulmonary metastases are treated according to the upper limit method described above. The mass of residual malignant or benign thyroid tissue and the effective half-time of ^{131}I in them are the two most important factors in determining success [127]. In one study, an 80% response was found in tumor deposits that received at least 8000 rad [41]. Lesions calculated to receive less than 3000 to 4000 rad despite reaching the calculated upper radiation limit should be considered for alternative therapy. Confounding factors of lesion-based dosimetry include estimation of the lesion mass, assumption of uniform distribution of ^{131}I in the lesion, and a lack of accounting for the importance of the dose rate as opposed to the total lesion dose [138].

3.1.4. *Renal insufficiency*

The kidney is the main pathway of iodine elimination, and is not adaptive or saturable [79]. Thus, safe and effective ^{131}I therapy and ablation in patients with renal insufficiency can be challenging, and dosimetry may be indispensable [139,159]. Dialysis patients are likely to have higher serumstable iodine concentrations that may be exacerbated by commonly used topical iodine containing skin cleansers. It is unknown how long a low-iodine diet should be implemented in these patients prior to ^{131}I therapy (≥ 4 weeks may be necessary), as their iodine half-life may be 4.5 times those with normal renal function [160]. Contamination of dialysis equipment and the local environment is minimal [159].

3.1.5. *Children*

Although mortality typically increases as age advances, death rates may be high in children under the age of 10 years [72,73] and recurrence rates are very high in patients diagnosed with DTC during the first 2 decades [20]. Empiric dose schemes for thyroid remnant ablation and therapy have been developed based on experience with adults. Guidelines for the treatment of children are more limited [71,73]. Modification of adult, empiric doses based on body weight or body surface area to create an equivalent absorbed dose has been proposed [84]. Some routinely treat distant metastases with $1 \, mCi \, kg^{-1}$ body weight in children [37], while others recommend quantitative blood and tumor dosimetry [84].

3.2. *Lithium*

This drug inhibits iodine release from the thyroid without impairing iodine uptake, thus enhancing ^{131}I retention in normal thyroid and tumor cells [161]. Given at a dosage of $10 \, mg \, kg^{-1}$ for 7 days, it has been shown to increase ^{131}I uptake in metastatic lesions, while only slightly increasing the uptake in normal thyroid tissue [161]. One study [162] found that the mean increase in the biological or retention half-life was 50% in tumors and 90% in thyroid remnants. The effect was greater in lesions with poor ^{131}I retention. In tumors with a biological half-life of less than 3 days, lithium prolonged the effective half-life of ^{131}I by more than 50%. The increase in accumulation of ^{131}I and the lengthening of the effective half-life together increased the estimated ^{131}I radiation dose in metastatic tumors to an average of more than twofold [162]. One approach is to prescribe lithium carbonate 300 mg orally twice per day in elderly or small-framed people, and 300 mg orally three times per day in the remainder. Blood lithium levels are measured at 48 h intervals initially and then in decreasing frequency. Patients should be warned that they will feel some effects of the lithium that are often a metallic taste, mild ataxia, or dysphoria. The serum level should be maintained in the mid-normal range where some patients still have severe side effects and dose reduction is necessary, while the uncommon patient will be intolerant to lithium despite normal or even subtherapeutic serum levels.

Once the patient is restarted on thyroid hormone, the clearance of lithium increases and serum lithium levels decrease. The necessary duration of continued lithium therapy after ^{131}I treatment is less certain and some have continued it for 5 days [106]; however, the mean biological half-life of ^{131}I may be 7 days when lithium has been given [161], making 2 weeks a reasonable empiric duration of time to continue the lithium after ^{131}I therapy.

3.3. *Elevated serum Tg levels and negative diagnostic ^{131}I scans*

The sensitivity of ^{131}I WBS for metastatic disease is about 50–80%, but the specificity is over 95% [36]. Patients with elevated serum Tg (typically $>10\,\text{ng}\,\text{mL}^{-1}$) and negative WBS (diagnostic or therapeutic) may have tumors that do not concentrate ^{131}I or have a tumor mass too small to visualize by scanning. It is important to exclude iodine contamination as the cause of a false-negative [131]I DxWBS. Management of this group of patients has created controversy [163]. Proponents of ^{131}I therapy suggest that enough ^{131}I per gram of functional tissue may be concentrated after a high dose to provide therapy (possibly requiring several treatments [164]), or at least provide localization of the metastases that may alter therapies such as surgery (possibly with an intraoperative probe [164]) or external beam radiation therapy.

In 1986, Schlumberger et al. [27] reported 14 patients with normal chest X-rays and pulmonary metastases seen on RxWBS after 100 mCi of ^{131}I, and not on the preceding 2 mCi DxWBS. Chest CT was abnormal in 5 of the 7 patients imaged prior to therapy. In follow-up, 100 mCi therapies were repeated to search for residual metastatic disease. Ten of these 14 patients had complete remissions defined by a negative RxWBS, negative DxWBS, and normal chest X-rays. Follow-up chest CT was abnormal in only 1 patient.

In 1987, Pacini et al. [165] reported negative 5 mCi rectilinear DxWBS, Tg positive ($>15\,\text{ng}\,\text{mL}^{-1}$) results in 13% of 135 patients with no other evidence of residual or metastatic tissue. [131]I therapy in these 17 patients with 75–140 mCi resulted in 16 positive RxWBS in the thyroid bed (3), neck or mediastinal lymph nodes (4), or lung (9). Follow-up-stimulated serum Tg at THW was reduced in 58% of the patients (lowest $10\,\text{ng}\,\text{mL}^{-1}$), some of whom had received an additional interval therapy.

In 1990, Ronga et al. [112] reported a series of 61 patients in which 19 patients (31%) were 2–4 mCi [131]I DxWBS negative, Tg positive (25 $>1000\,\text{ng}\,\text{mL}^{-1}$). Eleven patients were treated with 53–175 mCi ^{131}I and all seven (64%) with positive RxWBS had lung metastases.

In 1995, Pineda et al. [166] reported 17 DxWBS negative, Tg positive (8–480 ng mL^{-1}) patients treated with 150–300 mCi [131]I. Prior to therapy, all had negative radiological evaluations for metastases, although 5 had previously resected, nonfunctioning metastases and 9 had previous ^{131}I therapy for recurrence or metastases. RxWBS was positive in 16/17, 8/13, and 5/5 after the first, second, and third therapies with reductions of Tg in 81, 90, and 100%, respectively. In 50% of patients the Tg decreased to $\leqslant 5\,\text{ng}\,\text{mL}^{-1}$. RxWBS in the initial 17 patients showed uptake in the thyroid bed [6], neck or mediastinal lymph nodes [7], or lung [3].

In 2001, Pacini et al. [167] retrospectively compared a cohort of 42 treated and 28 untreated patients who were DxWBS-negative and serum-Tg-positive without clinical or radiological evidence of disease. Treated patients received 90–150 mCi ^{131}I and were followed for about 7 years. Thirty of the forty-two patients (71%) had a positive RxWBS (3 thyroid bed, 18 cervical lymph nodes, 9 pulmonary) and ^{131}I therapy was continued until the stimulated Tg was undetectable or the RxWBS became negative. At the end of the follow-up, 12 of 42 (29%) were in remission with negative scans and undetectable, stimulated Tg levels including patients originally with negative RxWBS (2/12), thyroid bed (1/3), lymph nodes metastases (6/18), and pulmonary metastases (3/9). Nine of 42 (21%) developed negative RxWBS with reduced but detectable Tg levels, 11 had continued positive RxWBS with detectable Tg levels (unreported if reduced or not), and 10 with originally negative RxWBS had detectable Tg levels (unreported if reduced or not) with the development of mediastinal metastases in 2 and death in another. At the end of the follow-up of the untreated cohort all had negative DxWBS, 19 of 28 (69%) were in remission with undetectable, stimulated Tg levels, 6 of 28 (21%) had reduced Tg levels, and 3 (11%) had stable or increased Tg levels with the development of pulmonary metastases in 1 of them. Thus, 90% of untreated patients appeared to improve over time compared with 50% for treated patients. These finding may be confounded by the changing of the serum Tg assay partway through the follow-up period of the untreated group, an event that did not occur for the treated group. Analysis of the serum Tg levels between the two groups suggests milder disease in the untreated group. Serum Tg was suppressible to undetectable levels in ~60% of treated patients compared with 86% of the untreated group. The median-stimulated Tg was ~55 ng mL^{-1} in the treated group compared with 9.5 ng mL^{-1} in the untreated group, a level below the current 10 ng mL^{-1} NCCN guideline cutoff to recommend consideration of ^{131}I therapy [15]. In this study, the authors partially discount the favorable effects of no treatment and suggest that all DxWBS-negative, Tg-positive patients receive ^{131}I therapy with further management based on the RxWBS findings.

Most recently, Fatourechi et al. [168] reported their experience with ^{131}I therapy in DxWBS-negative, Tg-positive patients. Twenty-four patients were treated with 199–300 mCi (mean 207 mCi), 4 had no identifiable tumor, 7 had micrometastases, and 13 had macrometastases. Follow-up was not available in 3 patients: 1 was lost to follow-up and two died. RxWBS showed no pathologic uptake in 19 (including the 4 patients without identifiable tumor), thyroid bed [2], lungs [2], or possible neck uptake [1]. Follow-up serum Tg levels during T4 suppression in 2 evaluable patients without identifiable tumor showed a reduction from 5.0 to 3.2 ng mL^{-1}, while the other 2 had excisions of recurrent neck disease. There was no change in patients with micrometastases as a group, while a reduction was seen in 1 individual patient. A rise in serum Tg was found in patients with macrometastases and their disease progressed despite palliative surgical excisions or external radiotherapy in 50% of the patients.

One algorithm that can be derived from these studies is that patients with detectable serum Tg during T4 suppression, or a rise in Tg to >2 ng mL^{-1} after rhTSH stimulation, undergo a search for residual resectable disease. This may be best accomplished by neck ultrasonography by a physician experienced in thyroid cancer and ultrasound-guided FNA. With the physician's confidence, FNA can be limited to questionable lesions that would alter the surgical intervention and can be avoided in lesions with obvious metastases. A helical chest CT is also obtained. Therapeutic ^{131}I with lithium is administered in fixed doses (150–300 mCi) or after dosimetry to patients with unresectable disease and a ~7 day RxWBS is obtained. Further ^{131}I therapy is given to patients who demonstrate a reduction in LT4-suppressed serum Tg levels if the disease persists. Unfortunately, most DxWBS-negative, Tg-positive patients are not rendered disease-free by ^{131}I therapy, although the tumor burden may be diminished, a benefit that appears inversely related to the starting focal tumor mass. Patients not benefited from this therapy are considered for experimental trials, keeping in mind that patients without bulky residual disease may have prolonged survival without clinical recurrence [169]. The relationship between the tumor mass and response to therapy in DxWBS-negative, Tg-positive disease is consistent with the fact that small tumor deposits may concentrate a percentage of ^{131}I such that the total amount concentrated per gram of tissue after a diagnostic dose is below the camera detection level, whereas after therapy it is both detectable and therapeutic [164]. For a large tumor to not be visualized on a DxWBS implies that its ^{131}I concentrating ability per gram of tissue is very low and hence a lack of response to ^{131}I therapy may be anticipated.

3.4. *CNS or vertebral metastases*

Brain metastases from all types of thyroid carcinoma have an extremely poor prognosis [170]. In one study, the median survival after the discovery of brain metastases from DTC was 12 months [170]. Patients who underwent surgical resection of 1 or more lesions survived 22 months compared with 4 months for patients who had no surgery. [131]I uptake occurred in 17% who underwent WBS, while neurological complications during THW or after ^{131}I were common. No evidence of a survival benefit from ^{131}I, external beam radiotherapy, or chemotherapy was found [170]. While controlled studies are lacking, inoperable CNS metastases should probably be treated with gamma knife rather than whole brain radiotherapy if possible [15,170]. Arterial embolization of bone metastases with pain and/or signs of spinal cord compression may be of benefit and may be combined with other therapeutic modalities. The technique is relatively easy and safe to perform and may offer immediate relief of symptoms [171,172], and greater reduction in serum Tg compared with ^{131}I alone [172].

When ^{131}I therapy is utilized for CNS metastases, vertebral metastases, or tumor located in a potentially critical or painful limited space, most experts suggest adjunctive corticosteroids to prevent potentially rapid, painful, or devastating consequences from peri-tumoral edema [113,144,149,150,170,173]. Luster et al. [142] administered dexamethasone 8 mg orally twice per day or prednisone 80 mg orally once per day. However, there has been no well-designed, randomized trial to confirm the efficacy of this therapy [142], and *in vitro* data suggests dexamethasone-induced NIS down-regulation [174] that may be expected to reduce ^{131}I trapping.

3.5. ^{125}I

^{131}I has been the isotope of choice for thyroid cancer therapy because of its long half-life (8.1 days), its short path length β emission, and its relatively low cost. The mean and maximal ranges of the ^{131}I β emission in soft tissue are 0.4 and 2 mm, respectively, so that its optimal tumor size to treat is 2.6–5.0 mm [113]. With favorable conditions, ^{131}I can deliver greater than 500 Gy to thyroid cancer tissue, compared with 70 Gy for external beam radiation therapy [113]. However, small lesions of 0.1 or 1.0 mm in diameter receive relative doses of 8.6 or 56%, respectively, compared with doses of a 5 mm tumor [175]. Thus, smaller lesions such as pulmonary micro-metastases may be better treated with ^{125}I, whose energy is an Auger electron with a path length of 0.012 mm [176,177].

3.6. *Retinoic acid*

Retinoic acid partly redifferentiates thyroid carcinoma *in vitro* and may benefit a few patients [178,179]. Given orally for at least 2 months, retinoic acid-induced significant ^{131}I uptake in 2 of the 12 patients with DTC, untreatable by other modalities [179]. Four of 36 (11%) patients had tumor size regression after 5 weeks of retinoic acid and ^{131}I with 3–10 Gbq in a multicenter pilot study [180]. However, others have not convincingly reproduced this benefit.

4. Conclusion

^{131}I has been critical in the management of DTC for more than half a century; however, most aspects of its use remain controversial or at least open to refinement. It is disappointing that more data have not been developed regarding therapies using ^{125}I, while alternative, more potent radionuclides like ^{211}At are being explored. It is also unfortunate that a randomized, controlled trial of high- versus low-dose therapy for patients with distant metastases has not been done. It is startling that better data are not available about the ideal magnitude of TSH needed for ^{131}I administration, although this may become moot when the use of rhTSH for remnant ablation and therapy is developed. It is an exciting time in the field of thyroid cancer that mandatory, symptomatic hypothyroidism may soon be a historical caveat and no longer a necessary burden of treatment. While the fine points of ^{131}I ablation and therapy can be improved, the absence of ^{131}I uptake in disease that is unresectable or not amenable to external beam radiation therapy offers a much greater challenge and opportunity for improvement [26,181]. For these patients, no alternative therapy exists and the probability of eventual death from disease correlates to its bulk. The possibility of gene therapy for these patients to allow ^{131}I therapy and/or suicide gene therapy needs to be explored urgently, as do new chemotherapy agents. Currently, patients with incurable diseases are reassured that a relatively long duration of survival is possible, but for a large number of patients, this does not amount to a normal life span.

References

[1] N.A. Samaan, P.N. Schultz, R.C. Hickey, T.P. Haynie, D.A. Johnston, N.G. Ordonez, Well-differentiated thyroid carcinoma and the results of various modalities of treatment. A retrospective review of 1599 patients, J. Clin. Endocrinol. Metab. 75 (1992) 714–720.

[2] B. Cady, R. Rossi, An expanded view of risk-group definition in differentiated thyroid carcinoma, Surgery 104 (1988) 947–953.

[3] M.L. Carcangiu, G. Zampi, A. Pupi, A. Castagnoli, J. Rosai, Papillary carcinoma of the thyroid. A clinicopathologic study of 241 cases treated at the University of Florence, Italy, Cancer 55 (1985) 805–828.

[4] G. Crile Jr., A.R. Antunez, C.B. Esselstyn Jr., W.A. Hawk, P.G. Skillern, The advantages of subtotal thyroidectomy and suppression of TSH in the primary treatment of papillary carcinoma of the thyroid, Cancer 55 (1985) 2691–2697.

[5] S.K.G. Grebe, I.D. Hay, Follicular cell-derived thyroid carcinomas, in: A. Arnold (Ed.), Endocrine Neoplasms, Kluwer Academic Publishers, 1997, pp. 91–140.

[6] I.D. Hay, C.S. Grant, J.A. van Heerden, J.R. Goellner, J.R. Ebersold, E.J. Bergstralh, Papillary thyroid microcarcinoma: a study of 535 cases observed in a 50-year period, Surgery 112 (1992) 1139–1147.

[7] I.D. Hay, Papillary thyroid carcinoma, Endocrinol. Metab. Clin. North Am. 19 (1990) 545–576.

[8] S.F. Dinneen, M.J. Valimaki, E.J. Bergstralh, J.R. Goellner, C.A. Gorman, I.D. Hay, Distant metastases in papillary thyroid carcinoma: 100 cases observed at one institution during 5 decades, J. Clin. Endocrinol. Metab. 80 (1995) 2041–2045.

[9] J.J. Ruegemer, I.D. Hay, E.J. Bergstralh, J.J. Ryan, K.P. Offord, C.A. Gorman, Distant metastases in differentiated thyroid carcinoma: a multivariate analysis of prognostic variables, J. Clin. Endocrinol. Metab. 67 (1988) 501–558.

[10] E.L. Mazzaferri, Thyroid remnant ^{131}I ablation for papillary and follicular thyroid carcinoma, Thyroid 7 (1997) 265–271.

[11] L. Wartofsky, S.I. Sherman, J. Gopal, M. Schlumberger, I.D. Hay, The use of radioactive iodine in patients with papillary and follicular thyroid cancer, J. Clin. Endocrinol. Metab. 83 (1998) 4195–4199.

[12] C.J.H. Van De Velde, J.F. Hamming, B.M. Goslings, et al., Report of the consensus development conference on the management of differentiated thyroid cancer in the Netherlands, Eur. J. Cancer Clin. Oncol. 24 (1988) 287–292.

[13] L. Baldet, J.C. Manderscheid, D. Glinoer, C. Jaffiol, B. Coste Seignovert, C. Percheron. The management of differentiated thyroid cancer in Europe in 1988. Results of an international survey, Acta Endocrinol. (Copenh.) 120 (1989) 547–558.

[14] B.L. Solomon, L. Wartofsky, K.D. Burman, Current trends in the management of well differentiated papillary thyroid carcinoma, J. Clin. Endocrinol. Metab. 81 (1996) 333–339.

[15] E.L. Mazzaferri, NCCN thyroid carcinoma practice guidelines, Oncology 13 (1999) 391–442.

[16] J.B. Wong, M.M. Kaplan, K.B. Meyer, S.G. Pauker, Ablative radioactive iodine therapy for apparently localized thyroid carcinoma. A decision analytic perspective, Endocrinol. Metabol. Clin. North Am. 19 (1990) 741–760.

[17] P.E. Voutilainen, M.M. Multanen, A.K. Leppaniemi, C.H. Haglund, R.K. Haapiainen, K.O. Franssila, Prognosis after lymph node recurrence in papillary thyroid carcinoma depends on age, Thyroid 11 (10) (2001) 953–957.

[18] J.P. Massin, J.C. Savoie, H. Garnier, G. Guiraudon, F.A. Leger, F. Bacourt, Pulmonary metastases in differentiated thyroid carcinoma. Study of 58 cases with implications for the primary tumor treatment, Cancer 53 (1984) 982–992.

[19] L.J. DeGroot, E.L. Kaplan, M. McCormick, F.H. Straus, Natural history, treatment, and course of papillary thyroid carcinoma, J. Clin. Endocrinol. Metab. 71 (1990) 414–424.

[20] E.L. Mazzaferri, R.T. Kloos, Clinical review 128: current approaches to primary therapy for papillary and follicular thyroid cancer, J. Clin. Endocrinol. Metab. 86 (4) (2001) 1447–1463.

[21] E.L. Mazzaferri, S.M. Jhiang, Long-term impact of initial surgical and medical therapy on papillary and follicular thyroid cancer, Am. J. Med. 97 (1994) 418–428.

[22] K. Segal, E. Raveh, E. Lubin, A. Abraham, J. Shvero, R. Feinmesser, Well-differentiated thyroid carcinoma, Am. J. Otolaryngol. 6 (1996) 401–406.

[23] P. Pujol, J.P. Daures, N. Nsakala, L. Baldet, J. Bringer, C. Jaffiol, Degree of thyrotropin suppression as a prognostic determinant in differentiated thyroid cancer, J. Clin. Endocrinol. Metab. 81 (1996) 4318–4323.

[24] F. Pacini, M. Capezzone, R. Elisei, C. Ceccarelli, D. Taddei, A. Pinchera, Diagnostic 131-iodine whole-body scan may be avoided in thyroid cancer patients who have undetectable stimulated serum Tg levels after initial treatment, J. Clin. Endocrinol. Metab. 87 (4) (2002) 1499–1501.

[25] A.F. Cailleux, E. Baudin, J.P. Travagli, M. Ricard, M. Schlumberger, Is diagnostic iodine-131 scanning useful after total thyroid ablation for differentiated thyroid cancer?, J. Clin. Endocrinol. Metab. 85 (1) (2000) 175–178.

[26] M. Schlumberger, C. Challeton, F. De Vathaire, et al., Radioactive iodine treatment and external radiotherapy for lung and bone metastases from thyroid carcinoma, J. Nucl. Med. 37 (1996) 598–605.

[27] M. Schlumberger, M. Tubiana, F. De Vathaire, et al., Long-term results of treatment of 283 patients with lung and bone metastases from differentiated thyroid carcinoma, J. Clin. Endocrinol. Metab. 63 (1986) 960–967.

[28] E.L. Mazzaferri, R.T. Kloos, Is diagnostic iodine-131 scanning with recombinant human TSH (rhTSH) useful in the follow-up of differentiated thyroid cancer after thyroid ablation?, J. Clin. Endocrinol. Metab. 87 (4) (2002) 1490–1498.

[29] M.D. Morocco, R.T. Kloos, H. Nagaraja, Predicting the serum thyroglobulin level attributable to the post-operative thyroid tissue remnant. 73rd Annual Meeting of the American Thyroid Association, Program #127, 2001, p. 215 (Abstract).

[30] R.J. Robbins, R.M. Tuttle, R.N. Sharaf, et al., Preparation by recombinant human thyrotropin or thyroid hormone withdrawal are comparable for the detection of residual differentiated thyroid carcinoma, J. Clin. Endocrinol. Metab. 86 (2) (2001) 619–625.

[31] J.I. Torrens, H.B. Burch, Serum thyroglobulin measurement: utility in clinical practice, Endocrinologist 6 (1996) 125–144.

[32] C.A. Spencer, M. Takeuchi, M. Kazarosyan, et al., Serum thyroglobulin autoantibodies: prevalence, influence on serum thyroglobulin measurement, and prognostic significance in patients with differentiated thyroid carcinoma, J. Clin. Endocrinol. Metab. 83 (1998) 1121–1127.

[33] M. Ozata, S. Suzuki, T. Miyamoto, R.T. Liu, F. Fierro-Renoy, L.J. DeGroot, Serum thyroglobulin in the follow-up of patients with treated differentiated thyroid cancer, J. Clin. Endocrinol. Metab. 79 (1994) 98–105.

[34] F. Pacini, R. Lari, S. Mazzeo, L. Grasso, D. Taddei, A. Pinchera, Diagnostic value of a single serum thyroglobulin determination on and off thyroid suppressive therapy in the follow-up of patients with differentiated thyroid cancer, Clin. Endocrinol. 23 (1985) 405–411.

[35] B.R. Haugen, F. Pacini, C. Reiners, et al., A comparison of recombinant human thyrotropin and thyroid hormone withdrawal for the detection of thyroid remnant or cancer, J. Clin. Endocrinol. Metab. 84 (1999) 3877–3885.

[36] M. Franceschi, Z. Kusic, D. Franceschi, L. Lukinac, S. Roncevic, Thyroglobulin determination, neck ultrasonography and iodine-131 whole-body scintigraphy in differentiated thyroid carcinoma, J. Nucl. Med. 37 (1996) 446–451.

[37] M.J. Schlumberger, Medical progress—papillary and follicular thyroid carcinoma, N. Engl. J. Med. 338 (1998) 297–306.

[38] C.A. Spencer, C.C. Wang, Thyroglobulin measurement—techniques, clinical benefits, and pitfalls, Endocrinol. Metabol. Clin. North Am. 24 (1995) 841–863.

[39] B.R. Haugen, E.C. Ridgway, B.A. McLaughlin, M.T. McDermott, Clinical comparison of whole-body radioiodine scan and serum thyroglobulin after stimulation with recombinant human thyrotropin, Thyroid 12 (1) (2002) 37–43.

[40] C.A. Spencer, Recoveries cannot be used to authenticate thyroglobulin (Tg) measurements when sera contain Tg autoantibodies, Clin. Chem. 42 (1996) 661–663.

[41] H.R. Maxon, E.E. Englaro, S.R. Thomas, et al., Radioiodine-131 therapy for well-differentiated thyroid cancer—a quantitative radiation dosimetric approach: outcome and validation in 85 patients, J. Nucl. Med. 33 (1992) 1132–1136.

[42] L.A. Burmeister, R.P. duCret, C.N. Mariash, Local reactions to radioiodine in the treatment of thyroid cancer, Am. J. Med. 90 (1991) 217–222.

[43] F. Pacini, R. Elisei, M. Capezzone, et al., Contralateral papillary thyroid cancer is frequent at completion thyroidectomy with no difference in low- and high-risk patients, Thyroid 11 (9) (2001) 877–881.

[44] B. Cady, Our AMES is true: how an old concept still hits the mark: or, risk group assignment points the arrow to rational therapy selection in differentiated thyroid cancer, Am. J. Surg. 174 (1997) 462–468.

[45] A.R. Shaha, T.R. Loree, J.P. Shah, Prognostic factors and risk group analysis in follicular carcinoma of the thyroid, Surgery 118 (1995) 1131–1138.

[46] E.L. Mazzaferri, Treating differentiated thyroid carcinoma: where do we draw the line?, Mayo Clin. Proc. 66 (1991) 105–111.

[47] K.D. Newman, T. Black, G. Heller, et al., Differentiated thyroid cancer: determinants of disease progression in patients <21 years of age at diagnosis—a report from the Surgical Discipline Committee of the Children's Cancer Group, Ann. Surg. 227 (1998) 533–541.

[48] P. Miccoli, A. Antonelli, C. Spinelli, M. Ferdeghini, P. Fallahi, L. Baschieri, Completion total thyroidectomy in children with thyroid cancer secondary to the Chernobyl accident, Arch. Surg. 133 (1998) 89–93.

[49] I.D. Hay, C.S. Grant, E.J. Bergstralh, G.B. Thompson, J.A. van Heerden, Unilateral total lobectomy: Is it sufficient surgical treatment for patients with AMES low-risk papillary thyroid carcinoma?, Surgery 124 (1998) 958–966.

[50] J.L. Pasieka, N.W. Thompson, M.K. McLeod, R.E. Burney, M. Macha, The incidence of bilateral well-differentiated thyroid cancer found at completion thyroidectomy, World J. Surg. 16 (1992) 711–716.

[51] R. Arem, S.J. Padayatty, A.H. Saliby, S.I. Sherman, Thyroid microcarcinoma: prevalence, prognosis, and management, Endocrine Practice 5 (3) (1999) 148–156.

[52] J.C. Furlan, Y. Bedard, I.B. Rosen, Biologic basis for the treatment of microscopic, occult well-differentiated thyroid cancer, Surgery 130 (6) (2001) 1050–1054.

[53] M.D. Allo, W. Christianson, D. Doivunen, Not all 'occult' papillary carcinomas are 'minimal', Surgery 104 (1988) 971–976.

[54] M.O. Bernier, L. Leenhardt, C. Hoang, et al., Survival and therapeutic modalities in patients with bone metastases of differentiated thyroid carcinomas, J. Clin. Endocrinol. Metab. 86 (4) (2001) 1568–1573.

[55] E. Baudin, J.P. Travagli, J. Ropers, et al., Microcarcinoma of the thyroid gland—The Gustave-Roussy Institute Experience, Cancer 83 (1998) 553–559.

[56] J. Tourniaire, M.H. Bernard, M.H. Bizollon-Roblin, M. Bertholon-Gregoire, N. Berger-Dutrieux, Thyroid papillary microcarcinoma: 179 cases since 1973, Presse Med. 27 (1998) 1467–1469.

[57] M. Moosa, E.L. Mazzaferri, Occult thyroid carcinoma, Cancer J. 10 (1997) 180–188.

[58] L.A. Akslen, V.A. LiVolsi, Prognostic significance of histologic grading compared with subclassification of papillary thyroid carcinoma, Cancer 88 (8) (2000) 1902–1908.

[59] S. Prendiville, K.D. Burman, M.D. Ringel, et al., Tall cell variant: an aggressive form of papillary thyroid carcinoma, Otolaryngol. Head Neck Surg. 122 (3) (2000) 352–357.

[60] L.D. Thompson, J.A. Wieneke, E. Paal, R.A. Frommelt, C.F. Adair, C.S. Heffess, A clinicopathologic study of minimally invasive follicular carcinoma of the thyroid gland with a review of the English literature, Cancer 91 (3) (2001) 505–524.

[61] A. Machens, R. Hinze, C. Lautenschlager, O. Thomusch, H. Dralle, Prophylactic completion thyroidectomy for differentiated thyroid carcinoma: prediction of extrathyroidal soft tissue infiltrates, Thyroid 11 (4) (2001) 381–384.

[62] G.F.W. Scheumann, H. Seeliger, T.J. Musholt, et al., Completion thyroidectomy in 131 patients with differentiated thyroid carcinoma, Eur. J. Surg. 162 (1996) 677–684.

[63] W.H. Beierwaltes, R.H. Nishiyama, N.W. Thompson, J.E. Copp, A. Kubo, Survival time and 'cure' in papillary and follicular thyroid carcinoma with distant metastases: statistics following University of Michigan therapy, J. Nucl. Med. 23 (1982) 561–568.

[64] J.Y. Cho, S. Xing, X. Liu, et al., Expression and activity of human Na + /I– symporter in human glioma cells by adenovirus-mediated gene delivery, Gene Ther. 7 (9) (2000) 740–749.

[65] O.H. Beahrs, D.E. Henson, R.V.P. Hutter, M.H. Myers (Eds.), Manual for Staging of Cancer, J.B. Lippincott, Philadelphia, 1992, pp. 53–54.

[66] I.D. Hay, E.J. Bergstralh, J.R. Goellner, J.R. Ebersold, C.S. Grant, Predicting outcome in papillary thyroid carcinoma: development of a reliable prognostic scoring system in a cohort of 1779 patients surgically treated at one institution during 1940 through 1989, Surgery 114 (1993) 1050–1058.

[67] S.I. Sherman, Clinicopathologic and prognostic staging for thyroid carcinomas, Thyroid Today XXIII (3) (2000) 1–9.

[68] J.D. Brierley, T. Panzarella, R.W. Tsang, M.K. Gospodarowicz, B. O'Sullivan, A comparison of different staging systems predictability of patient outcome—thyroid carcinoma as an example, Cancer 79 (1997) 2414–2423.

[69] K.C. Loh, F.S. Greenspan, L. Gee, T.R. Miller, P.P.B. Yeo, Pathological tumor-node-metastasis (pTNM) staging for papillary and follicular thyroid carcinomas: a retrospective analysis of 700 patients, J. Clin. Endocrinol. Metab. 82 (1997) 3553–3562.

[70] S.A. Hundahl, I.D. Fleming, A.M. Fremgen, H.R. Menck, A national cancer data base report on 53,856 cases of thyroid carcinoma treated in the US, 1985–1995, Cancer 83 (1998) 2638–2648.

[71] M.E. Dottorini, A. Vignati, L. Mazzucchelli, G. Lomuscio, L. Colombo, Differentiated thyroid carcinoma in children and adolescents: a 37-year experience in 85 patients, J. Nucl. Med. 38 (1997) 669–675.

[72] H.R. Harach, E.D. Williams, Childhood thyroid cancer in England and Wales, Br. J. Cancer 72 (1995) 777–783.

[73] W. Hung, Well-differentiated thyroid carcinomas in children and adolescents: a review, Endocrinologist 4 (1994) 117–126.

[74] P. Hannequin, J.C. Liehn, M.J. Delisle, Multifactorial analysis of survival in thyroid cancer. Pitfalls of applying the results of published studies to another population, Cancer 58 (1986) 1749–1755.

[75] M. Lakshmanan, A. Schaffer, J. Robbins, J. Reynolds, J. Norton, A simplified low iodine diet in I-131 scanning and therapy of thyroid cancer, Clin. Nucl. Med. 2 (1988) 866–868.

[76] J. Maruca, S. Santner, K. Miller, R.J. Santen, Prolonged iodine clearance with a depletion regimen for thyroid carcinoma: concise communication, J. Nucl. Med. 25 (1984) 1089–1093.

[77] H.R. Maxon, T.A. Boehringer, J. Drilling, Low iodine diet in I-131 ablation of thyroid remnants, Clin. Nucl. Med. 8 (1983) 123–126.

[78] L. Guljord, Collection of Low-Iodine Recipes, 2 ed., http://www.thyca.org/: ThyCa:Thyroid Cancer Survivors' Association, 2000.

[79] P. Verger, A. Aurengo, B. Geoffroy, B. Le Guen, Iodine kinetics and effectiveness of stable iodine prophylaxis after intake of radioactive iodine: a review, Thyroid 11 (4) (2001) 353–360.

[80] R.R. Cavalieri, I.R. McDougall, In vivo isotopic tests and imaging, in: L.E. Braverman, R.D. Utiger (Eds.), Werner and Ingbar's the Thyroid: A Fundamental and Clinical Text, J.B. Lippincott Co., Philadelphia, 1991, pp. 437–462.

[81] K.F. Koral, R.S. Adler, J.E. Carey, W.H. Beierwaltes, Iodine-131 treatment of thyroid cancer: absorbed dose calculated from post-therapy scans, J. Nucl. Med. 27 (1986) 1207–1211.

[82] D.S. Cooper, Treatment of thyrotoxicosis, in: L.E. Braverman, R.D. Utiger (Eds.), Werner and Ingbar's the Thyroid: A Fundamental and Clinical Text, J.B. Lippincott Co., Philadelphia, 1991, pp. 887–916.

[83] A. Taurog, Hormone synthesis: thyroid iodine metabolism, in: L.E. Braverman, R.D. Utiger (Eds.), Werner and Ingbar's the Thyroid: A Fundamental and Clinical Text, J.B. Lippincott Co., Philadelphia, 1991, pp. 51–97.

[84] H.R. Maxon, Quantitative radioiodine therapy in the treatment of differentiated thyroid cancer, Q. J. Nucl. Med. 43 (4) (1999) 313–323.

[85] A.J. Laurie, S.G. Lyon, E.C. Lasser, Contrast material iodides: potential effects on radioactive iodine thyroid uptake, J. Nucl. Med. 33 (2) (1992) 237–238.

[86] B. Nygaard, T. Nygaard, L.I. Jensen, et al., Iohexol: effects on uptake of radioactive iodine in the thyroid and on thyroid function, Acad. Radiol. 5 (6) (1998) 409–414.

[87] C.R. Christensen, J.V. Glowniak, P.H. Brown, K.A. Morton, The effect of gadolinium contrast media on radioiodine uptake by the thyroid gland, J. Nucl. Med. Technol. 28 (1) (2000) 41–44.

[88] K. Mann, J. Rendl, R. Busley, et al., Systemic iodine absorption during endoscopic application of radiographic contrast agents for endoscopic retrograde cholangiopancreaticography, Eur. J. Endocrinol. 130 (5) (1994) 498–501.

[89] W.J. Fassbender, C. Vogel, W. Doppl, H. Stracke, R.G. Bretzel, H.U. Klor, Thyroid function, thyroid immunoglobulin status, and urinary iodine excretion after enteral contrast-agent administration by endoscopic retrograde cholangiopancreatography, Endoscopy 33 (3) (2001) 245–252.

[90] H. Monig, T. Arendt, S. Eggers, S. Kloehn, U.R. Folsch, Iodine absorption in patients undergoing ERCP compared with coronary angiography, Gastrointest. Endosc. 50 (1) (1999) 79–81.

[91] G. Hintze, O. Blombach, H. Fink, U. Burkhardt, J. Kobberling, Risk of iodine-induced thyrotoxicosis after coronary angiography: an investigation in 788 unselected subjects, Eur. J. Endocrinol. 140 (3) (1999) 264–267.

[92] C.J. Edmonds, S. Hayes, J.C. Kermode, B.D. Thompson, Measurement of serum TSH and thyroid hormones in the management of treatment of thyroid carcinoma with radioiodine, Br. J. Radiol. 50 (1977) 799–807.

[93] M.S. Torres, L. Ramirez, P.H. Simkin, L.E. Braverman, C.H. Emerson, Effect of various doses of recombinant human thyrotropin on the thyroid radioactive iodine uptake and serum levels of thyroid hormones and thyroglobulin in normal subjects, J. Clin. Endocrinol. Metab. 86 (4) (2001) 1660–1664.

[94] W.H. Beierwaltes, The treatment of thyroid carcinoma with radioactive iodine, Semin. Nucl. Med. 8 (1978) 79–94.

[95] H.R. Maxon, S.R. Thomas, V.S. Hertzberg, et al., Relation between effective radiation dose and outcome of radioiodine therapy for thyroid cancer, N. Engl. J. Med. 309 (1983) 937–941.

[96] S.V. Hilts, D. Hellman, J. Anderson, J. Woolfenden, J. Van Antwerp, D. Patton, Serial TSH determination after T3 withdrawal or thyroidectomy in the therapy of thyroid carcinoma, J. Nucl. Med. 20 (1979) 928–932.

[97] J.M. Goldman, B.R. Line, R.L. Aamodt, J. Robbins, Influence of triiodothyronine withdrawal time on 131-I uptake postthyroidectomy for thyroid cancer, J. Clin. Endocrinol. Metab. 50 (1980) 734–739.

[98] M. Schlumberger, P. Charbord, P. Fragu, J. Lumbroso, M. Tubiana, Circulating thyroglobulin and thyroid hormones in patients with metastases of differentiated thyroid carcinoma: relationship to serum thyrotropin levels, J. Clin. Endocrinol. Metab. 51 (1980) 513–519.

[99] A.B. Schneider, B.R. Line, J.M. Goldman, J. Robbins, Sequential serum thyroglobulin determinations, 131I scans and 131I uptakes after triiodothyronine withdrawal in patients with thyroid cancer, J. Clin. Endocrinol. Metab. 53 (1981) 1199–1206.

[100] V. Guimaraes, L.J. DeGroot, Moderate hypothyroidism in preparation for whole body 131I scintiscans and thyroglobulin testing, Thyroid 6 (1996) 69–73.

[101] H.R. Maxon, Detection of residual and recurrent thyroid cancer by radionuclide imaging, Thyroid - 9 (5) (1999) 443–446.

[102] C.L. Maini, R. Sciuto, A. Tofani, TSH suppression by octreotide in differentiated thyroid cancer, Clinical Endocrinol. 40 (1994) 335–339.

[103] V. Giovanni, L.G. Arianna, C. Antonio, et al., The use of recombinant human TSH in the follow-up of differentiated thyroid cancer: experience from a large patient cohort in a single centre, Clin. Endocrinol. (Oxf.) 56 (2) (2002) 247–252.

[104] F. Pacini, E. Molinaro, F. Lippi, et al., Prediction of disease status by recombinant human TSH-stimulated serum Tg in the postsurgical follow-up of differentiated thyroid carcinoma, J. Clin. Endocrinol. Metab. 86 (12) (2001) 5686–5690.

[105] M. Schlumberger, M. Ricard, F. Pacini, Clinical use of recombinant human TSH in thyroid cancer patients, Eur. J. Endocrinol. 143 (5) (2000) 557–563.

[106] J.C. Reynolds, J. Robbins, The changing role of radioiodine in management of differentiated thyroid cancer, Semin. Nucl. Med. 27 (1997) 152–164.

[107] L.F. Morris, A.D. Waxman, G.D. Braunstein, The nonimpact of thyroid stunning: remnant ablation rates in I-131 scanned and nonscanned individuals, J. Clin. Endocrinol. Metab. 86 (8) (2001) 3507–3511.

[108] G.H. Daniels, Radioiodine and thyroid cancer: some questions, controversies, and considerations, Endocrine Practice 7 (4) (2001) 320–323 Ref Type: Journal (Full).

[109] V. Fatourechi, I.D. Hay, B.P. Mullan, et al., Are posttherapy radioiodine scans informative and do they influence subsequent therapy of patients with differentiated thyroid cancer?, Thyroid 10 (7) (2000) 573–577.

[110] S.I. Sherman, E.T. Tielens, S. Sostre, M.D. Wharam Jr., P.W. Ladenson, Clinical utility of post-treatment radioiodine scans in the management of patients with thyroid carcinoma, J. Clin. Endocrinol. Metab. 78 (1994) 629–634.

[111] W.G. Spies, C.H. Wojtowicz, S.M. Spies, A.Y. Shah, A.M. Zimmer, Value of post-therapy whole-body I-131 imaging in the evaluation of patients with thyroid carcinoma, Clin. Nucl. Med. 14 (1989) 793–800.

[112] G. Ronga, A. Fiorentino, E. Paserio, et al., Can iodine-131 whole-body scan be replaced by thyroglobulin measurement in the post-surgical follow-up of differentiated thyroid carcinoma?, J. Nucl. Med. 31 (1990) 1766–1771.

[113] C. Reiners, J. Farahati, 131I therapy of thyroid cancer patients, Q. J. Nucl. Med. 43 (4) (1999) 324–335.

[114] R.W. Rawson, J.E. Rall, W. Peacock, Limitations in the treatment of cancer of the thyroid with radioactive iodine, J. Clin. Endocrinol. Metab. 11 (1951) 1128–1142.

[115] H.M. Park, O.W. Perkins, J.W. Edmondson, R.B. Schnute, A. Manatunga, Influence of diagnostic radioiodines on the uptake of ablative dose of iodine-131, Thyroid 4 (1994) 49–54.

[116] F.A. Leger, M. Izembart, F. Dagousset, et al., Decreased uptake of therapeutic doses of iodine-131 after 185- MBq iodine-131 diagnostic imaging for thyroid remnants in differentiated thyroid carcinoma, Eur. J. Nucl. Med. 25 (1998) 242–246.

[117] J.P. Muratet, A. Daver, J.F. Minier, F. Larra, Influence of scanning doses of iodine-131 on subsequent first ablative treatment outcome in patients operated on for differentiated thyroid carcinoma, J. Nucl. Med. 39 (1998) 1546–1550.

[118] J.P. Muratet, P. Giraud, A. Daver, J.F. Minier, E. Gamelin, F. Larra, Predicting the efficacy of first iodine-131 treatment in differentiated thyroid carcinoma, J. Nucl. Med. 38 (1997) 1362–1368.

[119] A. Waxman, L. Ramanna, N. Chapman, et al., The significance of I-131 scan dose in patients with thyroid cancer: determination of ablation: concise communication, J. Nucl. Med. 22 (10) (1981) 861–865.

[120] S.J. Mandel, L.K. Shankar, F. Benard, A. Yamamoto, A. Alavi, Superiority of iodine-123 compared with iodine-131 scanning for thyroid remnants in patients with differentiated thyroid cancer, Clin. Nucl. Med. 26 (1) (2001) 6–9.

[121] A.S. Alzahrani, S. Bakheet, M. Al Mandil, A. Al Hajjaj, A. Almahfouz, A. Al Haj, 123I isotope as a diagnostic agent in the follow-up of patients with differentiated thyroid cancer: comparison with post 131I therapy whole body scanning, J. Clin. Endocrinol. Metab. 86 (11) (2001) 5294–5300.

[122] S.P. Cholewinski, K.S. Yoo, P.S. Klieger, R.E. O'Mara, Absence of thyroid stunning after diagnostic whole-body scanning with 185 MBq 131I, J. Nucl. Med. 41 (7) (2000) 1198–1202.

[123] R.M. McMenemin, T.E. Hilditch, M.F. Dempsey, N.S. Reed, Thyroid stunning after (131)I diagnostic whole-body scanning, J. Nucl. Med. 42 (6) (2001) 986–987.

[124] H.W. Yeung, J.L. Humm, S.M. Larson, Radioiodine uptake in thyroid remnants during therapy after tracer dosimetry, J. Nucl. Med. 41 (6) (2000) 1082–1085.

[125] D.C. Hodgson, J.D. Brierley, R.W. Tsang, T. Panzarella, Prescribing [131]iodine based on neck uptake produces effective thyroid ablation and reduced hospital stay, Radiother. Oncol. 47 (1998) 325–330.

[126] C. Bal, A.K. Padhy, S. Jana, G.S. Pant, A.K. Basu, Prospective randomized clinical trial to evaluate the optimal dose of ^{131}I for remnant ablation in patients with differentiated thyroid carcinoma, Cancer 77 (1996) 2574–2580.

[127] J. Brierley, H.R. Maxon, Radioiodine and external radiation therapy, in: J.A. Fagin (Ed.), Thyroid Cancer, Kluwer Academic Publishers, Boston/Dordrecht, London, 1998, pp. 285–317.

[128] J.A. Siegel, Tracking the origin of the NRC 30-mCi rule, J. Nucl. Med. 41 (10) (2000) 10N–16N.

[129] P.W. Grigsby, B.A. Siegel, S. Baker, J.O. Eichling, Radiation exposure from outpatient radioactive iodine (^{131}I) therapy for thyroid carcinoma, JAMA 283 (17) (2000) 2272–2274.

[130] J.M. de Klerk, 131I therapy: inpatient or outpatient?, J. Nucl. Med. 41 (11) (2000) 1876–1878.

[131] L.F. Morris, M.S. Wilder, A.D. Waxman, G.D. Braunstein, Reevaluation of the impact of a stringent low-iodine diet on ablation rates in radioiodine treatment of thyroid carcinoma, Thyroid 11 (8) (2001) 749–755.

[132] J.R. Hurley, Management of thyroid cancer: radioiodine ablation, 'stunning,' and treatment of thyroglobulin-positive, ^{131}I scan-negative patients, Endocrine Practice 6 (5) (2000) 401–406.

[133] F. Grünwald, C. Menzel, R. Fimmers, P.O. Zamora, H.J. Biersack, Prognostic value of thyroglobulin after thyroidectomy before ablative radioiodine therapy in thyroid cancer, J. Nucl. Med. 37 (1996) 1962–1964.

[134] R.D. Leeper, The effect of ^{131}I therapy on survival of patients with metastatic papillary or follicular thyroid carcinoma, J. Clin. Endocrinol. Metab. 36 (6) (1973) 1143–1152.

[135] W. Wang, S.M. Larson, R.M. Tuttle, et al., Resistance of [18F]-fluorodeoxyglucose-avid metastatic thyroid cancer lesions to treatment with high-dose radioactive iodine, Thyroid 11 (12) (2001) 1169–1175.

[136] W. Wang, S.M. Larson, M. Fazzari, et al., Prognostic value of [18F]fluorodeoxyglucose positron emission tomographic scanning in patients with thyroid cancer, J. Clin. Endocrinol. Metab. 85 (3) (2000) 1107–1113.

[137] M. Gattellari, K.J. Voigt, P.N. Butow, M.H. Tattersall, When the treatment goal is not cure: are cancer patients equipped to make informed decisions?, J. Clin. Oncol. 20 (2) (2002) 503–513.

[138] D. Van Nostrand, F. Atkins, F. Yeganeh, E. Acio, R. Bursaw, L. Wartofsky, Dosimetrically determined doses of radioiodine for the treatment of metastatic thyroid carcinoma, Thyroid 12 (2) (2002) 121–134.

[139] E.L. Mazzaferri, R.T. Kloos, Using recombinant human TSH in the management of well-differentiated thyroid cancer: current strategies and future directions, Thyroid 10 (9) (2000) 767–778.

[140] M.D. Ringel, P.W. Ladenson, Diagnostic accuracy of ^{131}I scanning with recombinant human thyrotropin versus thyroid hormone withdrawal in a patient with metastatic thyroid carcinoma and hypopituitarism, J. Clin. Endocrinol. Metab. 81 (1996) 1724–1725.

[141] A.Z. Rudavsky, L.M. Freeman, Treatment of scan-negative, thyroglobulin-positive metastatic thyroid cancer using radioiodine ^{131}I and recombinant human thyroid stimulating hormone, J. Clin. Endocrinol. Metab. 82 (1997) 11–14.

[142] M. Luster, M. Lassmann, H. Haenscheid, U. Michalowski, C. Incerti, C. Reiners, Use of recombinant human thyrotropin before radioiodine therapy in patients with advanced differentiated thyroid carcinoma, J. Clin. Endocrinol. Metab. 85 (10) (2000) 3640–3645.

[143] G. Mariani, M. Ferdeghini, C. Augeri, et al., Clinical experience with recombinant human thyrotrophin (rhTSH) in the management of patients with differentiated thyroid cancer, Cancer Biother. Radiopharm. 15 (2) (2000) 211–217.

[144] P. Perros, Recombinant human thyroid-stimulating hormone (rhTSH) in the radioablation of well-differentiated thyroid cancer: preliminary therapeutic experience, J. Endocrinol. Invest. 22, Suppl. to No. 11 (11) (1999) 30–34.

[145] F. Lippi, M. Capezzone, F. Angelini, et al., Radioiodine treatment of metastatic differentiated thyroid cancer in patients on L-thyroxine, using recombinant human TSH, Eur. J. Endocrinol. 144 (1) (2001) 5–11.

[146] G. Pellegriti, C. Scollo, D. Giuffrida, R. Vigneri, S. Squatrito, V. Pezzino, Usefulness of recombinant human thyrotropin in the radiometabolic treatment of selected patients with thyroid cancer, Thyroid 11 (11) (2001) 1025–1030.

[147] M. Adler, H. Macapinlac, R. Robbins, Radioiodine treatment of thyroid cancer with the aid or recombinant human thyrotropin, Endocrine Practice 4 (1998) 282–286.

[148] G.E. Vargas, H. Uy, C. Bazan, T.A. Guise, J.M. Bruder, Hemiplegia after thyrotropin alfa in a hypothyroid patient with thyroid carcinoma metastatic to the brain, J. Clin. Endocrinol. Metab. 84 (1999) 3867–3871.

[149] R.J. Robbins, E. Voelker, W. Wang, H.A. Macapinlac, S.M. Larson, Compassionate use of recombinant human thyrotropin to facilitate radioiodine therapy: case report and review of literature, Endocrine Practice 6 (6) (2000) 460–464.

[150] M. Braga, M.D. Ringel, D.S. Cooper, Sudden enlargement of local recurrent thyroid tumor after recombinant human TSH administration, J. Clin. Endocrinol. Metab. 86 (11) (2001) 5148–5151.

[151] A.M. Samuel, B. Rajashekharrao, D.H. Shah, Pulmonary metastases in children and adolescents with well-differentiated thyroid cancer, J. Nucl. Med. 39 (1998) 1531–1536.

[152] E.L. Mazzaferri, Carcinoma of follicular epithelium: radioiodine and other treatment outcomes, in: L.E. Braverman, R.D. Utiger (Eds.), The Thyroid: A Fundamental and Clinical Text, Lippencott-Raven Publication, Philadelphia, 1996, pp. 922–945.

[153] C. Menzel, F. Grünwald, A. Schomburg, et al., 'High-dose' radioiodine therapy in advanced differentiated thyroid carcinoma, J. Nucl. Med. 37 (1996) 1496–1503.

[154] V. Rufini, M. Salvatori, I. Saletnich, et al., Disseminated bone marrow metastases of insular thyroid carcinoma detected by radioiodine whole-body scintigraphy, J. Nucl. Med. 37 (1996) 633–636.

[155] R.S. Benua, N.R. Cicale, M. Sonenberg, et al., The relation of radioiodine dosimetry to results and complications in the treatment of metastatic thyroid cancer, AJR 87 (1962) 171–178.

[156] H. Maxon III, H.S. Smith, Radioiodine-131 in the diagnosis and treatment of metastatic well differentiated thyroid cancer, Endocrinol. Metabol. Clin. North Am. 19 (1990) 685–718.

[157] D.L. Bushnell, M.A. Boles, G.E. Kaufman, M.A. Wadas, W.E. Barnes, Complications, sequela and dosimetry of iodine-131 therapy for thyroid carcinoma, J. Nucl. Med. 33 (1992) 2214–2221.

[158] M.E.A. O'Connell, M.A. Flower, P.J. Hinton, C.L. Harmer, V.R. McCready, Radiation dose assessment in radioiodine therapy. Dose-response relationships in differentiated thyroid carcinoma using quantitative scanning and PET, Radiother. Oncol. 28 (1993) 16–26.

[159] R.G. Jimenez, A.S. Moreno, E.N. Gonzalez, et al., Iodine-131 treatment of thyroid papillary carcinoma in patients undergoing dialysis for chronic renal failure: a dosimetric method, Thyroid 11 (11) (2001) 1031–1034.

[160] N. Howard, M. Glasser, Iodine 131 ablation therapy for a patient on maintenance haemodialysis, Br. J. Radiol. 54 (639) (1981) 259.

[161] F. Pons, I. Carrio, M. Estorch, M. Ginjuame, J. Pons, R. Milian, Lithium as an adjuvant of iodine-131 uptake when treating patients with well-differentiated thyroid carcinoma, Clin. Nucl. Med. 8 (1987) 644–647.

[162] S.S. Koong, J.C. Reynolds, E.G. Movius, et al., Lithium as a potential adjuvant to ^{131}I therapy of metastatic, well differentiated thyroid carcinoma, J. Clin. Endocrinol. Metab. 84 (1999) 912–916.

[163] S.I. Sherman, J. Gopal, Thyroglobulin positive, RAI negative thyroid cancers: the role of conservative management, J. Clin. Endocrinol. Metab. 83 (1998) 4199–4200.

[164] M. Schlumberger, F. Mancusi, E. Baudin, F. Pacini, 131-I Therapy for elevated thyroglobulin levels, Thyroid 7 (1997) 273–276.

[165] F. Pacini, F. Lippi, N. Formica, R. Elisei, S. Anelli, C. Ceccarelli, Therapeutic doses of iodine-131 reveal undiagnosed metastases in thyroid cancer patients with detectable serum thyroglobulin levels, J. Nucl. Med. 28 (1987) 1888–1891.

[166] J.D. Pineda, T. Lee, K. Ain, J. Reynolds, J. Robbins, Iodine-131 therapy for thyroid cancer patients with elevated thyroglobulin and negative diagnostic scan, J. Clin. Endocrinol. Metab. 80 (1995) 1488–1492.

[167] F. Pacini, L. Agate, R. Elisei, et al., Outcome of differentiated thyroid cancer with detectable serum Tg and negative diagnostic (131)I whole body scan: comparison of patients treated with high (131)I activities versus untreated patients, J. Clin. Endocrinol. Metab. 86 (9) (2001) 4092–4097.

[168] V. Fatourechi, I.D. Hay, H. Javedan, G.A. Wiseman, B.P. Mullan, C.A. Gorman, Lack of impact of radioiodine therapy in tg-positive, diagnostic whole-body scan-negative patients with follicular cell-derived thyroid cancer, J. Clin. Endocrinol. Metab. 87 (4) (2002) 1521–1526.

[169] M. Tubiana, M. Schlumberger, P. Rougier, et al., Long-term results and prognostic factors in patients with differentiated thyroid carcinoma, Cancer 55 (1985) 794–804.

[170] A.C. Chiu, E.S. Delpassand, S.I. Sherman, Prognosis and treatment of brain metastases in thyroid carcinoma, J. Clin. Endocrinol. Metab. 82 (1997) 3637–3642.

[171] J.W. Smit, G.J. Vielvoye, B.M. Goslings, Embolization for vertebral metastases of follicular thyroid carcinoma, J. Clin. Endocrinol. Metab. 85 (3) (2000) 989–994.

[172] K.M. van Tol, J.M. Hew, P.L. Jager, A. Vermey, R.P. Dullaart, T.P. Links, Embolization in combination with radioiodine therapy for bone metastases from differentiated thyroid carcinoma, Clin. Endocrinol. (Oxf.) 52 (5) (2000) 653–659.

[173] M.L. Adler, A. Macapinlac, R.J. Robbins, Radioiodine treatment of thyroid cancer with the aid of recombinant human thyrotropin, Endo. Pract. 4 (1998) 282–286.

[174] C. Spitzweg, W. Joba, J.C. Morris, A.E. Heufelder, Regulation of sodium iodide symporter gene expression in FRTL-5 rat thyroid cells, Thyroid 9 (8) (1999) 821–830.

[175] T. Schlesinger, M.A. Flower, V.R. McCready, Radiation dose assessments in radioiodine (131I) therapy. 1. The necessity for in vivo quantitation and dosimetry in the treatment of carcinoma of the thyroid, Radiother. Oncol. 14 (1989) 35–41.

[176] J.C. Sisson, D.A. Jamadar, E.A. Kazerooni, T.J. Giordano, J.E. Carey, S.A. Spaulding, Treatment of micronodular lung metastases of papillary thyroid cancer: are the tumors too small for effective irradiation from radioiodine?, Thyroid 8 (3) (1998) 215–221.

[177] H.R. Maxon, S.R. Thomas, R.C. Samaratunga, Dosimetric considerations in the radioiodine treatment of macrometastases and micrometastases from differentiated thyroid cancer, Thyroid 7 (2) (1997) 183–187.

[178] F. Grünwald, E. Pakos, H. Bender, et al., Redifferentiation therapy with retinoic acid in follicular thyroid cancer, J. Nucl. Med. 39 (1998) 1555–1558.

[179] F. Grünwald, C. Menzel, H. Bender, et al., Redifferentiation therapy-induced radioiodine uptake in thyroid cancer, J. Nucl. Med. 39 (1998) 1903–1906.

[180] C. Schmutzler, J. Kohrle, Retinoic acid redifferentiation therapy for thyroid cancer, Thyroid 10 (5) (2000) 393–406.

[181] D. Casara, D. Rubello, G. Saladini, et al., Different features of pulmonary metastases in differentiated thyroid cancer: natural history and multivariate statistical analysis of prognostic variables, J. Nucl. Med. 34 (1993) 1626–1631.

[182] T.W. Tsang, J.D. Brierley, W.J. Simpson, T. Panzarella, M.K. Gospodarowicz, S.B. Sutcliffe, The effects of surgery, radioiodine, and external radiation therapy on the clinical outcome of patients with differentiated thyroid carcinoma, Cancer 82 (1998) 375–388.

[183] T. Taylor, B. Specker, J. Robbins, et al., Outcome after treatment of high-risk papillary and non-Hurthle-cell follicular thyroid carcinoma, Ann. Intern. Med. 129 (1998) 622–627.

[184] M.P. Cunningham, R.B. Duda, W. Recant, J.S. Chmiel, J.A. Sylvester, A. Fremgen, Survival discriminants for differentiated thyroid cancer, Am. J. Surg. 160 (1990) 344–347.

[185] L.J. DeGroot, E.L. Kaplan, F.H. Straus, M.S. Shukla, Does the method of management of papillary thyroid carcinoma make a difference in outcome?, World J. Surg. 18 (1994) 123–130.

[186] N.A. Samaan, Y.K. Maheshwari, S. Nader, et al., Impact of therapy for differentiated carcinoma of the thyroid: an analysis of 706 cases, J. Clin. Endocrinol. Metab. 56 (1983) 1131–1138.

[187] S.L. Sugg, S. Ezzat, I.B. Rosen, J.L. Freeman, S.L. Asa, Distinct multiple RET/PTC gene rearrangements in multifocal papillary thyroid neoplasia, J. Clin. Endocrinol. Metab. 83 (1998) 4116–4122.

[188] R. Vassilopoulou-Sellin, M.J. Klein, T.H. Smith, et al., Pulmonary metastases in children and young adults with differentiated thyroid cancer, Cancer 71 (1993) 1348–1352.

[189] M. Schlumberger, O. Arcangioli, J.D. Piekarski, M. Tubiana, C. Parmentier, Detection and treatment of lung metastases of differentiated thyroid carcinoma in patients with normal chest X-rays, J. Nucl. Med. 29 (1988) 1790–1794.

[190] T.C. Chao, L.B. Jeng, J.D. Lin, M.F. Chen, Completion thyroidectomy for differentiated thyroid carcinoma, Otolaryngol. Head Neck Surg. 118 (1998) 896–899.

[191] L.J. DeGroot, E.L. Kaplan, Second operations for 'completion' of thyroidectomy in treatment of differentiated thyroid cancer, Surgery 110 (1991) 936–940.

[192] G.T. Emerick, Q.-Y. Duh, A.E. Siperstein, G.N. Burrow, O.H. Clark, Diagnosis, treatment, and outcome of follicular thyroid carcinoma, Cancer 72 (1993) 3287–3295.

[193] C. Mettlin, F. Lee, J. Drago, G.P. Murphy, The American Cancer Society National Prostate Cancer Detection Project, Cancer 67 (12) (1991) 2929–2958.

[194] L.J. Auguste, J.N. Attie, Completion thyroidectomy for initially misdiagnosed thyroid cancer, Otolaryngol. Clin. North Am. 23 (1990) 429–439.

[195] S.A. De Jong, J.G. Demeter, A.M. Lawrence, E. Paloyan, Necessity and safety of completion thyroidectomy for differentiated thyroid carcinoma, Surgery 112 (1992) 734–737.

[196] R.J. Robbins, R.M. Tuttle, M. Sonenberg, et al., Radioiodine ablation of thyroid remnants after preparation with recombinant human thyrotropin, Thyroid 11 (9) (2001) 865–869.

Chapter 5

Thyroglobulin measurements in thyroid cancer evaluation and surveillance

Carole Spencer[a], Shireen Fatemi[b]

[a]*University of Southern California, Edmondson Building, Room 111, 1840 North Soto Street, Los Angeles, CA 90032*
[b]*13652 Cantara Street, Medical 10, Panorama City, CA 91402*

Thyroglobulin (Tg) is a large (660 kDa) glycoprotein that is synthesized and secreted by all normal thyroid follicular cells and most well-differentiated thyroid carcinomas (DTC) [1]. The thyroid-specific origin of Tg in the circulation is the reason that serum Tg measurements are useful as a tumor-marker test for patients diagnosed with DTC [1–4].

It is critical that serum Tg values are interpreted with respect to both patient-specific pathology and treatment, as well as the technical limitations of the Tg methodology used. Patient-specific factors include tumor type and staging, the degree of surgery, radioiodine ablative therapy, and TSH status. Methodologic factors include the class of Tg method [radioimmunoassay (RIA) or immunometric assay (IMA)], as well as methodologic bias, sensitivity, specificity, precision, strategies for eliminating 'hook' problems and most importantly the method's propensity for Tg autoantibody (TgAb) interference. This chapter will discuss the impact of patient and methodologic factors on the clinical interpretation of serum Tg values.

1. Thyroglobulin physiology

Thyroglobulin is the precursor protein for synthesizing the thyroid hormones, thyroxine (T4) and triiodothyronine (T3). Specifically, thyroid hormones are formed from iodination and coupling of tyrosine residues within the backbone of Tg molecules stored in the follicular lumen, a process catalyzed by the thyroid peroxidase (TPO) enzyme that is localized on the apical surface of follicular cells [1,5]. After endocytosis and lysosomal digestion of iodinated Tg molecules, a process dependent on the degree of TSH receptor stimulation, thyroid hormones are liberated into the circulation [6]. As a consequence of thyroid hormone secretion some intact Tg

ADVANCES IN MOLECULAR AND CELLULAR ENDOCRINOLOGY
VOLUME 4   ISSN 1569-2566/DOI 10.1016/S1569-2566(04)04005-0

molecules and also some Tg mRNAs are co-released. In fact, Tg should be detectable in the serum of all normal subjects with an intact thyroid gland [4,7,8]. The failure to detect Tg in 100% of normal euthyroid subjects is a hallmark of Tg assay insensitivity and suggests that this method will be too insensitive to detect recurrence in patients with DTC [9,10].

The amount of Tg entering the circulation reflects three principal factors: (1) the mass of differentiated thyroid tissue present (normal tissue and/or tumor); (2) any inflammation or injury to thyroid tissue, such as following fine needle aspiration (FNA), thyroid surgery, radioiodine therapy or thyroiditis; and (3) most importantly, degree of stimulation of the TSH receptors (by TSH, endogenous or recombinant, the high human chorionic gonodotrophin (hCG) of pregnancy or the thyroid-stimulating immunoglobulins of Graves' disease) [2]. It follows that an elevated serum Tg is a non-specific finding associated with virtually any thyroid pathology.

2. Clinical utility of serum Tg measurement

Most patients with elevated serum Tg concentrations have benign thyroid conditions. Specifically, serum Tg is elevated in any patient with an increase in thyroid mass (i.e. goiter) and with most hyperthyroid conditions involving excessive thyroid stimulation including those of an autoimmune or destructive nature [2,4]. It follows that a low serum Tg concentration is a useful test for confirming the diagnosis of thyrotoxicosis factitia [11]. Serum Tg measurement is also used to investigate the etiology of congenital hypothyroidism and for epidemiologic population studies of iodine deficiency [12,13]. In the setting of DTC, the clinical utility of serum Tg measurement begins preoperatively, that is after the diagnosis of DTC has been established and before thyroidectomy. Under these circumstances, serum Tg concentration reflects the mass of thyroid tissue (tumor or normal remnant), the capacity of the tumor to synthesize and secrete Tg and any thyroid injury TSH receptor stimulation [endogenous or recombinant human TSH(rhTSH)] [2,4]. Since TSH is the major regulator of the serum Tg concentration both in normal and neoplastic tissue, it is difficult to interpret serum Tg values without knowing the TSH status of the patient.

3. Serum Tg reference range values[1]

The typical mean serum Tg concentration for a cohort of normal euthyroid subjects approximates $13.5 \mu g \, L^{-1}$ [9,14]. This suggests that 1 g of normal thyroid tissue gives rise to ~ 1 to $2 \mu g \, L^{-1}$ Tg in the circulation when TSH is within normal limits

---

[1]The serum Tg values given in this chapter are appropriate for a Tg method having a mean value for normal euthyroid volunteers of $13.5 \mu g \, L^{-1}$ and a normal reference range of $3–40 \mu g \, L^{-1}$ [14]. When using a different Tg method, it is necessary to proportionally adjust the serum Tg cut-off values according to the mean normal value for that method, relative to the mean normal value of $13.5 \mu g \, L^{-1}$ for the method referenced [17].

$(0.5–2.5 \, \text{mIU L}^{-1})$ [4]. It should be noted that when TSH is suppressed to subnormal levels ($<0.1 \, \text{mIU L}^{-1}$), serum Tg concentrations fall by $\sim 50\%$ [15]. Although there is no 'normal Tg reference range' for DTC patients following surgery, the normal relationships between thyroid mass and serum Tg concentrations as well as between serum Tg and TSH concentrations provide important reference information for interpreting the serum Tg values of an individual DTC patient. Also, the pattern of change of serial serum Tg measurements made over time is more informative than an isolated serum Tg value. However, it is possible to judge the clinical significance of an isolated Tg value by knowing the normal reference range of the Tg assay, the extent of thyroid surgery, and the serum TSH level (at steady state) (Fig. 1).

Thus, as shown in Fig. 1, the normal reference range $3–40 \, \mu\text{g L}^{-1}$ only applies to normal subjects with intact thyroid glands who are euthyroid (TSH, $\sim 1.5 \, \text{mU L}^{-1}$). When such normal subjects are placed on high dose L-T4 therapy to suppress TSH below $0.1 \, \text{mU L}^{-1}$, serum Tg is expected to fall by 50% to a new upper normal reference limit of $20 \, \mu\text{g L}^{-1}$ [15]. These reference landmarks can then be used to interpret post-surgical serum Tg values in TgAb-negative DTC patients. Specifically, DTC patients who have one normal lobe remaining after lobectomy and who are receiving L-T4 suppression therapy (TSH $<0.1 \, \text{mIU L}^{-1}$) are expected to have serum Tg values not higher than $\sim 40 \, \mu\text{g L}^{-1}$ if no tumor is present. Higher serum Tg values in such patients suggest the possibility of multicentric disease, which is present in 66% patients with papillary thyroid carcinoma [16]. DTC patients who have had a near-total thyroidectomy usually have not more than 1–2 g of normal thyroid remnant remaining. In these patients, serum Tg concentrations during L-T4 therapy (TSH $<0.1 \, \text{mIU L}^{-1}$) are not expected to exceed $2 \, \mu\text{g L}^{-1}$. In contrast, when thyroidectomy and radioiodine has rendered the patient truly athyreotic, serum Tg should be undetectable irrespective of whether TSH is high or suppressed.

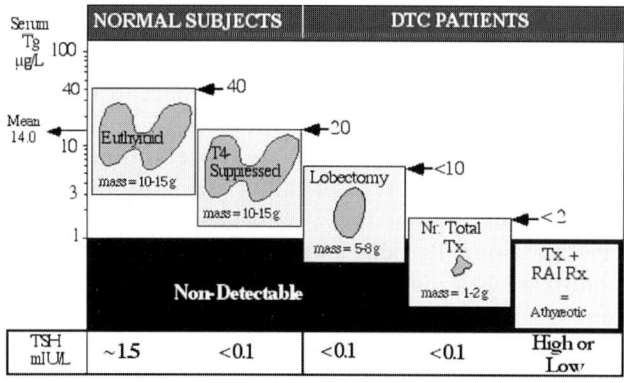

Fig. 1. Relationships between serum Tg, thyroid tissue mass and serum TSH based on a Tg assay with a normal reference range of $3–40 \, \mu\text{g L}^{-1}$ and the assumptions that the mass of normal thyroid tissue is 10–15 g; 1 g of normal thyroid tissue secretes $\sim 1 \, \mu\text{g L}^{-1}$ Tg into the circulation when TSH is normal and $\sim 0.5 \, \mu\text{g L}^{-1}$ Tg when TSH is $<0.1 \, \text{mU L}^{-1}$. (Adapted from the NACB Thyroid Monograph (www.nacb.org).)

4. Clinical utility of serum Tg in different stages of managing DTC

Serum Tg measurements are useful in all phases of managing patients with DTC. (1) A pre-operative serum Tg measurement, made before or >2 weeks after FNA, will give information on the ability of the tumor to secrete Tg and confirm the efficacy of using serial serum Tg measurements as a post-operative tumor marker test. (2) Acute serum Tg measurements (first 6 months following surgery) give information on the completeness of surgery and may help to determine the need for radioiodine therapy. (3) Serum Tg levels during L-T4 therapy in the early (6–24 months) post-operative period can be used for long-term recurrence-risk assessment. (4) When serum Tg is *detectable* during L-T4 therapy (low TSH), long-term monitoring of serial serum Tg measurements can be used to assess the efficacy of treatment without the need for TSH stimulation. (5) When serum Tg is *undetectable* during L-T4 therapy, rhTSH-stimulated serum Tg measurements can be used to enhance the sensitivity of serum Tg testing for detecting clinically significant diseases.

4.1. *Pre-operative serum Tg measurements*

The biosynthesis and processing of Tg molecules within normal follicular cells is complex. The formation of a mature Tg molecule involves chaperone proteins that regulate the trafficking of newly synthesized Tg from the endoplasmic reticulum to the Golgi for site-specific glycosylation, before targeting glycosylated Tg molecules to the follicular lumen for enzymatic iodination by the thyroid peroxidase enzyme localized on the apical cell membrane [18,19]. Given the complexity of the process for producing mature Tg molecules, it is not surprising that Tg molecular processing in tumor cells may become dysregulated. A number of studies suggest that DTC-derived Tg is poorly iodinated and some of the thyroid tumors lack the ability to synthesize and/or secrete conformationally normal Tg molecules [20–22].

Abnormalities in Tg molecular processing leading to impaired iodination and colloid storage, and dysregulated Tg secretion may explain why a large percentage of DTC patients have elevated pre-operative serum Tg concentrations [23]. As shown in Fig. 2, the highest pre-operative serum Tg values are seen with follicular tumors; however, the median pre-operative serum Tg concentrations is elevated in both Hurthle and Papillary DTC. The type of tumor seems to impact the pre-operative serum Tg value more than tumor mass, as evidenced by the lack of correlation between pre-operative serum Tg value and the presence of metastases. This suggests that thyroid tumors are heterogeneous with respect to their capability for Tg secretion. One gram of normal thyroid tissue secretes $\sim 1\,\mu g\,L^{-1}$ Tg into the circulation when TSH is normal, and $\sim 0.5\,\mu g\,L^{-1}$ Tg when TSH is $<0.1\,mU\,L^{-1}$ (Fig. 1). It follows that a 2 cm thyroid nodule would only be expected to elevate the pre-operative serum Tg value by $\sim 2\,\mu g\,L^{-1}$ and that an elevated pre-operative serum Tg likely represents excessive secretion of Tg per gram of tumor tissue as compared with normal. The study of Tegler and colleagues supports the contention that many thyroid tumors secrete an excessive amount of Tg pre gram of tumor tissue [24]. The finding of an elevated pre-operative serum Tg concentration has positive significance

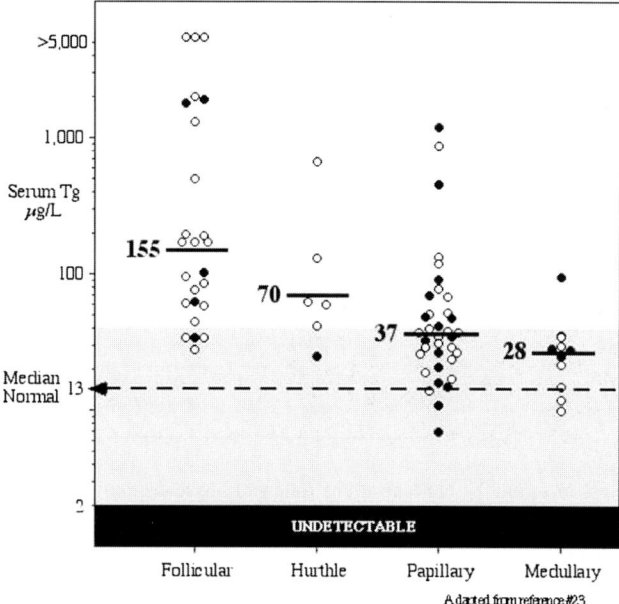

Fig. 2. Pre-operative serum Tg values in different types of DTC. Median values are indicated by horizontal bars. Patients with metastatic disease are denoted by solid symbols. The normal reference range (median normal value of $14\,\mu g\,L^{-1}$) is indicated by shading. (Data is taken from Ericsson et al. [23].)

for the use of serum Tg measurement as a post-operative tumor marker test. In fact, the pre-operative serum Tg concentration is the key for the interpretation of post-operative serum Tg values. Specifically, an undetectable post-operative serum Tg value is less reassuring if the pre-operative serum Tg was within normal limits. This is because in the absence of an elevated pre-operative Tg value, there is no indication that the tumor is capable of secreting Tg. Conversely, a detectable post-operative serum Tg value in a patient with a non-elevated pre-operative serum Tg could represent a large amount of low Tg-secreting tumor. If an elevated pre-operative serum Tg reflects neoplasmic Tg secretion, it follows that the sensitivity of post-operative serum Tg monitoring will be highest when the tumor is relatively small (<2 cm diameter) and the pre-operative serum Tg value is high. (FNA elevates serum Tg concentrations within hours. Pre-operative specimens for serum Tg measurement should be drawn either before FNA and held to await the cytologic diagnosis, or drawn >2 weeks following FNA [25].)

4.2. *Acute post-operative period (first 6 months)*

Estimates vary, but the half-life of Tg in the circulation is approximately 3–4 days [26–28]. Surgical margins that leak Tg should largely heal within the first 2 months following surgery. During the early post-surgical period, the mass of thyroid tissue remaining (normal remnant + any tumor) together with the prevailing TSH

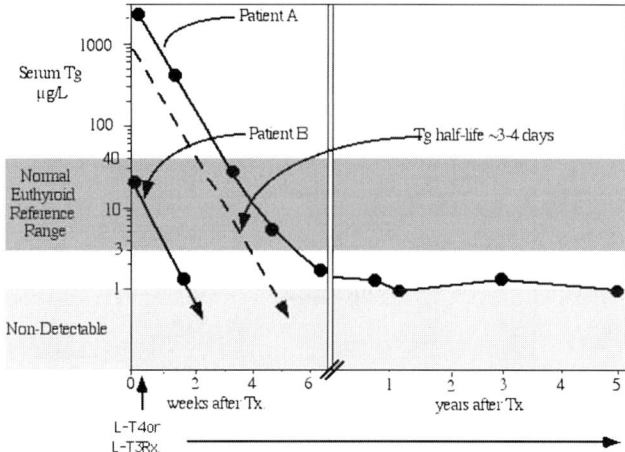

Fig. 3. Acute changes in serum Tg concentrations following thyroidectomy (Tx) if thyroid hormone is given to prevent a rise in TSH. Serum Tg concentrations plateau after 6–8 weeks in patients with elevated pre-operative serum Tg concentrations (Patient A), and after 2–3 weeks in patients with non-elevated pre-operative serum Tg concentrations (Patient B), assuming a Tg half-life of ~4 days.

concentration will be the dominant influences on serum Tg concentrations [29]. As shown in Fig. 3, if thyroid hormone therapy (L-T4 or L-T3) is initiated immediately after surgery to prevent the expected rise in TSH, the serum Tg concentration is expected to stabilize by 6–8 weeks at a level that reflects (1) the size of the normal thyroid remnant remaining; (2) any local or metastatic tumor; and (3) the ability of the tumor to secrete Tg (as suggested by the pre-operative serum Tg concentration). As discussed above, the normal thyroid remnant remaining after a successful near-total thyroidectomy typically approximates 2 g of tissue, and give rise to a serum Tg concentration $< 2\,\mu g\,L^{-1}$ when serum TSH is maintained below $0.1\,mU\,L^{-1}$. A serum Tg concentration below $2\,\mu g\,L^{-1}$ is a good prognostic sign during the first few weeks after surgery, especially if the pre-operative serum Tg was elevated above the upper normal limit, suggesting that the tumor was an efficient Tg-secretor [30].

4.3. *Early post-operative period (6–24 months)*

Most recurrences or persistent tumor are detected during the first 5 years [31]. Risk stratification based on prognostic factors, surgical findings, together with pre- and acute post-operative serum Tg measurements provide critical information during the early post-operative period. A recent study has reported that the 2-year post-operative serum Tg concentration is a good indicator of long-term recurrence risk [32]. Specifically, TgAb-negative patients who developed serum Tg below $2\,\mu g\,L^{-1}$ by the second post-operative year, while receiving a stable dose of L-T4 therapy, had a significantly lower risk of recurrence after 10 years of follow-up compared with patients whose serum Tg remained $> 2\,\mu g\,L^{-1}$ after 2 years (6.6 versus 71.1%, respectively). The efficacy of long-term serial Tg monitoring was shown even for the low Tg patients who had recurrence, 8/13 of whom exhibited a rise in Tg above $2 \mu g L^{-1}$ either the year before or when recurrence was detected [32].

4.4. *Long-term monitoring*

4.4.1. *TgAb-negative patients with detectable serum Tg on L-T4 treatment*
During long-term monitoring on a stable dose of L-T4 therapy, the serum Tg concentration will reflect the integrated effects of the mass of normal thyroid remnant remaining, the presence of any tumor, the efficiency of tumor Tg secretion, and the degree of TSH stimulation. Most patients with DTC are successfully treated with thyroidectomy $\pm$ radioiodine therapy [31]. Steadily decreasing serial serum Tg concentrations and serum TgAb concentrations (if detected), are usually the hallmark of successful treatment (Figs. 4 and 5). It is the *pattern* of serial serum Tg measurements during L-T4 therapy (when TSH is stable) that is more clinically useful than an isolated Tg value. As shown in Fig. 4a progressively decreasing Tg pattern is typical of patients judged to be disease-free, whereas a persistently detectable Tg or a rising Tg pattern is more typical of patients judged to have persistent or recurrent disease [2]. The slowly declining serum Tg seen in radioiodine-treated patients who become disease-free likely reflects the slow die-off of thyroid cells whose replication was damaged by the radioiodine therapy [33]. However, a progressive decline in serum Tg concentrations is often also seen in patients who did not receive radioiodine therapy, presumably reflecting a decrease in thyroid tissue mass secondary to impairment of TSH-dependent replication [34].

A rise in serum Tg (Fig. 4b) and/or a rise in the TgAb concentration of a TgAb-positive patient (Fig. 5a) during serial monitoring is often the first sign of recurrence [35]. Increase in serum Tg reflects either an increase in tumor mass (when TSH is stable) or increased TSH stimulation (when thyroid tissue mass is stable). Many well-differentiated thyroid tumors are exquisitely sensitive to the TSH concentration

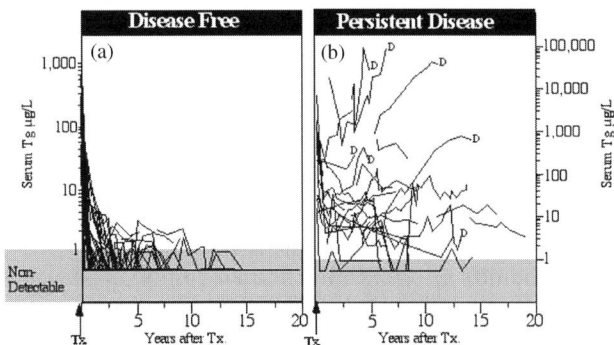

Fig. 4. Serial serum Tg patterns in TgAb-negative patients either judged disease-free at the end of the follow-up period (a) or with evidence of persistent or recurrent disease (b). The patients who died from DTC are indicated by the letter 'D'. Undetectable values are indicated by shading. (Adapted from Spencer and Wang [2].)

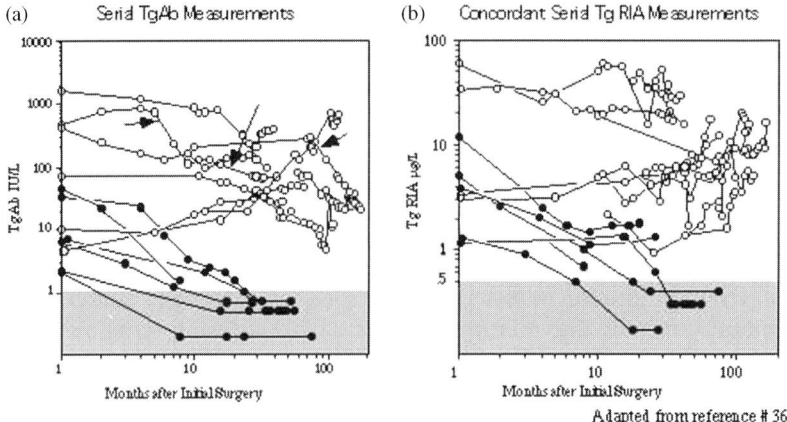

Fig. 5. Serial serum TgAb (a) (RIA methodology) and Tg RIA (b) measurements following initial thyroid surgery (month) for DTC. Patients were classified at their most recent follow-up visit as having persistent or recurrent disease (open symbols), or were judged to be disease-free (closed symbols). The shaded area represents undetectable values. Arrows indicate additional surgeries.

[2,36]. Before attributing a serum Tg rise to tumor recurrence it is important to ensure that the change is not secondary to non-compliance with L-T4 therapy. Non-compliance will not always be detected by a TSH measurement if the patient has resumed compliance immediately before the clinic visit, since the half-life of TSH in the circulation is much shorter than Tg (1 h ~4 days) [26–28,37]. Strategies that can be used to rule out a TSH-mediated serum Tg elevation include counselling the patient about compliance, ultrasound of the neck or testing for adequacy of the L-T4 dose used to suppress TSH. The latter can be done either by prescribing an increased L-T4 dose and rechecking serum Tg after 6–8 weeks, or by evaluating the serum Tg response to an oral 1 mg L-T4 loading dose (expect the serum Tg concentration to fall 30–50% after 8 days if the Tg rise was TSH-mediated) [2,15].

A rise in the serum Tg concentration in the face of an unchanged TSH will likely reflect an increase in tumor mass (since Tg secretion from normal remnant tissue mass would not be expected to increase in the absence of TSH stimulation). The clinical significance of small changes in serum Tg ($+1$–$3\,\mu g\,L^{-1}$) will be greater for tumors identified as a low Tg secretors by virtue of having a normal pre-operative serum Tg value. The magnitude of the rise in serum Tg in response to either endogenous TSH (thyroid hormone withdrawal) or rhTSH administration, may provide a gauge of the TSH sensitivity of the tumor [17,36]. Typically, TSH stimulation of normal thyroid remnants or well-differentiated tumor produces a 3–20-fold increase in serum Tg above basal (TSH-suppressed) levels when TgAb is negative. The serum Tg responses to endogenous TSH are typically greater than that for rhTSH [17,36,38,39]. Moreover, poorly differentiated tumors, display a blunted (<3-fold) increase in serum Tg in response to TSH stimulation [40].

Serial monitoring of serum Tg and TgAb concentrations is only useful if the same methods are used throughout the follow-up period. As shown in Fig. 6, serum Tg

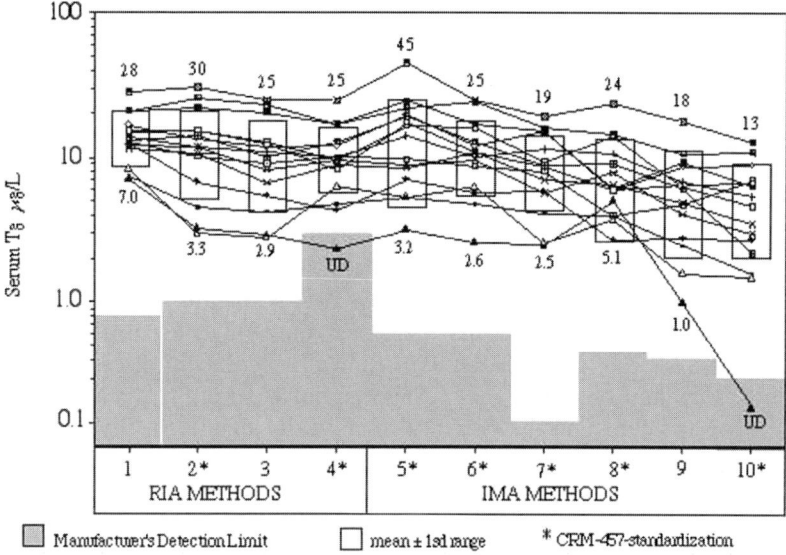

Fig. 6. Mean ± Sd values for TgAb-negative sera from 20 normal euthyroid subjects measured by 10 different Tg methods. Method 1 = Diagnostic Systems Laboratories, Webster, TX, USA; Method 2 = University of Southern California RIA, Los Angeles, CA, USA; RIA 3 = Kronus RIA, Boise ID, USA; Method 4 = Endocrine Sciences RIA, Calabasas, CA, USA; Method 5 = Nichols Institute Diagnostics ICMA, San Juan Capistrano, CA, USA; Method 6 = Endocrine Sciences ICMA, Calabasas, CA, USA; Tarzana, CA, USA; Method 7 = Sanofi Pasteur IRMA, Marnes-La-Coquette, France; Method 8 = Kronus OptiQuant IRMA, Boise ID, USA; Method 9 = Brahms DynoTest TgS IRMA, Berlin, Germany; Method 10 = Diagnostic Products Immulite ICMA, Los Angeles, CA, USA. The shaded area represents the manufacturer's stated sensitivity limit. The asterisk denotes assays claiming CRM-457 standardization. (Adapted from the NACB Thyroid Monograph (www.nacb.org).)

concentrations measured by different methods can vary more than 3-fold [4,9]. If the laboratory changes the Tg assay to one with a negative bias, lower serum Tg values will be reported and may mask a clinically significant serum Tg rise. Similarly, a change in Tg assay to one with a positive bias will lead to the reporting of higher values and prompt unnecessary concerns about recurrence. The new National Academy of Clinical Biochemistry (NACB) guidelines dictate that laboratories should consult their physician-users *before* implementing any change in the Tg or TgAb method [4]. It is recommended that laboratories should offer to re-baseline patients if the bias between the old and proposed new Tg method exceeds 10% [4].

4.4.2. *Use of rhTSH for TgAb-negative patients with undetectable serum Tg on L-T4 treatment*

When serum Tg is detectable during long-term monitoring on L-T4 therapy, TSH-stimulated serum Tg measurements are unnecessary, since Tg will predictably increase 3–20-fold in response to a high TSH [17,36]. However, an *undetectable* serum Tg during long-term monitoring on L-T4 therapy does not guarantee the absence of disease [14,39,41–45]. A number of studies have now reported that clinical recurrences and even metastatic disease can be present when patients have undetectable post-operative serum Tg values while receiving L-T4 therapy [14,39,41–45]. The paradoxical inability to detect Tg in such patients may either reflect the insensitivity of the Tg assay used and/or the presence of tumor cells with an impaired capacity to secrete Tg (as suggested by a non-elevated pre-operative serum Tg value) [10]. Many patients with undetectable serum Tg during L-T4 therapy and documented disease display detectable serum Tg values above $2\,\mu g\,L^{-1}$ when TSH becomes elevated following thyroid hormone withdrawal or rhTSH administration [14,39,41–45]. Thus an undetectable serum Tg during L-T4 therapy should not be used to rule out the presence of disease that may be revealed by TSH-stimulated serum Tg testing. In contrast, a rhTSH-stimulated serum Tg values below $2\,\mu g\,L^{-1}$ in low-risk TgAb-negative patients is rarely associated with clinically significant disease [45].

There is growing consensus that TSH-stimulated serum Tg measurements are more sensitive for detecting the presence of clinically significant thyroid tissue than either Tg measured during L-T4 therapy, or low-dose ^{131}I-imaging studies [14,39,41–46]. This consensus has arisen from a number of studies reporting a high rate of false-negative ^{131}I scans for patients with documented disease [45]. The high frequency of false-negative low-dose scans (withdrawal or rhTSH) for a cohort of patients with positive post-treatment scans is shown in Fig. 7. Specifically, both low-dose scanning protocols (withdrawal and rhTSH) were associated with higher false-negatives (~20 and ~30%, respectively) compared with a positive TSH-stimulated serum Tg using a cut-off of $2\,\mu g\,L^{-1}$ (~3 versus ~8%, respectively, for endogenous versus recombinant TSH stimulation). Thus, since TSH-stimulated serum Tg values are rarely misleading when using the $2\,\mu g\,L^{-1}$ cut-off rhTSH-stimulated serum Tg

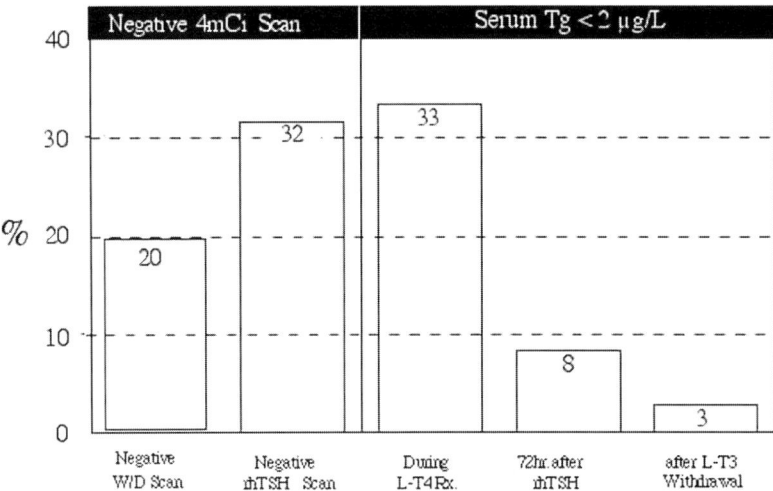

Fig. 7. False-negative tests in 44 patients with positive post-treatment (> 100 mCi) scans. Scans (4 mCi) were made either following thyroid hormone withdrawal (W/D) or after rhTSH administration using the standard protocols [17]. Serum Tg analysis was made on 41 TgAb-negative patients using the standard Tg cut-off value of $2\,\mu g\,L^{-1}$ [17].

measurements are clearly superior in sensitivity for detecting disease than either low-dose scanning regimen.

The $2 \mu g L^{-1}$ serum Tg cut-off was derived from the Phase III Thyrogen® study which analyzed the sensitivity of different serum Tg values for detecting the presence of disease [17]. The $2 \mu g L^{-1}$ serum Tg cut-off value was determined from measurements made by both an in-house Tg RIA and a commercially available Tg ICMA method, both methods having a mean normal range value approximating $14 \mu g L^{-1}$ and a normal euthyroid reference range approximating 3–$40 \mu g L^{-1}$ [17]. Given the large between-method biases shown in Fig. 6, it is clear that it is necessary to adjust the $2 \mu g L^{-1}$ Tg cut-off value when using a Tg method that has a significant bias ($\pm > 10\%$) relative to the reference methods used in the Phase III study report [17]. A method-specific rhTSH-stimulated serum Tg cut-off equivalent to the reference method value of $2 \mu g L^{-1}$ can be calculated from the ratio between the mean normal value of the test method and that of the reference method [14]). [For example, if the mean normal value of the test method is $9 \mu g L^{-1}$, the method-specific cut-off value for rhTSH testing equivalent to the reference method value of $2 \mu g L^{-1}$ would be $2(9/14) = 1.3 \mu g L^{-1}$.]

4.4.3. *Serial monitoring of TgAb-positive patients*

In all, 20–30% of DTC patients have serum TgAb detected when a sensitive TgAb immunoassay is used [35,47,48]. Even very low levels of TgAb can interfere with Tg measurement when made by IMA methodology, causing undetectable serum Tg values that may mask the presence of disease [35,49,50]. A *detectable* serum Tg IMA value in a TgAb-positive patient is good evidence that some Tg is present, albeit maybe underestimated, but an *undetectable* serum Tg IMA value is unreliable and should not be considered in clinical assessment. While the influence of TgAb on different RIA methods relates to the assay design, Tg RIA measurements in general appear to be less prone to TgAb interference [35,51]. As shown in Fig. 5b, some RIA methods that appear to give clinically useful information in the presence of TgAb, evident from the parallel decline in serial serum Tg RIA and TgAb concentrations in patients judged disease-free at the end of follow-up and the maintenance of detectable Tg RIA values in patients with documented disease [35]. These findings have led some laboratories to adopt RIA methodology for measuring serum Tg in TgAb-positive sera and limit the use of IMA methodology to TgAb-negative sera. Unfortunately, most laboratories do not have access to quality RIA methods and report only IMA values for both TgAb-negative and TgAb-positive patients. It is hoped that laboratories will change this strategy in accord with the new NACB guidelines that state:

'serum Tg values for TgAb-positive specimens should not be reported if the method gives inappropriately undetectable values in TgAb-positive DTC patients with documented disease' [4].

There is now consensus that serial TgAb measurements *per se* can be used as a surrogate tumor-marker test to assess the efficacy of therapy for TgAb-positive patients [35,52–54]. Specifically, TgAb-positive patients who are rendered disease-free by treatment typically display declining TgAb concentrations that become

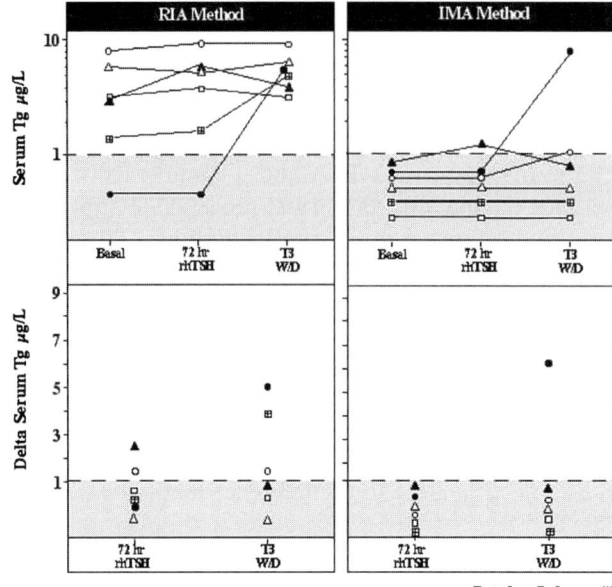

Fig. 8. Recombinant human TSH-stimulated serum Tg responses in six TgAb-positive patients with disease detected by ^{131}I scan measured by both a Tg RIA and Tg ICMA method. The shaded area represents undetectable values [17].

undetectable between 1 and 4 years (Fig. 5a). In contrast, TgAb concentrations will often plateau and remain stable for long periods of time when patients have persistent disease (Fig. 5a). A rise in TgAb is often the first sign of tumor growth in such patients [35]. However, it is important to expect a transient rise in TgAb in the first 6 months following ^{131}I treatment. This is likely an immune response to antigen (Tg) released by damaged tumor cells.

Unfortunately, rhTSH-stimulation testing does not resolve the problem of TgAb interference. As shown in Fig. 8, irrespective of the class of Tg assay used (IMA or RIA), TgAb-positive patients typically show an absent or blunted rhTSH-stimulated Tg response even when disease is present as evidenced by ^{131}I scan [17]. Most basal (low TSH) specimens exhibited the RIA/IMA discordance typical of TgAb-positive specimens (see below) and yet even when patients have detectable basal serum Tg RIA values, blunted or absent TSH-stimulated Tg responses are evident [36]. This paradoxical lack of response most likely reflects differences in clearance between free Tg and the Tg–TgAb complexes that are formed after TSH stimulates Tg release in the presence of TgAb.

5. Technical limitations of serum Tg measurement

The measurement of Tg in serum is technically challenging. A number of technical limitations currently impact the clinical utility and reliability of Tg testing [4,9].

(1) The class of Tg method (RIA or IMA) influences the degree and direction of TgAb interference. (2) Large between-method biases preclude the use of different Tg methods for serial monitoring of patients. (3) Inadequate sensitivity and suboptimal between-run precision impair the early detection of recurrence. (4) IMA methods are prone to 'hook' problems that can lead to an underestimation of the very high serum Tg values typical of metastatic disease.

Currently, IMA methodology is gaining popularity over RIA because IMA methods offer the practical advantage of shorter incubation times, an extended dynamic range of measurement and a more stable labeled antibody reagent that is less prone to labeling damage, as compared with RIA which employs antigen labeling [9,55]. Laboratories can now choose from a range of isotopic (immunoradiometric, IRMAs) and non-isotopic (primarily immunochemiluminometric, ICMA) IMA methods. Non-isotopic IMAs can be automated, which is the prime factor that most laboratories consider when selecting their Tg method.

5.1. *TgAb interference with serum Tg measurements*

TgAb is detected in a higher percentage of DTC patients than in the general population ($\sim$20 versus $\sim$10%, respectively) [35]. One disadvantage of IMA methodology is that it is more prone to interference by TgAb, which causes an underestimation of serum Tg concentrations that may mask the presence of clinically significant disease [35]. This has prompted some laboratories to restrict the use of IMA methods to TgAb-negative patients and adopt RIA for measuring serum Tg in TgAb-positive patients. However, no method whether IMA or RIA, can claim to be totally unaffected by TgAb interference in all cases. Consensus is growing that RIA methods are less prone to TgAb interference although some patients may still display inappropriately high or low Tg values. It is important to recognize that any TgAb present in the specimen has the potential to interfere with Tg measurement by any method [9,50]. In addition to its propensity for TgAb interference, IMA methodology is also prone to interference from heterophilic antibody (HAMA), which may result in inappropriately high Tg values that exhibit non-parallelism on dilution [56].

When sera containing TgAb are measured by both an RIA and IMA methods, an RIA:IMA discordance (Tg RIA = detectable, Tg IMA = undetectable) is frequently observed [4,9,36]. Because TgAb is heterogeneous, neither the measured TgAb concentration nor an exogenous Tg recovery test is 100% reliable for predicting whether the TgAb in a specimen will cause interference [35,50,57]. The finding of RIA:IMA discordance appears to be the most reliable characteristic of TgAb interference [4,9,35,50,57]. There is now a consensus that a Tg recovery test is an unreliable approach for detecting TgAb and should be eliminated [4,50]. Previous studies reporting that some sera displayed low recoveries in the absence of TgAb are now thought to be flawed by the insensitivity of early TgAb methods [35]. When a sensitive immunoassay is used, it is now apparent that TgAb is always detected when recoveries are low [4,35]. The reason why IMA methodology has a propensity to underestimate Tg concentrations appears to relate to its failure to quantify the Tg that is complexed with TgAb. In contrast, RIA methods appear to be capable of quantifying both the free Tg and the Tg–TgAb complexes, thereby producing higher total Tg values for most TgAb-positive specimens [35,36]. TgAb-mediated RIA:IMA discordances are most pronounced at low Tg concentrations, when more Tg is complexed with TgAb and is less available for IMA quantitation [4,36].

Although no Tg method is immune to TgAb interference, there is growing consensus that the RIA class of Tg method is less prone to TgAb interference, and produces more clinically valid serum Tg results for TgAb-positive patients than the IMA class of method [4,35,51]. However, it should be stressed that TgAb is heterogeneous and no RIA method can claim to be immune from TgAb interference in all cases. Clearly, the potential for and the direction (under- or overestimation) of TgAb interference with RIA measurements relates to the specificity of the assay reagents and to the incubation conditions used. Factors that determine the propensity of an RIA method for TgAb interference include the quality of the ^{125}I-Tg tracer, the specificity affinity of the Tg polyclonal antibody and the species-specificity of the second antibody reagents used [20,55,58–60].

The most clinically serious direction of TgAb interference is Tg underestimation, which has the potential to mask clinically significant and even metastatic disease [35]. Although RIA methods are not guaranteed free of TgAb interference, underestimation is rare with RIA measurement but common with IMA. The new NACB guidelines charge laboratories using IMA methodology to refrain from reporting undetectable serum Tg values for TgAb-positive patients [4]. Clearly, the class of Tg methods used will have an impact on the clinical decision-making in TgAb-positive patients when there is a significant RIA:IMA discordance of the magnitude RIA $= >2\,\mu g\,L^{-1}$: IMA $=$ undetectable [17]. Some laboratories now retain RIA methodology for measuring serum Tg in TgAb-positive sera, and limit the use of IMA methodology to TgAb-negative sera.

5.2. *TgAb measurement in DTC patients*

The sensitivity and specificity of different TgAb tests is highly variable [35]. The new NACB guidelines state that it is essential that the TgAb measurement be made by the laboratory performing the Tg testing, because *that* laboratory is responsible for selecting the TgAb method most suited for detecting TgAb interference with their selected Tg method [4]. Furthermore, recovery tests should not be used for detecting TgAb and should be eliminated [4,50]. TgAb should be measured concurrently with Tg on every specimen because the TgAb status of patients can change from positive to negative, and *vice versa*. The quality of the TgAb test is especially critical when laboratories measure serum Tg by IMA methodology since failure to detect the presence of TgAb can lead to the reporting of clinically misleading, undetectable serum Tg values [35]. Serum TgAb concentrations should be determined by a sensitive, quantitative immunoassay method, not a qualitative insensitive agglutination test because TgAb concentrations below the sensitivity limit of agglutination can interfere with serum Tg measurement [35]. It is possible for physicians to tell whether their laboratory uses quantitative immunoassay or insensitive agglutination by the units that are reported for the test. Specifically, TgAb immunoassays are standardized against an international standard (MRC 65/93) and reported in $IU\,mL^{-1}$ or $kIU\,L^{-1}$, whereas qualitative agglutination is reported as a titer (1:100, 1:400, etc) [35]. Also, as discussed above, when detected, serial quantitative TgAb measurements *per se* can be used as an independent surrogate tumor-marker test [35]. When TgAb-positive patients are monitored by serial Tg RIA and quantitative TgAb measurements, both the parameters give useful information. A progressive decline in both Tg RIA and TgAb concentrations is typical of successful treatment of tumor, whereas a rise in both parameters, or a disparity between the parameters (rising TgAb/falling Tg RIA), is an early sign of recurrence.

5.3. *Tg mRNA determinations in peripheral blood*

The reverse transcriptase–polymerase chain reaction (RT–PCR) amplification of tissue specific mRNA has been used to detect circulating cancer cells in the peripheral blood of patients with melanoma, prostate, and breast malignancies [61–63]. The use of RT–PCR to detect recurrent thyroid cancer was first reported in 1996 [64]. The availability of Tg-specific primers has prompted a number of groups to develop quantitative RT–PCR methods to detect Tg mRNA transcripts in blood [7,8,65–68]. Subsequently, the technique has been applied to cervical lymph-node metastases and has been found to be more sensitive than the measurement of Tg in the aspirate [69].

It is hoped that in future, Tg mRNA determinations in peripheral blood will prove useful for establishing the presence of disease, especially in TgAb-positive patients in whom the validity of the serum Tg measurement is questionable. However, the clinical value of Tg mRNA measurement has yet to be unequivocally established. Before Tg mRNA testing can be used to facilitate therapeutic decision-making for DTC patients, questions regarding the sensitivity and tissue specificity of Tg mRNA in peripheral blood need to be resolved [65–67]. Studies generally report detectable Tg mRNA for all normal subjects, but a poor correlation between quantitative Tg mRNA and serum Tg protein concentrations measured by immunoassay [7,8]. Correlations between Tg mRNA and tumor burden also differ. Some studies have reported that the amount of Tg mRNA correlates with the presence or absence of metastases while others report no such correlation [7,66,68]. These discrepancies probably reflect differences in the sensitivity and specificity of the Tg primers and RT–PCR systems used, differences in the sensitivity of the imaging techniques used to detect disease, differences in the sensitivity and specificity of the Tg immunoassays, as well as differences in the TSH status of the patient. It should be noted that specificity problems (false positives) are a recognized limitation of RT–PCR methodology and further studies are needed to determine whether the detectable Tg mRNA levels reported for athyreotic patients without known metastases reflect clinically occult disease, assay artifact, or illegitimate transcription [63,70].

A correlation between Tg mRNA test results and clinical recurrence, especially in patients with positive Tg mRNA and undetectable serum Tg levels, would need to be shown before the Tg mRNA test becomes widely used in clinical practice. Since the Tg mRNA test is more expensive than a serum Tg measurement, it is probable that even if Tg mRNA measurements are shown to be clinically useful that these tests will be reserved for high-risk or TgAb-positive patients in whom serum Tg measurements are diagnostically unreliable.

5.4. *Between-method biases*

As shown in Fig. 6, there can be 3-fold difference in the absolute Tg values reported by different methods despite the use of the international Tg standard CRM-457. These biases preclude the use of different Tg methods for serial monitoring DTC patients [9,71–73]. The degree of bias between methods is far greater than the percentage goal for maximum acceptable bias for Tg testing (16.8%) that is based on well-established concepts [4,74–77]. It was hoped that worldwide CRM-457, standardization would facilitate a better comparison of Tg values in published studies and improve the clinical use of serial Tg monitoring of DTC patients who sometimes have serum Tg measurements determined by different laboratories. Between-method biases that remain despite CRM-457 standardization probably reflect factors such as differences in epitope recognition by the Tg antibody reagents used by different manufacturers, and matrix effects resulting from the use of suboptimal Tg-free standard diluents. Matrix effects are likely to remain a problem because the ideal matrix (Tg-free or TgAb-free human serum) is not available in commercial quantities.

5.5. *Suboptimal sensitivity*

There is a growing recognition that the sensitivity of current Tg methods is suboptimal. The current 'first-generation' Tg methods display less than one order of magnitude (10-fold) difference between the assay functional sensitivity limit (typically ~ 0.1–$1.0 \, \mu g \, L^{-1}$) and the lower reference limit for normal euthyroid volunteers (typically ~ 0.5–$3.0 \, \mu g \, L^{-1}$). Some methods even report undetectable serum Tg values for some normal euthyroid subjects (Fig. 6). Recent data suggest that the clinical utility of serum Tg measurements made during L-T4 therapy would be enhanced, and rhTSH-stimulation testing perhaps rendered unnecessary, if 'third-generation' Tg assays could be developed which had two orders of magnitude more sensitivity (i.e., a functional sensitivity $< 0.01 \, \mu g \, L^{-1}$ for assays with a lower euthyroid reference limit $\sim 1 \, \mu g \, L^{-1}$) [78].

As manufacturers increasingly recognize that more sensitivity will enhance the clinical utility of serum Tg measurements made during L-T4 therapy, it is critical that the same scientific parameters are used to define functional sensitivity and not terms like 'ultrasensitive' and 'highly sensitive' are abandoned as they have been for TSH. The new NACB guidelines provide a specific protocol for determining Tg assay functional sensitivity based on the 20% CV of the between-run precision [4]. The primary difference between the Tg functional sensitivity protocol and that adopted for TSH is that the stipulation serum pools must be free of TgAb and that the test period for precision assessment be longer (6–12 months) in order to reflect the longer clinical interval used for assessing DTC patients in clinical practice [4].

5.6. *Between-run assay precision*

Within-run assay precision for immunoassay methodology is typically better than between-run precision, because measurements made within a single run are not subject to the variability introduced by changes in reagent lots, instrument calibrations, technical changes and a myriad of other poorly defined factors that change over time. Published studies are required to validate their Tg method by providing both the within- and between-run assay precision (% CV) assessed at three Tg levels covering the working range, using the recommended protocol [4]. Within-run precision is the relevant parameter for comparing basal and rhTSH-stimulated Tg specimens drawn 3–5 days apart and measured in the same run [17,36]. In contrast, within-run precision is not relevant to long-term serial monitoring during L-T4 therapy. Most recurrences occur during the first 5 years; however, recurrences can occur decades after thyroidectomy necessitating that patients carrying a diagnosis of DTC receive lifetime monitoring with serum Tg measurements and selected imaging studies [31]. Since typical thyroid neoplasms are slow growing, serial Tg monitoring of low-risk DTC patients is usually performed relatively infrequently (i.e., annually). It follows that the between-run precision across the typical clinical interval used (~12 months) will best describe assay precision in clinical practice. The suggested goal for maximum imprecision of serum Tg measurements for monitoring patients is <5% [4]. It is unlikely that current Tg assays can maintain such good precision over the 12-month clinical interval typically used for monitoring low-risk DTC patients. The new NACB guidelines suggest that laboratories archive specimen left after serum Tg measurement for at least 6 months [4]. Some laboratories choose to archive sera for longer periods. This allows concurrent re-measurement of the past and current specimens in the same run – a maneuver that eliminates the between-run error and improved the clinical sensitivity of the test [4,79].

5.7. *High-dose 'hook' effects*

High-dose 'hook' effects primarily impact IMA measurements [9,80]. Falsely low values caused by hooking are especially problematic for tumor-marker tests like Tg, and it is not unusual to encounter very high values ($>10,000\,\mu g\,L^{-1}$) when patients have advanced metastatic disease [23,40,81]. A hook effect occurs when an excessive amount of antigen overwhelms the binding capacity of the capture antibody. This results in an inappropriately low signal that translates into an inappropriately low or paradoxically normal range result for a patient with an excessively elevated serum Tg concentration ($>1000\,\mu g\,L^{-1}$) [9]. Manufacturers of IMA methods are aware of this problem and attempt to overcome it by a number of approaches which include the adoption of a two-step assay design whereby the specimen is first reacted with the capture antibody before unbound constituents are washed away and the labeled antibody is introduced, followed by a second incubation. Alternatively, a hook can be revealed by looking for lack of parallelism in measurements made of the specimen at two dilutions or other maneuvers [80]. Despite these safeguards, physicians should be aware that a 'hook' can still cause falsely low values for some very high

TgAb-negative specimens. When the reported serum Tg value appears inappropriately low for the clinical status of the patient, the physician should request that the laboratory rerun the specimen at 10- and 100-fold dilutions to check for hooking [9].

6. Summary

The quality of the Tg and TgAb methods selected by a laboratory will impact the clinical management of DTC patients using the tests. Since, no current Tg or TgAb method is 100% reliable, it is important for physicians managing patients with DTC to understand the technical limitations of Tg and TgAb measurements and carefully select an experienced laboratory to perform the tests. The use of quality Tg and TgAb methods for managing DTC patients improves the overall cost-effectiveness of management by minimizing costly imaging procedures. Even the best Tg and TgAb

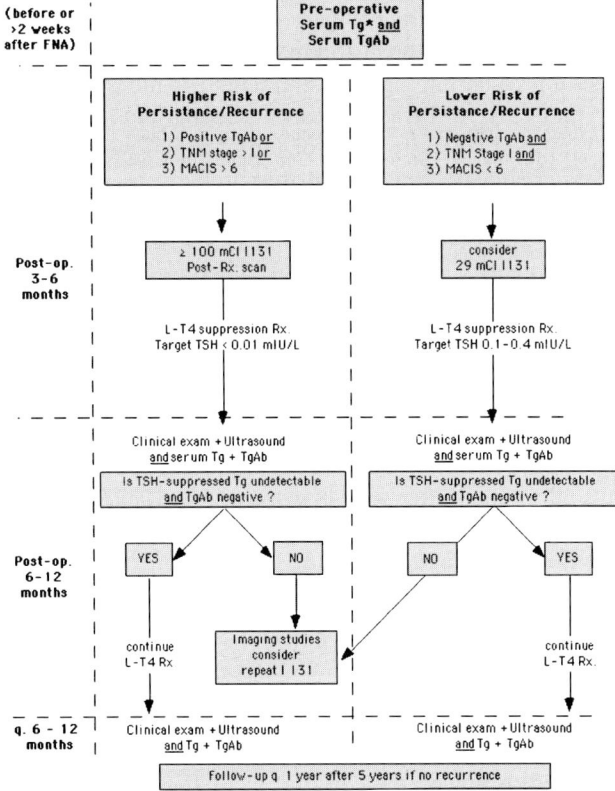

Fig. 9. Algorithm for using serum Tg measurements to monitor patients with differentiated thyroid carcinomas.

test results have to be interpreted relative to the patient-specific factors and the physiological factors that control Tg secretion. Fig. 9 provides an algorithm for using patient-specific factors and serum Tg and TgAb testing during the various stages of managing patients with DTC.

References

[1] C.A. Spencer, Thyroglobulin, in: B.L.A. Utiger (Ed.), The Thyroid, JB Lippincott, Philadelphia, PA, 2000.

[2] C.A. Spencer, C.C. Wang, Thyroglobulin measurement: - Techniques, clinical benefits, and pitfalls, Endocrinol. Metab. Clin. N. Am. 24 (1995) 841–863.

[3] J.I. Torrens, H.B. Burch, Serum thyroglobulin measurement. Utility in clinical practice, Endocrinol. Metab. Clin. N. Am. 30 (2001) 429–467.

[4] L.M. Demers, C.A. Spencer, Laboratory Support for the Diagnosis and Monitoring of Thyroid Disease, NACB, Washington DC, 2002.

[5] F. Bernier-Valentin, Z. Kostrouch, R. Rabilloud, B. Rousset, Analysis of the thyroglobulin internalization process using *in vitro* reconstituted thyroid follicles: evidence for a coated vesicle-dependent endocytic pathway, Endocrinology 129 (1991) 2194–2201.

[6] A.D. Dunn, H.E. Crutchfield, J.T. Dunn, Proteolytic processing of thyroglobulin by extracts of thyroid lysosomes, Endocrinology 128 (1991) 3073–3080.

[7] M.D. Ringel, P.L. Balducci-Silano, J.S. Anderson, C.A. Spencer, J. Silverman, Y.H. Sparling, G.L. Francis, K.D. Burman, L. Wartofsky, P.W. Ladenson, M.A. Levine, R.M. Tuttle, Quantitative reverse transcription-polymerase chain reaction of circulating thyroglobulin messenger ribonucleic acid for monitoring patients with thyroid carcinoma, J. Clin. Endocrinol. Metab. 84 (1998) 4037–4042.

[8] R.P. Biscolla, J.M. Cerutti, R.M. Maciel, Detection of recurrent thyroid cancer by sensitive nested reverse transcription-polymerase chain reaction of thyroglobulin and sodium/iodide symporter messenger ribonucleic acid transcripts in peripheral blood, J. Clin. Endocrinol. Metab. 85 (2000) 3623–3627.

[9] C.A. Spencer, M. Takeuchi, M. Kazarosyan, Current status and performance goals for serum thyroglobulin assays, Clin. Chem. 42 (1996) 164–173.

[10] L. Fugazzola, A. Mihalich, L. Persani, N. Cerutti, M. Reina, M. Bonomi, E. Ponti, D. Mannavola, E. Giammona, G. Vannucchi, A.M. Di Blasio, P. Beck-Peccoz, Highly sensitive serum thyroglobulin and circulating thyroglobulin mRNA evaluations in the management of patients with differentiated thyroid cancer in apparent remission, J. Clin. Endocrinol. Metab. 87 (2002) 3201–3208.

[11] J.H. Cohen, S.H. Ingbar, L.E. Braverman, Thyrotoxicosis due to ingestion of excess thyroid hormone, Endocrine Rev. 10 (1989) 113–124.

[12] N. Knudsen, I. Bulow, T. Jorgensen, H. Perrild, L. Oversen, P. Laurberg, Serum Tg - a sensitive marker of thyroid abnormalities and iodine deficiency in epidemiological studies, J. Clin. Endocrinol. Metab. 86 (2001) 3599–3603.

[13] T. Van den Briel, C.E. West, J.G. Hautvast, T. Vulsma, J.J. de Vijlder, E.A. Ategbo, Serum thyroglobulin and urinary iodine concentration are the most appropriate indicators of iodine status and thyroid function under conditions of increasing iodine supply in schoolchildren in Benin, J. Nutr. 131 (2001) 2701–2706.

[14] B.R. Haugen, E.C. Ridgway, B.A. McLaughlin, M.T. McDermott, Clinical comparison of whole-body radioiodine scan and serum thyroglobulin after stimulation with recombinant human thyrotropin, Thyroid 12 (2002) 37–43.

[15] D.F. Gardner, J. Rothman, R.D. Utiger, Serum thyroglobulin in normal subjects and patients with hyperthyroidism due to Graves' disease: effects of T3, iodide, ^{131}I, and antithyroid drugs, Clin. Endocrinol. 11 (1979) 585–594.

[16] F.W. Yip, T.S. Reeve, A.G. Poole, L. Delbridge, Thyroid nodules in childhood and adolescence, Aust. N. Z. J. Surg. 64 (1994) 676–678.

[17] B.R. Haugen, F. Pacini, C. Reiners, M. Schlumberger, P.W. Ladenson, S.I. Sherman, D.S. Cooper, K.E. Graham, L.E. Braverman, M.C. Skarulis, T.F. Davies, L.J. DeGroot, E.L. Mazzaferri, G.H. Daniels, D.S. Ross, M. Luster, M.H. Samuels, D.V. Becker, H.R. Maxon, R.R. Cavalieri, C.A. Spencer, K. McEllin, B.D. Weintraub, E.C. Ridgway, A comparison of recombinant human thyrotropin and thyroid hormone withdrawal for the detection of thyroid remnant or cancer, J. Clin. Endocrinol. Metab. 84 (1999) 3877–3885.

[18] B. Di Jesu, R. Pereira, E. Consiglio, S. Formisano, J. Satrustegui, I.V. Sandoval, Demonstration of a Ca^{2+} requirement for thyroglobulin dimerization and export to the golgi complex, Eur. J. Biochem. 252 (1998) 583–590.

[19] Z. Muresan, P. Arvan, Enhanced binding to the molecular chaperone BiP slow thyroglobulin export from the endoplasmic reticulum, Mol. Endocrinol. 12 (1998) 458–467.

[20] A. Schneider, K. Ikekubo, K. Kuma, Iodine content of serum thyroglobulin in normal individuals and patients with thyroid tumors, J. Clin. Endocrinol. Metab. 57 (1983) 1251–1256.

[21] R. Schulz, H. Bethauser, L. Stempka, B. Heilig, A. Moll, M. Hufner, Evidence for immunological differences between circulating and tissue-derived thyroglobulin in men, Eur. J. Clin. Invest. 19 (1989) 459–463.

[22] L. Druetta, K. Croizet, H. Bornet, B. Rousset, Analysis of the molecular forms of serum thyroglobulin from patients with Graves' disease, subacute thyroiditis or differentiated thyroid cancer by velocity sedimentation on sucrose gradient and Western blot, Eur. J. Endocrinol. 139 (1998) 498–507.

[23] U.B. Ericsson, L. Tegler, S. Lennquist, S.B. Christensen, E. Stahl, J.I. Thorell, Serum thyroglobulin in differentiated thyroid carcinoma, Acta Chir. Scand. 150 (1984) 367–375.

[24] L. Tegler, U.B. Ericsson, J. Gillquist, R. Lindvall, Basal and thyrotropin-stimulated secretion rates of thyroglobulin from the human thyroid gland during surgery, Thyroid 3 (1993) 213–217.

[25] M. Bayraktar, M. Ergin, A. Boyacioglu, S. Demir, A preliminary report of thyroglobulin release after fine needle aspiration biopsy of thyroid nodules, J. Int. Med. Res. 18 (1990) 253–255.

[26] U. Feldt-Rasmussen, P.H. Petersen, J. Date, C.M. Madsen, Serum thyroglobulin in patients undergoing subtotal thyroidectomy for toxic and nontoxic goiter, J. Endocrinol. Invest. 5 (1982) 161–164.

[27] M. Izumi, I. Kubo, M. Taura, S. Yamashita, I. Morimoto, S. Ohtakara, S. Okamoto, L.F. Kumagai, S. Nagataki, Kinetic study of immunoreactive human thyroglobulin, J. Clin. Endocrinol. Metab. 62 (1986) 410–412.

[28] M. Hocevar, M. Auersperg, L. Stanovnik, The dynamics of serum thyroglobulin elimination from the body after thyroid surgery, Eur. J. Surg. Oncol. 23 (1997) 208–210.

[29] G. Ronga, M. Filesi, G. Ventroni, A.R. Vestri, A. Signore, Value of the first serum thyroglobulin level after thyroidiectomy for the diagnosis of metastases from differentiated thyroid carcinoma, Eur. J. Nucl. Med. 26 (1999) 1448–1452.

[30] N. Lima, E. Cavaliere, E. Tomimori, M. Knobel, G. Medeieros-Neto, Prognostic value of serial serum thyroglobulin determinations after total thyroidectomy for differentiated thyroid cancer, J. Endocrinol. Invest. 25 (2002) 110–115.

[31] E.L. Mazzaferri, S.M. Jiang, Long-term impact of initial surgical and medical therapy on papillary and follicular thyroid cancer, Am. J. Med. 97 (1994) 418–428.

[32] S. Fatemi, J. Nicoloff, J. LoPresti, R. Guttler, C. Spencer, Use of 2 year post-Tx serum Thyroglobulin (Tg) to assess risk of recurrent/persistent (R/P) papillary thyroid cancer (PTC), Abstract, European Thyroid Association meeting, 2001.

[33] F. Pacini, L. Agate, R. Elisei, M. Capezzone, C. Ceccarelli, F. Lippi, E. Molinaro, A. Pinchera, Outcome of differentiated thyroid cancer with detectable serum Tg and negative diagnostic ^{131}I whole body scan; Comparison of patients treated with high ^{131}I activities versus untreated patients, J. Clin. Endocrinol. Metab. 86 (2001) 4092–4097.

[34] M. Ozata, S. Suzuki, T. Miyamoto, R.T. Liu, F. Fierro-Renoy, L.J. DeGroot, Serum thyroglobulin in the follow-up of patients with treated differentiated thyroid cancer, J. Clin. Endocrinol. Metab. 79 (1994) 98–105.

[35] C.A. Spencer, C. Wang, S. Fatemi, R.B. Guttler, M. Takeuchi, M. Kazarosyan, Serum Thyroglobulin Autoantibodies: Prevalence, influence on serum thyroglobulin measurement and prognostic

significance in patients with differentiated thyroid carcinoma, J. Clin. Endocrinol. Metab. 83 (1998) 1121–1127.

[36] C.A. Spencer, J.S. LoPresti, S. Fatemi, J.T. Nicoloff, Detection of residual and recurrent differentiated thyroid carcinoma by serum thyroglobulin measurement, Thyroid 9 (1999) 435–441.

[37] J. Weeke, H.J. Gundersen, Circadian and 30 minute variations in serum TSH and thyroid hormones in normal subjects, Acta Endocrinol. 89 (1978) 659–672.

[38] M. Schlumberger, M. Ricard, F. Pacini, Clinical use of recombinant human TSH in thyroid cancer patients, Eur. J. Endocrinol. 143 (2000) 557–563.

[39] F. Pacini, E. Molinaro, F. Lippi, M.G. Castagna, L. Agate, C. Ceccarelli, D. Taddei, R. Elisei, M. Capezzone, A. Pinchera, Prediction of disease status by recombinant human TSH-stimulated serum Tg in the postsurgical follow-up of differentiated thyroid carcinoma, J. Clin. Endocrinol. Metab. 86 (2001) 5686–5690.

[40] M. Schlumberger, P. Fragu, J. Lumbroso, C. Parmentier, M. Tubiana, Circulating thyrotropin and thyroid hormones in patients with metastases of differentiated thyroid carcinoma: relationship to serum thyrotropin levels, J. Clin. Endocrinol. Metab. 51 (1980) 513–519.

[41] A.F. Cailleux, E. Baudin, J.P. Travagli, M. Ricard, M. Schlumberger, Is diagnostic iodine-131 scanning useful after total thyroid ablation for differentiated thyroid cancer?, J. Clin. Endocrinol. Metab. 85 (2000) 175–178.

[42] R.J. Robbins, R.M. Tuttle, R.N. Sharaf, S.M. Larson, H.K. Robbins, R.A. Ghossein, A. Smith, W.D. Drucker, Preparation by recombinant human thyrotropin or thyroid hormone withdrawal are comparable for the detection of residual differentiated thyroid carcinoma, J. Clin. Endocrinol. Metab. 86 (2001) 619–625.

[43] G. Vitale, G.A. Lupoli, A. Ciccarelli, F. Fonderico, M. Klain, G. Squame, M. Salvatore, G. Lupoli, The use of recombinant human TSH in the follow-up of differentiated thyroid cancer: experience from a large patient cohort in a single centre, Clin. Endocrinol. 56 (2002) 247–252.

[44] R.J. Robbins, J.T. Chon, M. Fleisher, S.M. Larson, R.M. Tuttle, Is the serum thyroglobulin response to recombinant human thyrotropin sufficient, by itself, to monitor for residual thyroid carcinoma?, J. Clin. Endocrinol. Metab. 87 (2002) 3242–3247.

[45] E.L. Mazzaferri, R.T. Kloos, Is diagnostic iodine-131 scanning with recombinant human TSH useful in the follow-up of differentiated thyroid cancer after thyroid ablation?, J. Clin. Endocrinol. Metab. 87 (2002) 1490–1498.

[46] F. Pacini, M. Capezzone, R. Elisei, C. Ceccarelli, D. Taddei, A. Pinchera, Diagnostic 131-iodine whole-body scan may be avoided in thyroid cancer patients who have undetectable stimulated serum Tg levels after initial treatment, J. Clin. Endocrinol. Metab. 87 (2002) 1499–1501.

[47] S. Grant, B. Luttrell, T. Reeve, J. Wiseman, E. Wilmshurst, J. Stiel, D. Donohoe, R. Cooper, M. Bridgman, Thyroglobulin may be undetectable in the serum of patients with metastatic disease secondary to differentiated thyroid carcinoma, Cancer 54 (1984) 1625–1628.

[48] A. Kumar, D.H. Shah, U. Shrihari, S.R. Dandekar, U. Vijayan, S.M. Sharma, Significance of antithyroglobulin autoantibodies in differentiated thyroid carcinoma, Thyroid 4 (1994) 199–202.

[49] S. Mariotti, G. Barbesino, P. Caturegli, M. Marino, L. Manetti, F. Pacini, R. Centoni, A. Pinchera, Assay of thyroglobulin in serum with thyroglobulin autoantibodies: an unobtainable goal?, J. Clin. Endocrinol. Metab. 80 (1995) 468–472.

[50] C. Massart, D. Maugendre, Importance of the detection method for thyroglobulin antibodies for the validity of thyroglobulin measurements in sera from patients with Graves' disease, Clin. Chem. 48 (2002) 102–107.

[51] E.G. Black, R. Hoffenberg, Should one measure serum thyroglobulin in the presence of anti-thyroglobulin antibodies?, Clin. Endocrinol. 19 (1983) 597–601.

[52] D. Rubello, D. Casara, M.E. Girelli, M. Piccolo, B. Busnardo, Clinical meaning of circulating antithyroglobulin antibodies in differentiated thyroid cancer: a prospective study, J. Nucl. Med. 33 (1992) 1478–1480.

[53] F. Pacini, S. Mariotti, N. Formica, R. Elisei, Thyroid autoantibodies in thyroid cancer: Incidence and relationship with tumor outcome, Acta Endocrinol. 119 (1988) 373–380.

[54] P. Hjiyiannakis, J. Mundy, C. Harmer, Thyroglobulin antibodies in differentiated thyroid cancer, Clin. Oncol. 11 (1999) 240–244.

[55] C.A. Spencer, B.W. Platler, J.T. Nicoloff, The effect of 125-I thyroglobulin tracer heterogeneity on serum Tg RIA measurement, Clin. Chem. Acta 153 (1985) 105–115.

[56] L.J. Kricka, Human anti-animal antibody interference in immunological assays, Clin. Chem. 45 (1999) 942–956.

[57] C.A. Spencer, Recoveries cannot be used to authenticate thyroglobulin (Tg) measurements when sera contain Tg autoantibodies, Clin. Chem. 42 (1996) 661–663.

[58] A.B. Schneider, K. Ikekubo, Measurement of thyroglobulin in the circulation: clinical and technical considerations, Ann. Clin. Lab. Sci. 9 (1979) 230–235.

[59] C.A. Spencer, B. Platler, R.B. Guttler, J.T. Nicoloff, Heterogeneity of 125-I labelled thyroglobulin preparations, Clin. Chim. Acta 151 (1985) 121–132.

[60] U. Feldt-Rasmussen, A.K. Rasmussen, Serum thyroglobulin (Tg) in presence of thyroglobulin autoantibodies (TgAb). Clinical and methodological relevance of the interaction between Tg and TgAb *in vitro* and *in vivo*, J. Endocrinol. Invest. 8 (1985) 571–576.

[61] B. Smith, P. Selby, J. Southgate, K. Pittman, C. Bradley, G.E. Blair, Detection of melanoma cells in peripheral blood by means of reverse transcriptase and polymerase chain reaction, Lancet 338 (1991) 1227–1229.

[62] M. Luppi, M. Morselli, E. Bandieri, M. Federico, R. Marasca, P. Barozzi, M.G. Ferrari, M. Savarino, A. Frassoldati, G. Torelli, Sensitive detection of circulating breast cancer cells by reverse-transcriptase polymerase chain reaction of maspin gene, Ann. Oncol. 7 (1996) 619–624.

[63] R.A. Ghossein, S. Bhattacharya, Molecular detection and characterisation of circulating tumour cells and micrometastases in solid tumours, Eur. J. Cancer 36 (2000) 1681–1694.

[64] B.A. Ditkoff, M.R. Marvin, S. Yemul, Y.J. Shi, J. Chabot, C. Feind, P.L. Lo Gerfo, Detection of circulating thyroid cells in peripheral blood, Surgery 120 (1996) 959–965.

[65] M.J. Bugalho, R.S. Domingues, A.C. Pinto, A. Garrao, A.L. Catarino, T. Ferreira, E. Limbert, L. Sobrinho, Detection of thyroglobulin mRNA transcripts in peripheral blood of individuals with and without thyroid glands: evidence for thyroglobulin expression by blood cells, Eur. J. Endocrinol. 145 (2001) 409–413.

[66] R. Bellantone, C.P. Lombardi, M. Bossola, A. Ferrante, P. Princi, M. Boscherini, L. Maussier, M. Salvatori, V. Rufini, F. Reale, L. Romano, G. Tallini, G. Zelano, A. Pontecorvi, Validity of thyroglobulin mRNA assay in peripheral blood of postoperative thyroid carcinoma patients in predicting tumor recurrence varies according to the histologic type: results of a prospective study, Cancer 92 (2001) 2273–2279.

[67] J. Bojunga, S. Roddiger, M. Stanisch, K. Kusterer, R. Kurek, H. Renneberg, S. Adams, E. Lindhorst, K.H. Usadel, P.M. Schumm-Draeger, Molecular detection of thyroglobulin mRNA transcripts in peripheral blood of patients with thyroid disease by RT-PCR, Br. J. Cancer 82 (2000) 1650–1655.

[68] T. Takano, A. Miyauchi, H. Yoshida, Y. Hasegawa, K. Kuma, N. Amino, Quantitative measurement of thyroglobulin mRNA in peripheral blood of patients after total thyroidectomy, Br. J. Cancer 85 (2001) 102–106.

[69] F. Arturi, D. Russo, D. Giuffrida, et al., Early diagnosis by genetic analysis of differentiated thyroid cancer metastases in small lymph nodes, J. Clin. Endocrinol. Metab. 82 (1997) 1638–1641.

[70] J. Chelly, J.P. Concordet, J.C. Kaplan, A. Kahn, Illegitimate transcription: transcription of any gene in any cell type, Proc. Natl. Acad. Sci. USA 86 (1989) 2617–2621.

[71] U. Feldt-Rasmussen, M. Schlumberger, European interlaboratory comparison of serum thyroglobulin measurement, J. Endocrinol. Invest. 11 (1988) 175–181.

[72] U. Feldt-Rasmussen, C. Profilis, E. Colinet, E. Black, H. Bornet, P. Bourdoux, P. Carayon, U.B. Ericsson, D.A. Koutras, L. Lamas de Leon, P. DeNayer, F. Pacini, G. Palumbo, A. Santos, M. Schlumberger, C. Seidel, A.J. Van Herle, J.J.M. DeVijlder, Human thyroglobulin reference material (CRM 457) 2nd part: Physicochemical characterization and certification, Ann. Biol. Clin. 54 (1996) 343–348.

[73] U. Feldt-Rasmussen, Analytical and clinical performance goals for testing autoantibodies to thyroperoxidase, thyroglobulin and thyrotropin receptor, Clin. Chem. 42 (1996) 160–163.

[74] U. Feldt-Rasmussen, P.H. Petersen, O. Blaabjerg, M. Horder, Long-term variability in serum thyroglobulin and thyroid related hormones in healthy subjects, Acta Endocrinol. (Copenh) 95 (1980) 328–334.

[75] C.G. Fraser, Biological Variation: From Principles to Practice, AACC Press, Washington DC, 2001.

[76] C.G. Fraser, P.H. Petersen, Desirable standards for laboratory tests if they are to fulfill medical needs, Clin. Chem. 39 (1993) 1453–1455.

[77] E.K. Harris, Statistical principles underlying analytic goal-setting in clinical chemistry, Am. J. Clin. Pathol. 72 (1979) 374–382.

[78] C. Spencer, S. Fatemi, R.B. Guttler, J. LoPresti, P. Singer, J.T. Nicoloff, New insight into rhTSH-stimulated serum Tg testing as revealed by a recently developed second generation Tg assay, Abstract, American Thyroid Association, 2002.

[79] R.H. Cobin, H. Gharib, D.A. Bergman, O.H. Clark, D.S. Cooper, G.H. Daniels, R.A. Dickey, D.S. Duick, J.R. Garber, I.D. Hay, J.S. Kukora, H.M. Lando, A.B. Schorr, M.A. Zeiger, AACE/AAES Medical/Surgical Guidelines for Clinical Practice: Management of Thyroid Carcinoma, Endocrine Pract. 7 (2001) 203–220.

[80] T.G. Cole, D. Johnson, B.J. Eveland, M.H. Nahm, Cost-effective method for detection of 'hook effect' in tumor marker immunometric assays, Clin. Chem. 39 (1993) 695–696.

[81] M.J. Schlumberger, Papillary and Follicular Thyroid Carcinoma, NEJM 338 (1998) 297–306.

Chapter 6

The role of fluoro-deoxy glucose (FDG) positron emission tomography (PET) in the management of differentiated thyroid cancer

Richard J. Robbins, Chee-Yeung Chan, R. Michael Tuttle, Steven M. Larson

Endocrine and Nuclear Medicine Services, Departments of Medicine and Radiology, Memorial Sloan-Kettering Cancer Center, New York, NY 10021, USA

1. History of FDG-PET and thyroid cancer

Warburg [1] was one of the first to clearly show increased glucose consumption by malignant tumors. This was subsequently discovered to be due to the elevated membrane glucose transport [2], and increased intracellular glycolytic pathway activity [3]. The quantitative analysis of this phenomenon was established by Sokoloff et al. [4] using deoxyglucose and autoradiography. This was followed by the development of ^{18}F-fluoro-deoxy glucose (FDG) which could be regionally quantitated using positron emission tomography [5]. The use of FDG-PET in oncology has undergone an enormous expansion with thousands of papers being published over the past 10 years.

The first report on FDG localization of metastatic thyroid cancer was that of Joensuu and Ahonen in 1987 [6]. They made a number of seminal observations despite the fact that their report contained only three patients. First, they observed that some of the FDG-avid lesions also concentrated radioactive iodine (RAI), while others did not. Next, they observed that some of the RAI avid lesions did not concentrate FDG. This heterogeneity of tracer avidity could actually be demonstrated within single patients, suggesting that each metastatic lesion might have its own unique metabolic pattern. They also suggested that lesions that accumulated FDG were more aggressive in their growth pattern than those that only concentrated RAI. Feine et al. [7] reported the first series of 24 patients with differentiated thyroid carcinoma (DTC) and confirmed the observations of Joensuu and Ahonen that a reciprocal pattern of FDG and RAI avidity often occurred. In fact, they observed that every DTC distant metastatic lesion that did not take up RAI, did concentrate sufficient FDG to be visualized on a PET scan.

ADVANCES IN MOLECULAR AND CELLULAR ENDOCRINOLOGY
VOLUME 4   ISSN 1569-2566/DOI 10.1016/S1569-2566(04)04006-2

Sisson et al. [8] were the first to note that standard uptake values (SUV) readings in metastatic lesions were higher when the patient had an elevated serum TSH. The authors attributed this to the known induction of GLUT expression in thyroid cells by TSH [9].

2. Use of FDG-PET to detect occult metastases

The reports by Feine et al. [7,10] and Grünwald et al. [11] confirmed the initial impression of Joensuu and Ahonen, 8 years earlier, there was a reciprocal or 'flip–flop' relationship between FDG and radioiodine avidity. Well-differentiated thyroid cancers tended to concentrate RAI but not FDG while poorly differentiated, or anaplastic tumors, were highly FDG-avid but frequently did not concentrate RAI. Some disagreement has arisen regarding the value of FDG scanning for detecting cervical lymphadenopathy. Scott et al. [12] were the first to report FDG uptake by metastatic cervical nodes. Grünwald et al. [11] reported on 10 cases of FDG uptake by cervical nodes (one false-positive due to sarcoidosis). Our own experience has been that there is a high false-negative rate in small cervical nodes that harbor well-differentiated papillary thyroid carcinoma.

Dietlein et al. [13] found that FDG scanning was slightly less sensitive than RAI diagnostic scanning for the detection of residual thyroid carcinoma (50 vs. 61%), but when combined it had an 86% sensitivity to detect residual disease. Importantly, they also found in patients who had an elevated serum Thyroglobin (Tg) and a negative RAI scan, the FDG scan was 82% sensitive at localizing the occult disease. These findings were confirmed by Grünwald et al. [14], Altenvoerde et al. [15], Huang et al. [16], Jadvar et al. [17], Chung et al. [18], and Alnafisi et al. [19]. This collective experience has established the FDG scan as the test of choice when evaluating a thyroid cancer survivor, who has an elevated serum Tg but a negative diagnostic whole body RAI scan (see Figs. 1 and 2). Wang et al. [20] found that in the setting of a negative RAI scan and an elevated Tg, a FDG scan had a 93% positive predictive value and conversely in patients with a negative RAI scan and a low Tg, the FDG scan had a 93% negative predictive value (Table 1). This role for FDG-PET scanning in the evaluation of RAI-negative patients with suspected residual disease continues to solidify [21–23]. However, even the combination of a diagnostic whole body scan and an FDG scan is only 85–90% sensitive at detecting residual DTC. The majority of the cases that are missed are the patients with small volume cervical lymph nodes that are often detected by high-resolution neck ultrasonography (Fig. 3).

Hürthle cell thyroid carcinoma is a unique entity, which tends to be a more aggressive cancer if the initial lesion demonstrates extrathyroidal extension or size greater than 4 cm [24]. In our experience, metastases from Hürthle cell carcinoma exhibit the highest SUV readings of any type of thyroid cancer, except anaplastic carcinoma. This may be related to the extremely high concentration of mitochondria that are present in Hürthle cells. The ability of FDG scanning to detect recurrent Hürthle cell carcinoma is extremely high with a sensitivity of 92% and a negative predictive value of 80% [25].

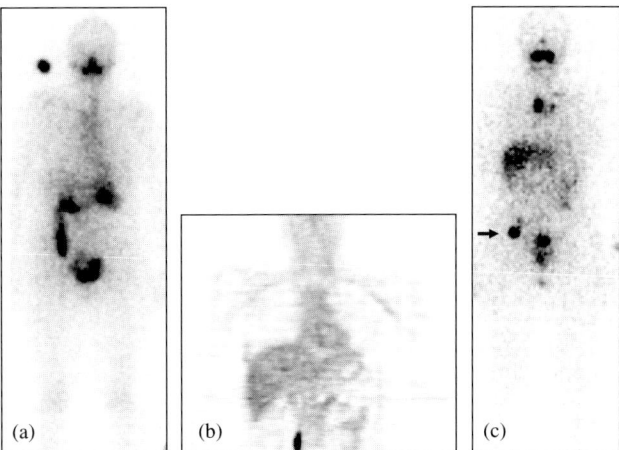

Fig. 1. A 42-year-old female with papillary thyroid cancer with persistently elevated Tg after surgery and ^{131}I ablation. DxWBS (a) and FDG-PET (b) were negative. She was given 230 mCi of [131]I. The RxWBS (c) showed focal uptake in the mediastinum and right ilium (arrow).

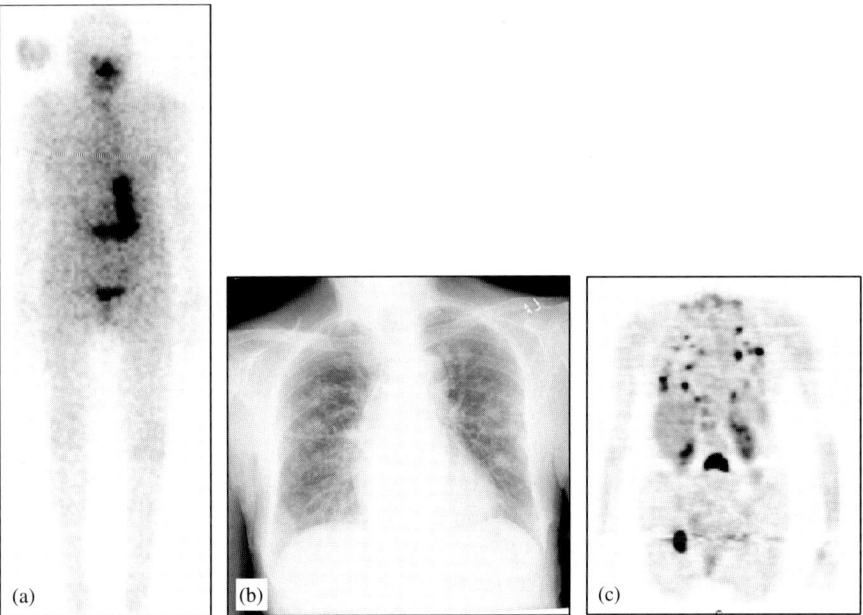

Fig. 2. A 77-year-old female with papillary thyroid cancer metastatic to lung and bone. Following total thyroidectomy and two ^{131}I therapies, her DxWBS (a) became negative. Her Tg was never elevated. The chest X-ray (b) and [18]FDG-PET (c) showed multiple abnormalities. On review of her pathology, there was an anaplastic component found in her original specimen.

Table 1
FDG-PET results in patients who have negative diagnostic RAI scans

	High Tg[a]			Low Tg		
	Positive[b]	Negative[b]		Positive[b]	Negative[b]	
PET positive	12	1	12/13(92%)[c]	2	3	2/5(40%)[c]
PET negative	5	0	0/5(0%)[d]	1	13	13/14(93%)[d]
	12/17(71%)[e]	0/1(0%)[f]		2/3(67%)[e]	13/16(81%)[e]	

From Wang et al. [20], with permission.
[a]Tg was considered 'High' if it was above 2 ng/ml when the TSH was suppressed or above 5 ng/ml if the TSH was elevated.
[b]Disease status.
[c]Positive predictive value.
[d]Negative predictive value.
[e]Sensitivity.
[f]Specificity.

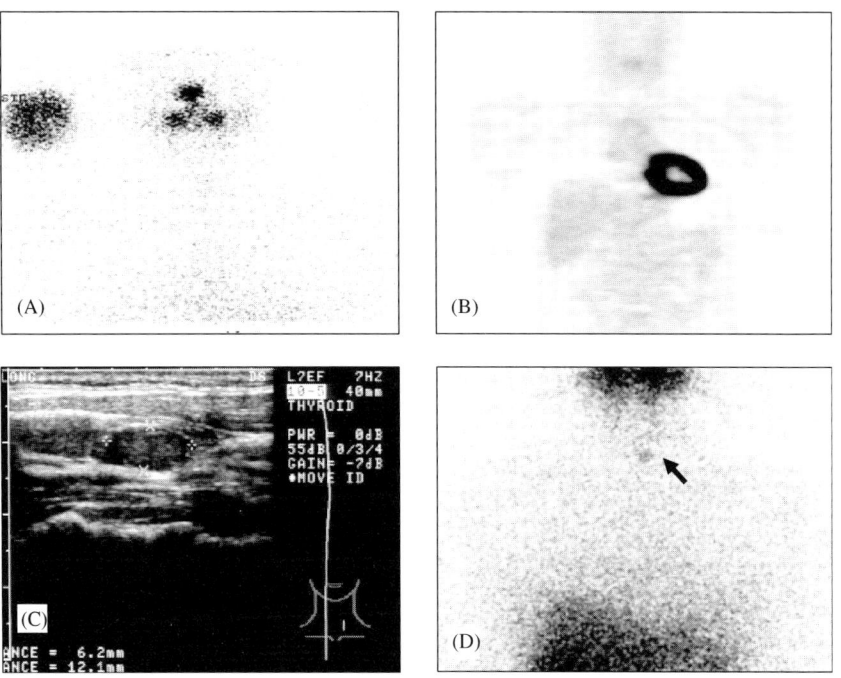

Fig. 3. A 45-year-female with papillary thyroid cancer. Following total thyroidectomy and ablation, her Tg was low and both DxWBS (A) and FDG-PET (B) were negative. Neck ultrasound was performed because of the suspicion of recurrence in the setting of positive TgAb. Three cervical lymph nodes were seen in the left neck (C) and biopsy showed thyroid cancer. She was given ^{131}I therapy with dose of 200 mCi and RxWBS demonstrated focal uptake in left lower neck (D) (arrow).

3. FDG-PET evaluation of thyroid nodules and incidentalomas

Adler and Bloom [26] were the first to study thyroid nodules with PET scanning. They evaluated nine individuals and found increased FDG uptake in seven. Pathology showed that only three of the seven were malignant. All the malignant lesions had higher standard uptake ratios (SUV) than the benign ones. Importantly, they were unable to distinguish the malignant nodules based on the visual pattern of uptake. A larger series of 19 patients, who all had surgical resection was reported by Adler and Bloom [27]. Twelve of nineteen patients in this series had solitary thyroid nodules while the remaining had multinodular goiters. The four malignant nodules were identified from the subset with solitary nodules (three papillary thyroid cancers and one follicular thyroid cancer). Again, Adler and Bloom were able to distinguish the malignant nodules by their higher SUVs without any overlap with the benign entities. However, in two patients sub-centimeter malignancies were identified on pathology that did not take up excess FDG.

Uematsu et al. [28] also evaluated preoperative FDG-PET scans in 11 individuals with nodular thyroid disease with a combination of static and dynamic PET over a period of 60 min. Four of the 11 patients had papillary thyroid cancer while five had benign follicular adenomas, one had a multinodular goiter, and one had thyroiditis without a stable nodule. The malignant lesions showed a pattern of increasing FDG uptake over 60 min, whereas all of the benign nodules showed gradual decrease of uptake over time. The SUV of the patient with thyroiditis was in the 'malignant' range.

FDG-PET is increasingly becoming accepted as a useful imaging tool in oncology. Recent studies suggest that thyroid cancers which concentrate FDG are more aggressive and are less likely to concentrate radioiodine. A number of reports have appeared describing the unexpected uptake of FDG by the thyroid, the 'thyroid incidentaloma'. The largest study to date, published by Cohen et al. [29] reviewed 4525 PET scans performed on cancer patients. Of 102 (2.3%), these scans revealed unexpected thyroid uptake and 71 exhibited focal uptake compared to 31 with diffuse patterns. Of the 102 individuals with thyroid uptake, 15 underwent biopsies. Seven (44%) had thyroid cancer, six (40%) had nodular hyperplasia, one had thyroiditis, and one had cells with atypia of undetermined significance. Of the patients with thyroid cancer, two had Hürthle cell variants, one had poorly differentiated thyroid cancer, one had poorly differentiated papillary thyroid cancer, and the remainder had papillary thyroid cancer. Although the average SUV for the malignant lesions were higher than the benign ones ($p = 0.04$) there was some overlap.

Van den Bruel et al. [30] evaluated eight patients who underwent FDG-PET scanning for various reasons and had thyroid incidentalomas. Of the eight, seven underwent thyroidectomy. Five had thyroid cancer, (three papillary and two medullary carcinomas), while the remainder were follicular adenomas. Of note, seven of the eight scans showed focal uptake in contrast to a diffuse pattern in a patient with a follicular adenoma and Hashimoto's thyroiditis.

Davis et al. [31] presented five cases of patients with no palpable thyroid disease, who had unexpected FDG thyroid uptake that was associated with occult carcinoma. The exact frequency of malignancy in this setting is still undefined, however, these authors echo the sentiment in the other publications by stating that any FDG thyroid 'incidentaloma' should be thoroughly evaluated with the knowledge that many herald occult malignancies.

4. Does the TSH level affect FDG-PET outcome?

Sisson [8] was the first to observe that the uptake of FDG was apparently higher in thyroid cancer metastases when the TSH level was elevated. Wang et al. [20] subsequently confirmed that an elevated TSH often led to finding more metastatic lesions in the same patient compared with a suppressed TSH. However, in their series, the new sites detected in the high TSH state did not reveal any new lesions that changed the clinical decision making. van Tol et al. [32] found that FDG scans revealed more lesions in eight patients who had scans done both on thyroid hormone suppression and subsequently, when hypothyroid. Moog et al. [33] found that the SUV of individual metastatic thyroid cancer lesions was significantly increased in the same patients after they were rendered hypothyroid compared to when they were on thyroxine with suppressed TSH. Petrich et al. [34] used recombinant human TSH (rhTSH) to elevate the circulating TSH level while the patients were euthyroid. Compared to the same patients when their TSH levels were suppressed, more patients were found to have metastatic lesions (19 compared to 9) and the total number of lesions discovered was 82, compared to 45 without rhTSH stimulation.

5. Does FDG-PET provide information about the biology of the tumor?

It is well established that metastases from thyroid carcinoma which do not concentrate radioiodine are more clinically aggressive [35,36]. If FDG scans can detect thyroid cancer metastases which do not concentrate radioiodine, one would hypothesize that the patients who harbored such lesions would have a less favorable prognosis. Wang et al. [37] directly tested this proposal by retrospectively evaluating survival in thyroid cancer survivors, who were being evaluated according to standard of care, with the addition of an FDG scan during the evaluation. They reported from a cohort of 125 patients that survival correlated with (1) the presence of distant metastases; (2) age over 45; (3) FDG positivity; (4) maximum SUV value; and, (5) the total volume of FDG disease, in univariate analysis. Survival was not affected by gender, histology, tumor grade, or radioiodine avidity. Multivariate analyses indicated that the FDG volume was the single strongest predictor of survival. Only 20% of individuals with a total tumor volume of over 125 ml survived for 3 years. Only 50% of those whose maximum SUV was greater than 10 survived at the 3 year mark (Fig. 4). It is possible that the FDG scanning could be used to re-define prognosis for thyroid cancer patients once distant metastases are discovered.

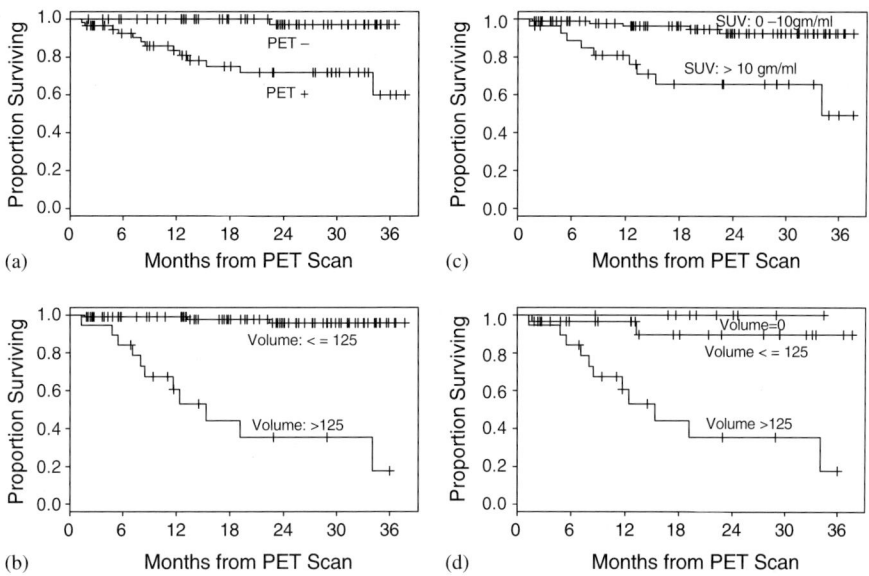

Fig. 4. Kaplan-Meier survival curves in thyroid cancer patients. (a) overall PET outcome; (b) aggregate tumor volume above or below 125 ml; (c) maximum standard uptake value above or below 10 gm/ml; (d) survival in only patients who had distant metastases. Volume = 0 implies a negative PET scan.

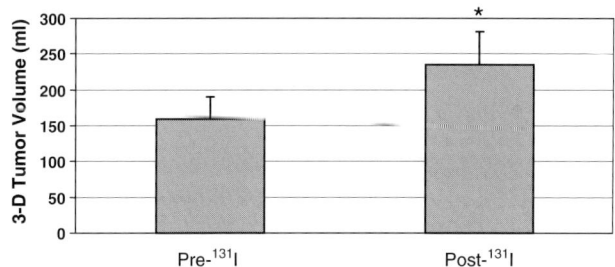

Fig. 5. Effect of ^{131}I on mean FDG volume.

6. Sensitivity of FDG-PET lesions to radioactive iodine therapy

Recent evidence clearly suggests a positive correlation between the FDG-avidity of a metastatic lesion and the level of dedifferentiation. There is ample evidence from the 'flip–flop' pattern that the less well-differentiated lesions do not concentrate radio-iodine very effectively. How then are clinicians to approach the therapy of RAI negative, FDG-positive lesion? A recent report from our unit examined the value of using very high dose ^{131}I therapy for such lesions [38]. We compared the 1 year outcome of a group of patients who had FDG-avid distant metastases with another group that had FDG-negative distant metastases. The FDG-positive group was administered a mean activity of 429 mCi of ^{131}I compared to 246 mCi for the FDG-negative group. Ten months later, on average, the FDG lesions had grown (Fig. 5), the maximum SUV had risen, and the serum Tg had increased by 32%. In the FDG-negative group the serum Tg fell to 38% of the baseline. We concluded that even high dose ^{131}I therapy was quite ineffective in treating FDG-positive metastatic lesions. To date, the only complete destruction of such lesions has been accomplished with surgical removal or external beam radiotherapy.

7. Summary

Despite the relatively good overall prognosis, approximately 1400 patients are expected to die of thyroid cancer in the United States alone in 2003 [39]. More than 70% of the deaths occur in individuals whose initial histology was well-differentiated thyroid carcinoma. The current prognostic scoring systems (e.g. MACIS, TNM, and AGES), which utilize clinical and pathological information obtained at the time of initial diagnosis, have served us well and have stood the test of time. The major limitation is their inability to predict the outcome of patients when, years later, they are discovered to harbor metastases. This is particularly important as it is well known that there is a highly variable trajectory of disease in such patients. Some will die within a year, where as others can survive for more than 30 years with stable metastases.

The recent use of FDG-PET scanning for evaluating patients with DTC has added a new dimension to our understanding of this protean disease. It appears that metastatic lesions that contain predominantly well-differentiated clones have functional NIS and transport RAI. The less well-differentiated clones cannot effectively trap iodine but appear to have much higher metabolic activity and have high FDG-avidity. This characteristic enables us to detect small deposits of the more metabolically active disease when the RAI scans are negative. Furthermore, it now appears, as expected, that the more metabolically active disease is associated with a poor prognosis. Preliminary reports suggest that the volume of FDG disease or the maximum SUV may be able to predict disease trajectory. It is conceivable that the FDG scan results may enable us to achieve real-time prognosis in patients after they are found to harbor residual or recurrent metastatic thyroid carcinoma.

However, FDG scanning is not perfect. It is expensive; it has poor specificity due to the high glycolytic rate of infectious or inflammatory processes; and, it has poor sensitivity at detecting well-differentiated clones of thyroid cancer cells, such as those commonly seen in cervical lymph nodes. The recent development of hybrid scanners that merge PET technology with computed tomography (PET/CT) or with magnetic resonance (PET/MRI) may reveal even more insights into the biology of thyroid cancer metastases, as we further integrate metabolism with detailed anatomy.

References

[1] O. Warburg, F. Wind, E. Neglers, On the metabolism of tumors in the body, in: O. Warburg (Ed.), Metabolism of Tumors, Constable, London, 1930, pp. 254–270.

[2] M. Hatanaka, Transport of sugars in tumor cell membranes, Biochim. Biophys. Acta 355 (1974) 77–104.

[3] G. Weber, Enzymology of cancer cells (second of two parts), N. Engl. J. Med. 296 (1977) 541–551.

[4] L. Sokoloff, M. Reivich, C. Kennedy, M.H. Des Rosiers, C.S. Patlak, K.D. Pettigrew, O. Sakurada, M. Shinohara, The [11C]deoxyglucose method for the measurement of local cerebral glucose utilization: theory, procedure, and normal values in the conscious and anesthetized albino rat, J. Neurochem. 28 (1977) 897–916.

[5] M. Reivich, A. Alavi, A. Wolf, J. Fowler, J. Russell, C. Arnett, R.R. MacGregor, C.Y. Shiue, H. Atkins, A. Anand, et al., Glucose metabolic rate kinetic model parameter determination in humans: the lumped constants and rate constants for [18F]fluorodeoxyglucose and [11C]deoxyglucose, J. Cereb. Blood Flow Metab. 5 (1985) 179–192.

[6] H. Joensuu, A. Ahonen, Imaging of metastases of thyroid carcinoma with fluorine-18 fluorodeoxyglucose, J. Nucl. Med. 28 (1987) 910–914.

[7] U. Feine, R. Lietzenmayer, J.P. Hanke, H. Wohrle, W. Muller-Schauenburg, [18FDG whole-body PET in differentiated thyroid carcinoma. Flipflop in uptake patterns of 18FDG and 131I], Nuklearmedizin 34 (1995) 127–134.

[8] J.C. Sisson, R.J. Ackermann, M.A. Meyer, R.L. Wahl, Uptake of 18-fluoro-2-deoxy-D-glucose by thyroid cancer: implications for diagnosis and therapy, J. Clin. Endocrinol. Metab. 77 (1993) 1090–1094.

[9] Y. Hosaka, M. Tawata, A. Kurihara, M. Ohtaka, T. Endo, T. Onaya, The regulation of two distinct glucose transporter (GLUT1 and GLUT4) gene expressions in cultured rat thyroid cells by thyrotropin, Endocrinology 131 (1992) 159–165.

[10] U. Feine, R. Lietzenmayer, J.P. Hanke, J. Held, H. Wohrle, W. Muller-Schauenburg, Fluorine-18-FDG and iodine-131-iodide uptake in thyroid cancer, J. Nucl. Med. 37 (1996) 1468–1472.

[11] F. Grünwald, A. Schomburg, H. Bender, E. Klemm, C. Menzel, T. Bultmann, H. Palmedo, J. Ruhlmann, B. Kozak, H.J. Biersack, Fluorine-18 fluorodeoxyglucose positron emission tomography in the follow-up of differentiated thyroid cancer, Eur. J. Nucl. Med. 23 (1996) 312–319.

[12] G.C. Scott, D.A. Meier, C.Z. Dickinson, Cervical lymph node metastasis of thyroid papillary carcinoma imaged with fluorine-18-FDG, technetium-99m-pertechnetate and iodine-131-sodium iodide, J. Nucl. Med. 36 (1995) 1843–1845.

[13] M. Dietlein, K. Scheidhauer, E. Voth, P. Theissen, H. Schicha, Fluorine-18 fluorodeoxyglucose positron emission tomography and iodine-131 whole-body scintigraphy in the follow-up of differentiated thyroid cancer, Eur. J. Nucl. Med. 24 (1997) 1342–1348.

[14] F. Grünwald, C. Menzel, H. Bender, H. Palmedo, P. Willkomm, J. Ruhlmann, T. Franckson, H.J. Biersack, Comparison of 18FDG-PET with 131iodine and 99mTc-sestamibi scintigraphy in differentiated thyroid cancer, Thyroid 7 (1997) 327–335.

[15] G. Altenvoerde, H. Lerch, T. Kuwert, P. Matheja, M. Schafers, O. Schober, Positron emission tomography with F-18-deoxyglucose in patients with differentiated thyroid carcinoma, elevated thyroglobulin levels, and negative iodine scans, Langenbecks Arch. Surg. 383 (1998) 160–163.

[16] T.S. Huang, P.U. Chieng, C.C. Chang, R.F. Yen, Positron emission tomography for detecting iodine-131 nonvisualized metastasis of well-differentiated thyroid carcinoma: two case reports, J. Endocrinol. Invest. 21 (1998) 392–398.

[17] H. Jadvar, I.R. McDougall, G.M. Segall, Evaluation of suspected recurrent papillary thyroid carcinoma with [18F]fluorodeoxyglucose positron emission tomography, Nucl. Med. Commun. 19 (1998) 547–554.

[18] J.K. Chung, Y. So, J.S. Lee, C.W. Choi, S.M. Lim, D.S. Lee, S.W. Hong, Y.K. Youn, M.C. Lee, B.Y. Cho, Value of FDG PET in papillary thyroid carcinoma with negative 131I whole-body scan, J. Nucl. Med. 40 (1999) 986–992.

[19] N.S. Alnafisi, A.A. Driedger, G. Coates, D.J. Moote, S.J. Raphael, FDG PET of recurrent or metastatic 131I-negative papillary thyroid carcinoma, J. Nucl. Med. 41 (2000) 1010–1015.

[20] W. Wang, H. Macapinlac, S.M. Larson, S.D. Yeh, T. Akhurst, R.D. Finn, J. Rosai, R.J. Robbins, [18F]-2-fluoro-2-deoxy-D-glucose positron emission tomography localizes residual thyroid cancer in patients with negative diagnostic (131)I whole body scans and elevated serum thyroglobulin levels, J. Clin. Endocrinol. Metab. 84 (1999) 2291–2302.

[21] P. Lind, E. Kresnik, G. Kumnig, H.J. Gallowitsch, I. Igerc, S. Matschnig, I. Gomez, 18F-FDG-PET in the follow-up of Thyroid Cancer, Acta Med. Austr. 30 (2003) 17–21.

[22] S.M. Larson, R. Robbins, Positron emission tomography in thyroid cancer management, Semin. Roentgenol. 37 (2002) 169–174.

[23] L. Hooft, O.S. Hoekstra, W. Deville, P. Lips, G.J. Teule, M. Boers, M.W. van Tulder, Diagnostic accuracy of 18F-fluorodeoxyglucose positron emission tomography in the follow-up of papillary or follicular thyroid cancer, J. Clin. Endocrinol. Metab. 86 (2001) 3779–3786.

[24] A. Stojadinovic, A. Hoos, R.A. Ghossein, M.J. Urist, D.H. Leung, R.H. Spiro, J.P. Shah, M.F. Brennan, B. Singh, A.R. Shaha, Hurthle cell carcinoma: a 60-year experience, Ann. Surg. Oncol. 9 (2002) 197–203.

[25] M. Plotkin, H. Hautzel, B.J. Krause, D. Schmidt, R. Larisch, F.M. Mottaghy, A.R. Boemer, H. Herzog, H. Vosberg, H.W. Muller-Gartner, Implication of 2-18fluor-2-deoxyglucose positron emission tomography in the follow-up of Hurthle cell thyroid cancer, Thyroid 12 (2002) 155–161.

[26] L.P. Adler, A.D. Bloom, Positron emission tomography of thyroid masses, Thyroid 3 (1993) 195–200.

[27] A.D. Bloom, L.P. Adler, J.M. Shuck, Determination of malignancy of thyroid nodules with positron emission tomography, Surgery 114 (1993) 728–734 [discussion 734–735].

[28] H. Uematsu, N. Sadato, T. Ohtsubo, T. Tsuchida, S. Nakamura, K. Sugimoto, A. Waki, N. Takahashi, Y. Yonekura, G. Tsuda, H. Saito, N. Hayashi, K. Yamamoto, Y. Ishii, Fluorine-18-fluorodeoxyglucose PET versus thallium-201 scintigraphy evaluation of thyroid tumors, J. Nucl. Med. 39 (1998) 453–459.

[29] M.S. Cohen, N. Arslan, F. Dehdashti, G.M. Doherty, T.C. Lairmore, L.M. Brunt, J.F. Moley, Risk of malignancy in thyroid incidentalomas identified by fluorodeoxyglucose-positron emission tomography, Surgery 130 (2001) 941–946.

[30] A. Van den Bruel, A. Maes, T. De Potter, L. Mortelmans, M. Drijkoningen, B. Van Damme, P. Delaere, R. Bouillon, Clinical relevance of thyroid fluorodeoxyglucose-whole body positron emission tomography incidentaloma, J. Clin. Endocrinol. Metab. 87 (2002) 1517–1520.

[31] P.W. Davis, N.D. Perrier, L. Adler, E.A. Levine, Incidental thyroid carcinoma identified by positron emission tomography scanning obtained for metastatic evaluation, Am. Surg. 67 (2001) 582–584.

[32] K.M. van Tol, P.L. Jager, D.A. Piers, J. Pruim, E.G. de Vries, R.P. Dullaart, T.P. Links, Better yield of (18)fluorodeoxyglucose-positron emission tomography in patients with metastatic differentiated thyroid carcinoma during thyrotropin stimulation, Thyroid 12 (2002) 381–387.

[33] F. Moog, R. Linke, N. Manthey, R. Tiling, P. Knesewitsch, K. Tatsch, K. Hahn, Influence of thyroid-stimulating hormone levels on uptake of FDG in recurrent and metastatic differentiated thyroid carcinoma, J. Nucl. Med. 41 (2000) 1989–1995.

[34] T. Petrich, A.R. Borner, D. Otto, M. Hofmann, W.H. Knapp, Influence of rhTSH on [(18)F]fluorodeoxyglucose uptake by differentiated thyroid carcinoma, Eur. J. Nucl. Med. Mol. Imaging 29 (2002) 641–647.

[35] J. Hoie, A. Stenwig, G. Kullmann, M. Lindegaard, Distant metastases in papillary thyroid cancer. A review of 91 patients, Cancer 61 (1988) 1–6.

[36] M. Schlumberger, Papillary and Follicular Thyroid Carcinoma, N. Engl. J. Med. 338 (1998) 297–306.

[37] W. Wang, S.M. Larson, M. Fazzari, S.K. Tickoo, K. Kolbert, G. Sgouros, H. Yeung, H. Macapinlac, J. Rosai, R.J. Robbins, Prognostic value of [18F]fluorodeoxyglucose positron emission tomographic scanning in patients with thyroid cancer, J. Clin. Endocrinol. Metab. 85 (2000) 1107–1113.

[38] W. Wang, S.M. Larson, R.M. Tuttle, H. Kalaigian, K. Kolbert, M. Sonenberg, R.J. Robbins, Resistance of [18f]-fluorodeoxyglucose-avid metastatic thyroid cancer lesions to treatment with high-dose radioactive iodine, Thyroid 11 (2001) 1169–1175.

[39] A. Jemal, T. Murray, A. Samuels, A. Ghafoor, E. Ward, M.J. Thun, Cancer statistics, CA. Cancer. J. Clin. 53 (2003) 5–26.

Chapter 7

Preclinical studies of chemotherapy for undifferentiated thyroid carcinoma

Sai-Ching Jim Yeung

Department of General Internal Medicine, Ambulatory Treatment and Emergency Care and Department of Endocrine Neoplasia and Hormonal Disorders, The University of Texas M. D. Anderson Cancer Center, Houston, TX 77030, USA

1. Introduction

For differentiated thyroid carcinomas that retain the ability to take up radioactive iodine, surgery and radioactive iodine remain the primary treatments. Poorly differentiated and anaplastic thyroid carcinomas do not take up radioactive iodine and are aggressive and usually fatal despite treatment [1,2]. Without radioactive iodine as an effective therapy against metastatic disease, external-beam radiation therapy and chemotherapy are usually the remaining options. Most poorly differentiated and anaplastic thyroid carcinomas are very resistant to chemotherapeutic agents, and *in vitro* chemosensitivity testing has been advocated to prevent the administration of ineffective agents [3]. The results of *in vitro* chemosensitivity testing appear to correctly predict clinical responses [4]. In this chapter, new chemotherapy agents and approaches for the treatment of poorly differentiated and anaplastic thyroid cancer will be discussed. The chapter is organized into sections on the basis of the mechanisms of action of the therapeutic agents.

2. DNA-damaging agents

Doxorubicin is a DNA-damaging agent via multiple mechanisms [5]. Doxorubicin-based combination chemotherapy or chemoradiotherapy is the most widely used therapy for poorly differentiated and anaplastic thyroid cancer [6–12]. Doxorubicin-based therapy is associated with partial response rates of 30–40%, but long-term remissions are rare [13].

Cisplatin is another DNA-damaging agent (formation of adducts to DNA) that is frequently used against thyroid cancer. In a study of 13 dogs with thyroid cancers (12 with follicular thyroid cancers) treated with cisplatin, one dog had a complete

ADVANCES IN MOLECULAR AND CELLULAR ENDOCRINOLOGY
VOLUME 4 ISSN 1569-2566/DOI 10.1016/S1569-2566(04)04007-4

remission, six had partial remissions, three had stable disease, and three had progressive disease [14].

Combinations of doxorubicin and cisplatin are commonly used against aggressive thyroid cancer in current clinical practice [12]. A case report described a 29-year-old man with extensive metastatic papillary thyroid carcinoma not demonstrable on whole-body radioiodine imaging, who was treated with cisplatin and doxorubicin. Repeat radioiodine scanning after three cycles of chemotherapy demonstrated significant reappearance of radioiodine uptake, and the patient was then treated with radioiodine (200 mCi) [15]. It appears that dedifferentiated noniodine-concentrating thyroid cancer may be able to take up iodine again after chemotherapy because of a differentiating effect of chemotherapy on the cancer cells, a selective cytotoxicity of the chemotherapy against poorly differentiated thyroid cancer cells or both [15].

Combinations of doxorubicin and cisplatin with new agents are under investigation, and some of these combinations will be discussed later in this chapter.

3. Antimetabolites

3.1. *Tezacitabine*

Tezacitabine (MDL-101731, KW-2331, FMdC) is an antimetabolite deoxycytidine analogue currently used in clinical trials for nonthyroidal tumors [16]. It irreversibly inhibits ribonucleotide reductase and is a DNA chain terminator. Tezacitabine deoxynucleotides are incorporated relatively efficiently into deoxycytidine sites [17]. Once incorporated, tezacitabine stops chain elongation by DNA polymerases, and the 3′ to 5′ exonuclease activity of DNA polymerase epsilon is unable to remove the incorporated tezacitabine. In cell culture, tezacitabine (10 nM) induces S- or G1-phase cell-cycle arrest, followed by apoptosis as exposure continues [17]. Inhibition of tezacitabine incorporation into DNA by aphidicolin diminished the cytotoxic effect of tezacitabine, indicating that its incorporation is a key event mediating this drug's cytotoxicity [17].

The effect of tezacitabine against three thyroid carcinoma cell lines [8505C (anaplastic), B-CPAP (papillary), and BHT-101 (anaplastic)] has been studied [18]. Tezacitabine at concentrations $< 0.1\,\mu M$ decreased both DNA synthesis and the growth of cancer cells, while the drug at concentrations $> 5\,\mu M$ showed only modest inhibition of the growth of the normal fibroblasts. Tezacitabine is a potent apoptosis-inducing drug against human thyroid cancer cells *in vitro* [18].

In nude mice bearing human cancer xenografts, tezacitabine was suggested to have a radiosensitizing effect [19]. Since external-beam radiation therapy plays an important part in the management of anaplastic thyroid cancer, the radiosensitizing effect of tezacitabine may warrant further investigation.

3.2. *Gemcitabine*

Gemcitabine (2′, 2′-difluorodeoxycytidine) is a fluorinated nucleoside analog that has an established and significant role in the treatment of a variety of solid tumors

[20–23]. The advantages of this drug are a relatively mild side-effect profile and a radiosensitizing effect. The mechanism of radiosensitization is thought to be simultaneous gemcitabine-induced deoxyadenosine triphosphate depletion and cell-cycle redistribution into the S-phase.

Gemcitabine has been evaluated against two poorly differentiated thyroid cancer cell lines (WRO and NPA) and an anaplastic thyroid cancer cell line (ARO). Each cell line was treated with gemcitabine (up to 3 mM) for 24, 48, and 72 h [24]. For all three cell lines, maximal reduction in cell viability as measured by a tetrazolium dye assay was seen after 72 h of gemcitabine exposure. NPA was the most sensitive cell line when evaluated after 24 and 48 h of exposure, but at 72 h, all three cell lines were similarly sensitive to gemcitabine. The values IC_{50} (50% inhibitory concentrations) for cell viability ranged from 0.7 to 1 µM for each cell line after 72 h of exposure [24].

Gemcitabine has been investigated in combination with cisplatin. The antineoplastic activity of gemcitabine alone, cisplatin alone, and the two drugs in combination (1- and 24-h drug exposure) was investigated in four anaplastic thyroid cancer cell lines (8505C, C643, HTh74, and SW1736) [25]. IC_{50} values were determined by biomass measurement using sulforhodamine B dye binding. Gemcitabine alone seemed to be active in anaplastic thyroid cancer, while cisplatin was only modestly active. Four different drug schedules were tested: a 1-h cisplatin treatment immediately followed by a 23-h gemcitabine treatment, a 1-h cisplatin treatment followed by a 1-h gemcitabine treatment 23 h later, a 23-h gemcitabine treatment immediately followed by a 1-h cisplatin treatment, and a 1-h gemcitabine treatment followed by a 1-h cisplatin treatment 23 h later. The drug combinations were additive when gemcitabine preceded cisplatin exposure, whereas the combinations were antagonistic when cisplatin preceded gemcitabine exposure [25].

3.3. *Multimeric gemcitabine monophosphate*

A novel multimeric form of gemcitabine monophosphate (2′-deoxy-2′, 2′-difluorocytidine-5′-*O*-monophosphate), $GemMP_{10}$, also has *in vitro* activity against thyroid cancer cells. The cytotoxicity of $GemMP_{10}$ was studied in three thyroid carcinoma cell lines [8505C (anaplastic), B-CPAP (papillary), and BHT-101 (anaplastic)]. $GemMP_{10}$ inhibited cancer cell growth at concentrations from 1 to 50 nM. These concentrations were 5–10-fold lower than those for monomeric gemcitabine. $GemMP_{10}$ induces apoptosis of thyroid cancer cells and S-phase cell-cycle arrest [26].

4. Antimicrotubule agents

4.1. *Paclitaxel*

Paclitaxel is derived from the Pacific yew tree (*Taxus brevifolia*). The drug's best-known mechanism of antitumor activity is the promotion of microtubule assembly [27], and thus an inhibition of mitotic spindle function. Recent studies have shown that paclitaxel affects the activities of several intracellular tyrosine and serine/threonine protein kinases [27,28]. Another report indicates that paclitaxel inhibits isoprenylation [29]. The paclitaxel-induced mitotic block triggers apoptosis via a p53 tumor suppressor gene-independent pathway [30–32]. Other intracellular signaling molecules (e.g., ERK [33–35], p38 mitogen-activated protein kinase [33], protein kinase C [36], protein kinase A-type II [36,37], and p34-cdc2 [36]) may also play a role in paclitaxel-induced apoptosis.

Dr. Kenneth Ain's group (Veterans Affairs Medical Center, Lexington, Kentucky, USA) demonstrated the antitumor activity of paclitaxel against six human anaplastic thyroid carcinoma cell lines (ARO, BHT-101, DRO, KAT-4, KAT-18, and SW-1736) [38]. Maximal inhibition was observed at a paclitaxel concentration of $0.05\,\mu M$. Paclitaxel delivered by subcutaneous injection was effective against xenografts of DRO, ARO, and KAT-4 cells in nude mice [38]. These results led to a phase II clinical trial of paclitaxel in anaplastic thyroid carcinoma patients with persistent or metastatic disease after surgery or external-beam radiation therapy [39]. One complete response and nine partial responses were seen among 19 evaluable patients (a 53% response rate). Weekly 1-h infusions were more efficacious than 96-h infusions every 3 weeks. Although paclitaxel appears to have significant clinical activity against anaplastic thyroid carcinoma, it does not improve the prognosis of this malignancy [39].

It was demonstrated in our laboratory that a farnesyl transferase inhibitor (FTI), manumycin, and paclitaxel enhanced each other's apoptotic effect in six anaplastic thyroid cancer cell lines (ARO, C643, DRO, Hth-74, KAT-4, and KAT-18) [40]. Enhancement of the cytotoxic action of paclitaxel by other FTIs (L-744832 [41] and SCH-66336 [42]) was also observed in other cancer cell lines. The combination of manumycin and paclitaxel was also studied in a nude mouse xenograft model, and the combination was observed to have increased antitumor activity compared with the activity of either drug alone [40,43].

4.2. *2-Methoxyestradiol*

2-Methoxyestradiol, a natural estrogen metabolite, depolymerizes microtubules and arrests cells in G_2/M-phase of the cell cycle [44]. Roswall et al. [45] reported that 2-methoxyestradiol inhibited five out of six human anaplastic thyroid cancer cell lines. It induced apoptosis, perhaps involving the p38-MAPK signaling pathway.

4.3. *Vinorelbine*

Vinorelbine is a semisynthetic vinca alkaloid derived from vinblastine. This second-generation vinca alkaloid affects microtubule dynamics in a manner different from that of the first-generation vinca alkaloids [46]. Vinblastine and other first-generation agents decrease the rate and extent of microtubule shortening, whereas vinorelbine decreases the rate and extent of microtubule lengthening. A study that compared the effects of vinblastine, vinorelbine, and vinflunine (another second-generation vinca alkaloid) on HeLa cells found that despite differences in the effects of the three drugs on microtubule dynamics, there are minimal morphological differences in their

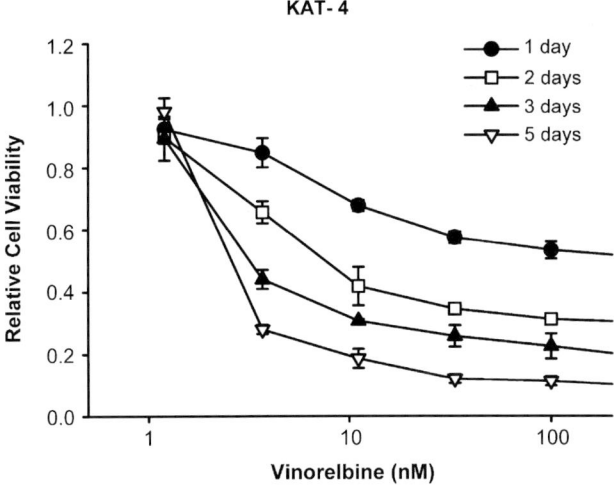

Fig. 1. Dose–response curves for vinorelbine at various durations of exposure in KAT-4 cells. The error bars represent 95% confidence intervals.

effects on the mitotic spindles [46]. Perhaps the overall suppression of microtubule dynamics is more important than specific effects on lengthening or shortening of the microtubules in blocking mitosis [46].

Vinorelbine has a radiation-sensitizing effect [47]. At a minimally toxic concentration (20 nM), moderate sensitization to radiation was observed in human non-small-cell lung cancer. The sensitization may be due to cell cycle arrest at the G_2/M-phase [47]. In patients with metastatic breast cancer, in whom treatment with anthracyclines and taxanes has failed, weekly vinorelbine is an effective salvage therapy [48]. These observations stir an interest in vinorelbine as a potential agent for the treatment of anaplastic thyroid cancer.

The cytotoxic effect of vinorelbine on two anaplastic thyroid cancer cell lines (ARO and KAT-4) *in vitro* has been tested in our laboratory. Using a tetrazolium dye assay (MTT) to measure the number of live cells, we calculated the viability of vinorelbine-treated cells relative to untreated control cells. The dose–response curves for various durations of drug treatment in KAT-4 cells are shown in Fig. 1. ARO cells showed similar response to vinorelbine (data not shown). Vinorelbine inhibited the two anaplastic thyroid cancer cell lines at nanomolar concentrations. Further investigation of vinorelbine against anaplastic thyroid carcinoma may be warranted.

5. Mitogenic signaling blockers

Mutations activating the mitogenic signaling pathway (e.g., mutations in *ras, ret/PTC3*, and c-*met*) have been found in differentiated thyroid carcinomas [49]. Undifferentiated and anaplastic thyroid cancer are thought to develop from preexisting differentiated thyroid carcinoma following a 'second hit' mutation (probably a *p53* tumor suppressor gene mutation) that leads to aggressive behavior [49]. In recent years, therapeutic agents aimed at disrupting the aberrant mitogenic signal caused by oncogenic mutations have attracted great interest in the cancer research community.

Tyrosine kinases play important roles in various aspects of tumor biology (growth, survival, metastasis, and angiogenesis) [50,51]. Small-molecule compounds have been discovered that selectively inhibit tyrosine kinases by competing for ATP binding at catalytic sites [52]. Inhibitors of protein kinases (e.g., MEK) downstream in the mitogenic signaling pathway have also been discovered. A large number of these small-molecule inhibitors of tyrosine kinases are being developed for use in cancer therapy.

5.1. *4,5-Dianilinophthalimide*

As mentioned in the preceding section, overexpression of c-*met* is common among thyroid cancers. Activation of Met is mitogenic in thyrocytes. The expression of Met and the degree of glycosylation of Met in human anaplastic thyroid carcinoma cell lines are variable. In one study, high Met expression (compared to the expression in normal human thyrocytes) was found in four of six anaplastic thyroid carcinoma cell lines, and activation of Met was ligand independent in all four cell lines [53]. A follow-up study indicated that activation of epidermal growth factor receptors (EGFRs) might be responsible for the overexpression and activation of Met in anaplastic thyroid carcinoma cells [54].

4,5-Dianilinophthalimide (CGP 54211 or DAPH) is a selective inhibitor of EGFR tyrosine kinase activity [55,56]. DAPH competes with ATP at its binding site [57]. Daily oral administration of DAPH inhibited EGFR phosphorylation, and inhibition of EGFR phosphorylation correlated with inhibition of tumor growth [58]. We have tested DAPH against six anaplastic thyroid cancer cell lines with 72-h incubations. The number of viable cells was measured using a tetrazolium dye assay (MTT), and the viability of the cells relative to that of untreated control cells was plotted against the concentration of DAPH (Fig. 2). Four of six anaplastic thyroid cancer cell lines were sensitive to DAPH. Further investigation is needed to find out whether overexpression of Met can predict tumor response to DAPH.

5.2. *Pyrazolo-pyrimidine PP1*

A pyrazolo-pyrimidine tyrosine kinase inhibitor, PP1, selectively inhibits the *src* tyrosine kinase family by binding to the ATP-binding site of the kinase. Crystal structure analysis suggests that a methylphenyl group on PP1 is inserted into an adjacent hydrophobic pocket at the ATP-binding site of the enzyme, effecting the inhibition of tyrosine kinase activity [59]. Chromosomal translocation leading to constitutively active chimeric Ret oncoproteins is important in the carcinogenesis of papillary thyroid carcinomas. Pyrazolo-pyrimidine PP1 was found to inhibit *ret*-derived tyrosine kinase as well [60]. PP1 reversed the malignant phenotype of *ret/PTC3*-transformed cells, and it inhibited two human papillary thyroid carcinoma

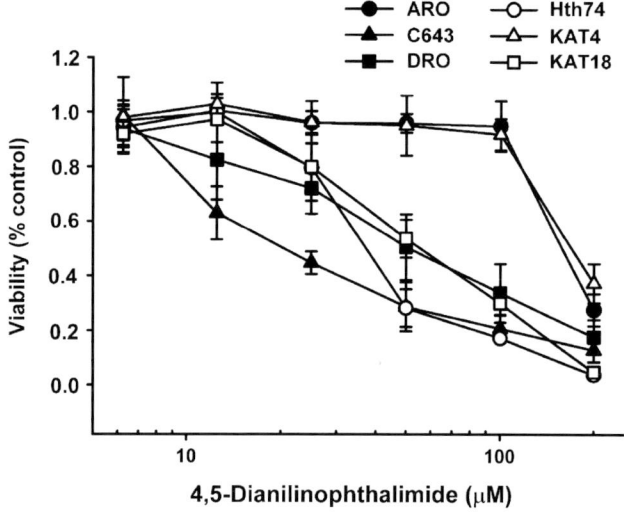

Fig. 2. Dose–response curves for 4,5-dianilinophthalimide in anaplastic thyroid cancer cell lines. Cells were exposed to the drug for 72 h. The error bars represent 95% confidence intervals.

cell lines that carry *ret/PTC1* rearrangements in the soft-agar clonogenic assay [60]. In a nude mouse model, PP1 inhibited tumor formation of NIH3T3 fibroblast cells transformed with the *ret/PTC3* chimeric gene [60]. Therefore, PP1 or other related tyrosine kinase inhibitors may be useful in the treatment of thyroid cancers with *ret*-derived chimeric oncoproteins.

5.3. *Manumycin*

Another mitogenic signaling blocker that may be effective against undifferentiated thyroid carcinoma is manumycin A, a natural product of *Streptomyces parvulus* identified as a farnesyl transferase inhibitor (FTI) in 1993 [61].

Research on *ras* oncogenes led to the development of FTIs to treat cancer [62–67]. As mentioned above, *ras* oncogenes are frequently found in thyroid cancers. Ras, the protein product of *ras* proto-oncogenes, is synthesized as a cytosolic precursor, and it requires posttranslational modification by conjugation of a farnesyl moiety (15-carbon isoprenyl group) to the C-terminus. After farnesylation, Ras is localized to the inner surface of the cell membrane and becomes functional in transducing the mitogenic signals of tyrosine kinase receptors. Inhibition of farnesyl transferase abolishes the function of Ras and blocks the mitogenic action of *ras* oncogenes. K-Ras and N-Ras can be alternately geranylgeranylated when farnesylation is inhibited [68,69], but nonfarnesylated oncogenic H-Ras can exert a dominant-negative effect and thus inhibit the function of membrane-bound Ras in some circumstances. Thus, even though inhibition of farnesyl transferase would be expected to affect only H-Ras, the dominant-negative effect would inhibit the Ras-transforming pathway.

Since wild-type Ras does not display the dominant-negative phenotype, the observed inhibition would be selective for tumor cells.

FTIs induce apoptosis in cancer cells [40,70–74]. The antineoplastic activity of FTIs results, at least in part, from inhibition of farnesylation of proteins other than Ras [64,67]. In a cell culture study, 31 of 42 cancer cell lines of various tumor types and oncogenetic backgrounds (including wild-type *ras*) were sensitive to a peptido-mimetic FTI (L-744832) [75]. This suggests that FTIs may exert anticancer activity via mechanisms in addition to blocking the function of Ras. More than 10 unidentified isoprenylated proteins are affected by FTIs [76]. Among the known farnesylated proteins other than Ras, several may be relevant in intracellular signaling and apoptosis, including lamin A and B, Rap2, Rho, and inositol triphosphate 5-phosphatase type I. The roles of these proteins in the antineoplastic activity of FTIs are not clear.

Manumycin is a relatively selective inhibitor of farnesyl:protein transferase ($IC_{50} = 5\,\mu M$), but at high concentrations, manumycin also inhibits geranylgeranyl:protein transferase ($IC_{50} = 180\,\mu M$) [61]. The mechanism of action of this inhibition is competitive with farnesyl pyrophosphate groups [62,77]. Manumycin has been shown to have antitumor activity in cell culture [72,78,79] and in nude mouse xenograft models [40,43,80,81].

We investigated the effects of manumycin in combination with other drugs frequently used to treat anaplastic thyroid cancer in six human anaplastic thyroid cancer cell lines: ARO, C643, DRO, Hth-74, KAT-4, and KAT-18. Manumycin enhanced the effect of paclitaxel in all six of the cell lines. The mechanism of cell death was apoptosis as demonstrated by an increase in caspase-3 activity, specific cleavage of poly-(ADP-ribose)polymerase, and internucleosomal fragmentation of DNA [40]. In a subsequent study [82], we investigated the apoptosis pathway involved. Our results indicated that cytochrome *c* release was upstream of the activation of caspase-9, caspase-8, and caspase-3 and that the interaction between manumycin and paclitaxel occurred at or upstream of cytochrome *c*. The combination of manumycin with cisplatin resulted in enhanced cytotoxicity in two of six anaplastic thyroid cancer cell lines, and the combination of manumycin with doxorubicin resulted in enhanced cytotoxicity in three of six cell lines [40].

The *in vivo* antitumor effect and toxicity of the combination of manumycin and paclitaxel were evaluated in a nude mouse xenograft model using ARO and KAT-4 cells. Drugs were injected intraperitoneally on days 1 and 3 of a 7-day cycle for three cycles. Both manumycin ($7.5\,\mathrm{mg\,kg^{-1}\,dose^{-1}}$) and paclitaxel ($20\,\mathrm{mg\,kg^{-1}\,dose^{-1}}$) had significant inhibitory effects on tumor growth. Combined manumycin and paclitaxel treatments were as effective as manumycin against ARO cells and were more effective than either manumycin or paclitaxel alone against KAT-4 cells [40], Hth-74 cells [43] and KAT-18 cells [43]. The treatments caused no significant morbidity or mortality.

In summary, studies to date indicate that manumycin can inhibit the growth of anaplastic thyroid cancer both *in vitro* and *in vivo*. Manumycin plus paclitaxel has enhanced cytotoxic effects and increased apoptotic cell death in anaplastic thyroid cancer cells *in vitro* beyond the apoptotic cell death seen with either drug by itself.

Manumycin plus paclitaxel is also effective *in vivo*, and no significant toxicity has been observed with this combination [40,43].

5.4. *Lonafarnib (SCH66336)*

Lonafarnib (also known as SCH66336) is a tricyclic nonpeptidic farnesyl transferase inhibitor that competes with protein substrates for binding to farnesyl transferase. Crystallographic and thermodynamic studies of farnesyl transferase complexed with tricyclic inhibitors reveal that the tricyclic compound spans the enzyme's active site and interacts with both functional groups from the protein and the isoprenoid portion of bound farnesyl diphosphate [83]. Preclinical studies have demonstrated the activity of SCH66336 against tumors of pancreas, colon, prostate, lung and urinary bladder origin both in animal models and *in vitro* [74]. Enhanced antitumor effect was observed in animal models when SCH66336 was combined with cyclophosphamide, fluorouracil or vincristine [74]. In a study that used a soft-agar clonogenic assay to study the effect of a 14-day exposure to SCH66336, inhibitory response to SCH66336 (2.5 µM) was seen in three (50%) of six breast tumors, six (40%) of 15 ovarian tumors, and five (38%) of 13 non-small-cell lung tumors [84]. SCH66336 had activity in 27% of tumour specimens resistant to doxorubicin, 38% resistant to cisplatin, 33% resistant to paclitaxel, and 27% resistant to etoposide [84]. The combination of SCH66336 and paclitaxel has also resulted in improved antineoplastic activity in preclinical cancer models [42].

The activity of SCH66336 against drug-resistant solid tumors, the synergism of SCH66336 with paclitaxel, and our previous work with manumycin, another FTI [40,43,85], sparked our interest in SCH66336 as a chemotherapy agent against undifferentiated and anaplastic thyroid carcinoma. *In vitro*, SCH66336 inhibited the incorporation of ^{3}H-thymidine into trichloroacetic acid-precipitable materials in both ARO (Fig. 3) and KAT-4 cells (data not shown) when the cells were labeled with ^{3}H-thymidine for 2 h at the end of 48-h drug incubations.

We also tested the effect of SCH66336 on clonogenicity of anaplastic thyroid cancer cells in soft agar. The experiment started with the same number of cells in Petri dishes. Anaplastic thyroid cancer cells were incubated with different concentrations of SCH66336 or SCH66337 (an inactive isomer of SCH66336) in Petri dishes for 48 h. Then the attached cells were collected by trypsinization and combined with the detached cells collected by centrifugation, and the cell pellets were resuspended in equal volumes of culture medium. Then equal volumes of the cell suspensions were plated into soft agar in the absence of drugs. In ARO cells, the ability of the anaplastic thyroid cancer cells to form colonies depended on the concentration of SCH66336 to which the cells had been exposed (Fig. 4). Similar results were observed in KAT-4 cells (data not shown). The IC_{50} values for KAT-4 and ARO were about 5 µg ml^{-1} and 7 µg ml^{-1}, respectively. Treatment with the control drug SCH66337 caused a maximum decrease of about 8% in colonies. Since the structures of the two compounds are very similar, inhibition of proliferation of the anaplastic thyroid cancer cells was likely to be due to the ability of SCH66336 to inhibit farnesyl transferase.

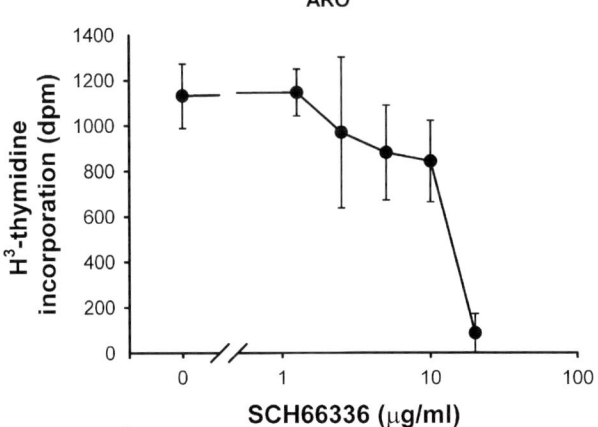

Fig. 3. Inhibition of ^{3}H-thymidine incorporation by SCH66336. The amount of ^{3}H-thymidine incorporated into trichloroacetic acid-precipitable material was plotted against the concentration of SCH66336. The error bars represent 95% confidence intervals.

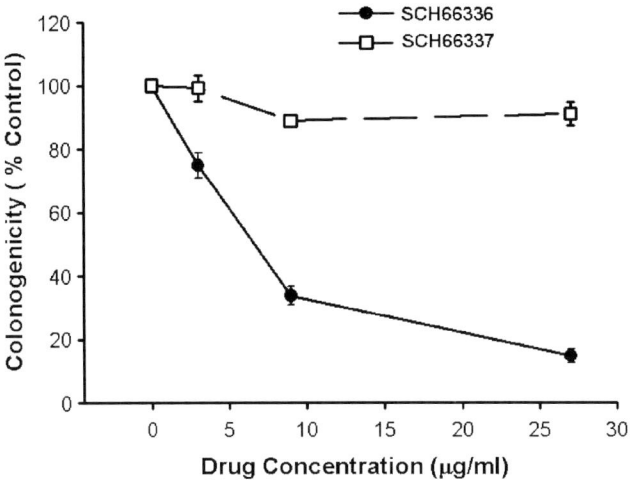

Fig. 4. Dose–response curve for SCH66336 using the soft-agar clonogenic assay. The number of colonies in treated plates was expressed as a percentage of the number of colonies in control plates, and the relative clonogenicity was plotted against drug concentration. The control compound is the inactive isomer SCH66337. Each data point represents the average of four plates. The error bars represent 95% confidence intervals.

Dr. Michael J. Demeure (University of Arizona Medical Center, Tucson, AZ, USA) and colleagues are organizing a multicenter-phase II trial of paclitaxel, carboplatin and lonafarnib (SCH66336) in patients with anaplastic thyroid cancer (M.J. Demeure, pers. Comm., 2002).

6. Angiogenesis inhibitors

Angiogenesis is an important step in cancer proliferation and metastasis [86,87]. Blood vessels supply oxygen and nutrients vital to the growth and survival of cancer cells. Solid tumors cannot grow beyond $1-2\,mm^3$ or metastasize without the development of new blood vessels. In general, antiangiogenic agents, on the basis of strategies used to block angiogenesis, can be classified into four groups (1) agents that block the factors that stimulate the formation of blood vessels, (2) natural inhibitors of angiogenesis, (3) agents that block molecules that allow newly formed blood vessels to invade surrounding tissue, and (4) agents that block the proliferation of endothelial cells.

Drugs that block factors that stimulate the formation of blood vessels include a monoclonal antibody to VEGF, Su5416, and interferon-α. Suramin and eriochrome black T belong to the group of polyanionic sequesters that bind heparin-binding angiogenic growth factors. Natural inhibitors of angiogenesis include platelet factor-4, interleukin-12, thrombospondin, endostatin, and angiostatin. Matrix metalloproteinase inhibitors are examples of drugs that block molecules that allow new blood vessels to invade the surrounding tissue. Matrix metalloproteinase inhibitors include marimastat, Bay 12-9566, AG3340, COL-3, and minocycline. Agents that block the proliferation of endothelial cells include methionine aminopeptidase-2 inhibitors, i.e., fumagillin and its derivative, TNP-470 (AGM-1470). There are also other compounds with antiangiogenic activities of unknown mechanisms, e.g., thalidomide and squalamine. Other chemotherapeutic agents such as the FTIs, which in addition to their antiproliferative and apoptotic effects on cancer cells also inhibit VEGF expression by cancer cells and/or proliferation/ differentiation of endothelial cells. For some cancers, combination therapy in which antiangiogenic strategies are combined with chemotherapeutic agents is known to be more effective than monotherapy [88,89]. Therefore, it will be interesting to further investigate antiangiogenic drugs like TNP-470 in combination with other cytotoxic chemotherapeutic agents.

Drugs with antiangiogenic effects that have been tested on anaplastic thyroid cancer cells are discussed below.

6.1. *TNP-470*

TNP-470 is a synthetic analogue of fumagillin. The antitumor activity of TNP-470 against human anaplastic thyroid carcinoma was evaluated using xenografts in nude mice [90]. The transplanted tumor line was established from a 78-year-old woman and retained anaplastic morphological characteristics of the original cancer. TNP-470 ($50\,mg\,kg^{-1}$) was given to xenografted nude mice intratumorally, peritumorally, subcutaneously, and intraperitoneally. Intratumoral administration completely inhibited tumor growth, and peritumoral administration was also effective. Possible clinical application of TNP-470 to anaplastic thyroid carcinoma was suggested [90].

6.2. Combretastatin A-4 phosphate

Combretastatin A-4 is a tubulin-binding chemotherapy drug that is structurally related to colchicine [91]. This drug was discovered and isolated from the African bush willow, *Combretum caffrum*. The more soluble phosphate form is cleaved by endogenous phosphatases to the original compound, which is then taken up into cells. In animal models, combretastatin A-4 phosphate selectively prevents the blood flow in established tumor blood vessels [91]. In a published phase I trial [92], a single patient with anaplastic thyroid cancer had a complete 'response' and survived more than 30 months after treatment. Recent preliminary preclinical data also fueled the interest to further investigate this agent in the treatment of anaplastic thyroid cancer [93]. Combretastatin A-4 phosphate inhibited growth of four anaplastic thyroid cancer cell lines xenografted in nude mice [93].

6.3. Manumycin

Evidence suggests that manumycin also functions as an angiogenesis inhibitor with a potential role in the treatment of undifferentiated or anaplastic thyroid carcinoma [43].

Many angiogenic factors have been discovered, the two most important of which are VEGF and basic fibroblast growth factor [94]. VEGF, an important mitogen for angiogenesis, binds to two endothelial cell tyrosine kinase receptors: the fms-like tyrosine kinase [95] and the kinase domain receptor (KDR) tyrosine kinase [96]. Although expressed at very low levels in quiescent tissue, VEGF mRNA is temporarily upregulated by various external stimuli and is persistently upregulated in many cancer cell lines. Oncogenic-activated tyrosine kinases and Ras proteins induce a 6–16-fold increase in VEGF mRNA and cause VEGF mRNA to become more stable [97].

The upregulation of VEGF by activated H-*ras* in HaCaT cells can be reversed by an FTI [98]. Feldkemp et al. [99] found that the FTI L-744832 inhibited the synthesis and secretion of VEGF in the astrocytoma cell line U373 under hypoxic conditions. Gu et al. [100] found that another peptidomimetic FTI, A-170634, decreased VEGF secretion from HCT116 colon cancer cells and decreased vascularization in and around xenografted tumors.

In the course of our investigation of combined manumycin (an FTI) and paclitaxel (a taxane microtubule inhibitor) against anaplastic thyroid carcinoma [40,43] (see Section 4.1), we observed that manumycin-treated tumors looked paler than both control and paclitaxel-treated tumors. We hypothesized that angiogenesis inhibition mediated part of the *in vivo* effect of manumycin. This hypothesis was supported by the findings that (i) manumycin significantly inhibited angiogenesis in Matrigel (a solubilized basement membrane preparation extracted from the Engelbreth–Holm–Swarm mouse sarcoma) implanted into mice (ii) manumycin decreased VEGF in hypoxic anaplastic thyroid cancer cells (ARO and KAT-4) [43], and (iii) both manumycin and paclitaxel inhibited endothelial cell proliferation [43]. The combination of manumycin and paclitaxel also resulted in enhanced inhibition of endothelial tubule formation in Matrigel [43].

As angiogenesis and tumor growth are continuous processes, we investigated the effect of sustained delivery of manumycin. We found that paclitaxel plus the slow-released manumycin ($13.25 \, \mathrm{mg \, kg^{-1} \, week^{-1}}$) inhibited anaplastic thyroid cancer xenografts more than paclitaxel plus intermittent manumycin ($15 \, \mathrm{mg \, kg^{-1} \, week^{-1}}$). Inhibition of angiogenesis plays a role in the antineoplastic effect of manumycin plus paclitaxel [43].

6.4. *Imatinib mesylate (STI571, Gleevec®, CGP 57148B)*

Imatinib, a tyrosine kinase inhibitor well known for its inhibitory effect on c-Abl and c-Kit, potently inhibits α- and β-platelet-derived growth factor receptors (PDGFR) but not other closely related tyrosine kinase receptors [101]. In cancers, PDGF signaling may be involved in autocrine stimulation of cancer proliferation, paracrine interactions between the cancer cells and the stroma, and angiogenesis [102]. β-PDGFR are present in blood vessels and stroma. Imatinib was shown to decrease the interstitial pressure in tumors and facilitate capillary-to-interstitium transport (103), and similar effects were observed with an anti-β-PDGF oligonucleotide aptamer [103]. The treatment of anti-β-PDGF oligonucleotide aptamer or imatinib mesylate decreased tumor interstitial pressure and enhanced the uptake of paclitaxel, resulting in increased antineoplastic effect against xenografts of KAT-4 cells (anaplastic thyroid cancer cell line) in SCID mice [104].

7. Gene therapy

Gene therapy for cancer has made remarkable advances in pace with the leaping advances in molecular and cell biology. As mentioned earlier in this chapter, mutations in *ras*, *ret/PTC3*, c-*met*, c-*myc*, c-*fos*, and *p53* have been found in thyroid carcinomas [49]. Several different gene therapy strategies are being investigated in undifferentiated and anaplastic thyroid cancer. One strategy is to induce expression of tumor suppressor genes that have been inactivated by mutation. Another strategy is to express the enzymes that confer selective susceptibility to toxic effects of a drug. A third strategy is to allow replication-competent viruses to replicate selectively in proliferating cancerous cells and kill those cells selectively. A fourth strategy is to express apoptosis-inducing genes (e.g., *bax*) in a tissue-specific manner. In thyroid cancer, the first three strategies have been studied.

7.1. *Adenovirus expressing wild-type p53*

The tumor suppressor *p53* is a transcription factor that regulates cell cycling, DNA repair and apoptosis. *p53* mutations are present in 14% of thyroid cancers overall and are much more frequent in poorly differentiated and anaplastic tumors [105].

Infection of replication-deficient recombinant adenovirus vector expressing wild-type *p53* led to a dose-dependent reduction in viability in both normal and cancerous thyroid cells (ARO, FRO, NPA, and WRO) in culture [106]. Overexpression of wild-type *p53* induced apoptosis in all the cell lines and improved the sensitivity of two cell lines (FRO and NPA) to doxorubicin and the sensitivity of one cell line (FRO) to fluorouracil. Direct intratumoral injection of adenovirus expressing wild-type *p53* [1×10^9 plaque-forming units (pfu) per tumor] into subcutaneous FRO and NPA cell xenografts in nude mice completely inhibited growth of the xenografts [106].

SCH58500 is a replication-deficient adenovirus expressing wild-type p53. We tested the effect of SCH58500 (48-h incubation) on DNA content, protein biomass, and number of trypan blue dye-excluding viable cells in two anaplastic thyroid cancer cell lines (ARO and KAT-4). The DNA and protein contents of cell samples treated with SCH58500 both decreased in a dose-dependent manner, and the decrease correlated very well with the dose-dependent decrease in the number of viable cells (as counted under the microscope using a hemocytometer with trypan blue) (Fig. 5).

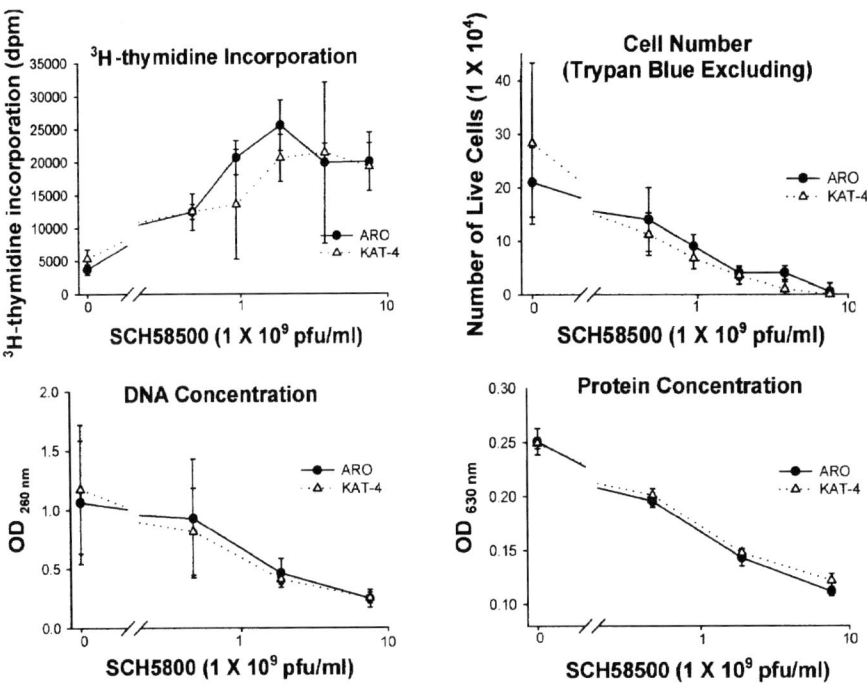

Fig. 5. Effects of SCH58500 on ARO and KAT-4 anaplastic thyroid carcinoma cells. **Upper panel: left,** effect of SCH58500 on incorporation of ^{3}H-thymidine into trichloroacetic acid-precipitable material; **right,** number of live cells that excluded trypan blue counted under the microscope using a hemocytometer. **Lower panel: left,** absorbance at wavelength 260 nm (OD 260), which is proportional to the concentration of DNA purified from the cell samples; **right,** absorbance at wavelength 630 nm (OD = 630) after the Lowry reaction, a measure of the protein concentration of the cell lysates. The error bars represent 95% confidence intervals.

Paradoxically, SCH58500 increased the incorporation of ^{3}H-thymidine into trichloroacetic acid–precipitable materials. We speculated that this paradoxical increase was due to the induction of DNA repair by wild-type p53.

The ability of the anaplastic thyroid cancer cells to form colonies depended on the concentration of SCH58500 that the cells had been exposed to. Anaplastic thyroid cancer cells (starting with the same number of cells per group) were infected with different concentrations of SCH58500 in Petri dishes for 48 h. The attached cells were collected by trypsinization and combined with the detached cells collected by centrifugation, and the cell pellets were resuspended in equal volumes of culture medium. Then equal volumes of the cell suspensions were plated into soft agar. Dose-dependent inhibition of colony formation was observed in both the KAT-4 (data not shown) and ARO cell lines (Fig. 6).

Adenoviral expression of wild-type p53 augments the antineoplastic effects of other chemotherapeutic drugs. Three anaplastic thyroid carcinoma cell lines with nonfunctional p53 (BHT-101, SW-1736, and KAT-4) were infected with an adenovirus expressing wild-type *p53*, and all three cell lines were sensitive to killing by the adenovirus. KAT-4 cells were least sensitive, SW-1736 cells had intermediate sensitivity, and BHT-101 cells were most sensitive. All three cell lines also became 10 times more sensitive to doxorubicin after wild-type *p53* expression [107]. Intratumoral injection of adenovirus expressing wild-type p53 in combination with doxorubicin (4 mg kg^{-1}, three times per week) led to tumor regression in the nude mouse xenograft model [106]. These reports suggest that the strategy of combining

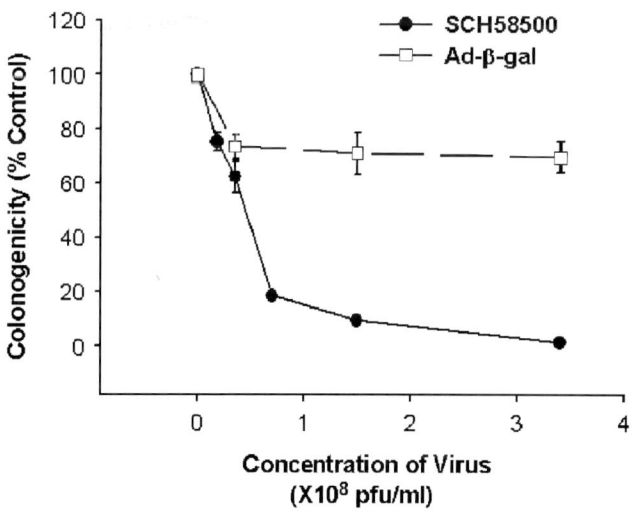

Fig. 6. Inhibition by SCH58500 of colony formation by ARO cells in soft agar. The number of colonies in treated plates was expressed as a percentage of the number of colonies in control plates. The graph shows the relative clonogenicity plotted against the virus concentration. The control virus expressing β-galactosidase is labeled as Ad-β-gal. Each data point represents the average of four plates. The error bars represent 95% confidence intervals.

wild-type *p53* gene therapy with cytotoxic chemotherapy has potential for clinical application in undifferentiated and anaplastic thyroid carcinoma.

7.2. *Thyroid-specific expression of prodrug/suicide genes*

Cell-type-specific gene therapy using the thyroglobulin gene (*TG*) promoter may be ideal for thyroid cancer. However, most poorly differentiated and anaplastic thyroid carcinomas do not express thyroglobulin and the thyroid-specific transcription factors [Pax-8, thyroid transcription factor-1 (*TTF-1*), and *TTF-2*]; thus they present a technical challenge. This problem may be solved by cotransfection of the *TTF-1*. *TTF-1* expression stimulated *TG* promoter activity in dedifferentiated thyroid cells but not in control cells from different tissue types. Cotransfection of AdTTF-1 (cytomegalovirus promoter and rat *TTF-1* cDNA) and AdTGTK (*TG* promoter-driven herpes simplex virus thymidine kinase gene) and ganciclovir treatment killed 90% or more of BHP15-3, BHP7-13 and BHP18-21v thyroid cancer cell lines, and FRT cells [108].

Another strategy to overcome lack of *TG* expression in undifferentiated or anaplastic thyroid cancer cells in the context of *TG*-promoter-driven gene therapy is to induce redifferentiation with histone deacetylase inhibitors. Treatment with the histone deacetylase inhibitors depsipeptide (FR9012228) and sodium butyrate resulted in enhanced expression of a drug susceptibility gene (herpes simplex virus thymidine kinase) driven by a *TG* promoter in anaplastic thyroid carcinoma cells [109].

These results suggest that adenoviral transfection of a *TG* promoter-controlled suicide gene and prodrug administration is a feasible strategy for poorly differentiated thyroid carcinoma cells lacking *TG* gene expression. Redifferentiation therapy with histone deacetylase inhibitors or cotransfection of the *TTF-1* gene may overcome the problems presented by the lack of *TG* expression.

7.3. *ONYX-015 (an E1B-defective adenovirus)*

ONYX-015 adenovirus does not have a functional *E1B* 55-kDa gene. Therefore, this adenovirus replicates only in cells with impaired p53 function and kills these cells with defective p53 tumor suppressor function. In cell culture, ONYX-015 is cytotoxic to ARO, KAT-4 and FRO cells (all anaplastic thyroid cancer cell lines) [110]. Synergism was observed in combinations with doxorubicin and paclitaxel against ARO and KAT-4 cells. In an athymic mice xenograft model, ARO xenografts were inhibited by ONYX-015 [110].

8. Redifferentiation therapy

Epigenetic inactivation of genes regulating cell growth is one characteristic of cancer cells [111]. An important difference between epigenetic inactivation of tumor suppressor genes and inactivation by genetic changes (mutation or deletion) is that epigenetic inactivation may be reversed by drugs. Combination treatments consisting of drugs that reactivate expression of silenced genes plus treatment modalities (radiation, DNA-damaging chemotherapy, etc.) that target or take advantage of the liberated genes may be feasible [112].

Disseminated progressive dedifferentiated thyroid carcinoma, which cannot concentrate therapeutic radioiodide, is often terminal. Since radioactive iodine is an effective therapy for differentiated thyroid cancer, a logical focus of research is on how to redifferentiate dedifferentiated, undifferentiated or anaplastic thyroid cancer and in doing so make these cancer cells to take up radioactive iodine.

8.1. *Azacitidine*

A natural focus of redifferentiation therapies is the human sodium-iodide symporter gene (*hNIS*), which is one of the genes required for iodide uptake. Analysis of *hNIS* mRNA expression in 23 thyroid tumor samples showed that *hNIS* expression is necessary but may not be sufficient for radioiodide uptake [113]. Reduced expression of nuclear factor(s) may contribute to reduced *hNIS* expression in some papillary thyroid cancers [114], and DNA methylation of the 5′-untranslated region within the first exon of *hNIS* may be involved in others [113].

Azacitidine restored *hNIS* expression in four of seven human thyroid cancer cell lines without *hNIS* expression and restored iodide transport in two of the cell lines [113]. Evaluation of methylation patterns in these cell lines showed that restoration of *hNIS* transcription correlated with demethylation of *hNIS* DNA in the untranslated region within the first exon. Restoration of *hNIS* transcription also correlated with restoration of expression of *TTF-1*. Azacitidine-induced DNA demethylation may restore susceptibility to therapeutic doses of radioiodide in dedifferentiated or undifferentiated thyroid carcinoma [113].

8.2. *Trichostatin A*

Trichostatin A is another agent that may be able to induce differentiation of dedifferentiated or undifferentiated thyroid carcinoma by promoting histone acetylation. Eukaryotic DNA is arranged into chromatin in which histone components of nucleosomes can be regulated by reversible acetylation. Histone acetylation is regulated by histone acetyltransferases and histone deacetylases (HDACs), which play important roles in transcription, DNA replication, and cell-cycle progression [115,116].

Trichostatin A, which inhibits HDAC reversibly at nanomolar concentrations by chelating zinc at the active site of HDAC with its hydroxamic acid group, stops cell cycling, induces differentiation, and reverses morphological changes seen in transformation [117]. The inhibitor activates the expression of *Waf-1/p21* without requiring the *p53* tumor suppressor gene. The cell-cycle arrest and antitumor activity of HDAC inhibitors are due to increased histone acetylation causing perturbations of regulators of cell cycling, differentiation, and apoptosis. Susceptibility to HDAC inhibitors may depend on DNA methylation status [118].

The antineoplastic effect of trichostatin A has been tested in cell lines derived from anaplastic thyroid carcinomas [119]. Trichostatin A induced apoptosis by activating the caspase cascade, and it induced cell-cycle arrest by decreasing cdk2- and cdk1-associated kinase activities. Trichostatin A has also been shown to potentiate retinoic acid-mediated gene expression [120]. Perhaps a combination of retinoids with trichostatin A may be tested for the ability to restore radioiodine uptake in dedifferentiated thyroid cancers.

8.3. *Retinoic acids*

In thyroid cancers, retinoic acid has an antiproliferative effect as well as a redifferentiating effect [121]. In thyroid carcinoma lines, retinoic acid treatment affects thyroid-specific genes (*hNIS,* type I 5'-deiodinase), adhesion (intercellular adhesion molecule-1, E-cadherin), growth, and tumorigenicity, and these changes suggest partial redifferentiation [122]. Data with follicular thyroid tumor cells also support similar conclusions that retinoic acid induces redifferentiation and inhibits proliferation [123].

There are also reports that therapy with 13-*cis*-retinoic acid resulted in significant radioiodine uptake in metastatic tumors that were initially unable to take up radioiodine [124]. In a pilot study, about 40% of the patients responded to 13-*cis*-retinoic acid treatment with increased radioiodide uptake [123]. In 20 patients treated with retinoic acid, eight showed a regression (four patients) or stabilization (four patients), as measured by tumor size and/or serum thyroglobulin levels, together with enhanced radioiodide uptake [125].

8.4. *Vitamin D analog*

1,25-Dihydroxycholecalciferol is known to induce differentiation in nonthyroid cell types [126,127]. The effects of 1,25-dihydroxycholecalciferol and a noncalciomimetic analog, EB1089, on thyroid carcinoma cell growth were studied in WRO and NPA cells. 1,25-Dihydroxycholecalciferol and EB1089 inhibited proliferation in a dose-dependent manner [128]. Vitamin D analogs are potentially useful in the treatment of thyroid cancers [128].

9. Miscellaneous agents

9.1. *Bovine seminal ribonuclease*

Bovine seminal ribonuclease (BS-RNase) is a dimeric RNase with selective cytotoxic effect against malignant cells and not normal cells [129]. BS-RNase enters cells from the extracellular matrix in endosomes. In malignant cells, BS-RNase enters the *trans*-Golgi network, but in normal cells, BS-RNase does not progress from the endosomes to the Golgi complex [130]. Degradation of intracellular RNA is the primary action causing cytotoxicity [131]. The ability of BS-RNase to dimerize is necessary for the cytotoxic effect because the dimeric structure protects the enzyme from the cytosolic RNase inhibitor [132]. BS-RNase has antitumor activity against a variety of human cancers [133–135].

BS-RNase may be useful in the treatment of anaplastic thyroid cancer [136]. The cytotoxic effect of BS-RNase was evaluated in thyroid cancer cell lines and non-malignant cells (human foreskin fibroblasts and retinal pigment epithelial cells). All the thyroid cancer cell lines were sensitive to BS-RNase, whereas none of the non-malignant cells were. BS-RNase induced apoptosis in the thyroid cancer cells. While not affecting the expressions of Fas and Fas-ligand, BS-RNase downregulated Bcl-2 [136].

In vivo antineoplastic effects of BS-RNase were evaluated on xenografts of 8505C (an anaplastic thyroid cancer cell line) in nude mice [136]. The mice received sub-cutaneous injections of BS-RNase ($12.5\,\mathrm{mg\,kg^{-1}\,day^{-1}}$ for 20 days). Significant tumor regression was observed after 20 days, and there were no apparent toxic effects. After cessation of therapy, tumor volume continued to decrease, and complete remission was achieved in all animals.

New modified formulations of BS-RNase may have improved activity. BS-RNase conjugated to water-soluble polymers (poly[*N*-(2-hydroxypropyl)methacrylamide]) may have activity against tumor growth and metastasis following intravenous administration [137], and BS-RNase conjugated to polyethylene glycol may drastically increase antitumoral activity compared to the free enzyme [138]. These new formulations of BS-RNase may be evaluated in undifferentiated and anaplastic thyroid cancer because the animal model data for BS-RNase were quite impressive [136].

9.2. *Apigenin*

Apigenin is a common dietary flavonoid with antitumor activity. Apigenin is present in large amounts in fruits and vegetables. The signal transduction mechanism mediating the antiproliferative effect of apigenin was investigated in an anaplastic thyroid cancer cell line (ARO). The inhibitory effect of apigenin was associated with inhibition of EGFR tyrosine phosphorylation and downstream mitogen-activated protein kinase phosphorylation. The effective concentration ranged from 12.5 to $50\,\mu\mathrm{M}$ [139]. Apigenin may have mechanisms of action in addition to interference with EGFR signaling [140–142]. It is a promising agent that should be further investigated against undifferentiated and anaplastic thyroid cancers [139].

9.3. *Troglitazone*

Peroxisome proliferator-activated receptors (PPAR) are nuclear receptors involved in tumor progression, cellular differentiation, and apoptosis [143]. Ligands for PPAR gamma (PPARγ) induce apoptosis and inhibit proliferation in various carcinoma cell lines [144–147].

Troglitazone is a PPARγ agonist. The antineoplastic effect of troglitazone was studied in six cell lines from patients with papillary thyroid carcinoma [148]. Three of the six samples of papillary thyroid carcinoma expressed more PPARγ than did adjacent normal thyroid tissue. PPARγ-positive thyroid cancer cells were incubated with the PPARγ agonists: troglitazone (10 μM), 15-deoxy-12,14-prostaglandin J2 (1 μg mL^{-1}), and BRL 49653 (10 μM). All three drugs inhibited ^{3}H-thymidine incorporation and induced apoptosis.

Troglitazone induced the expression of c-*myc* mRNA but had no effect on *bcl-2* and *bax* expression. Troglitazone (500 mg kg^{-1} daily) inhibited tumor growth and metastasis of papillary thyroid carcinoma xenografts in nude mice. These results suggest that troglitazone can inhibit tumor growth of some papillary thyroid cancers that express PPARγ [148].

9.4. *Tumor necrosis factor-related apoptosis inducing ligand (TRAIL)*

In an *in vitro* study with a number of thyroid cancer cell lines (TPC-1, NPA, SW579, and two anaplastic cell lines ARO and FRO), TRAIL triggered significant apoptosis and was more effective than TNF-α and Fas [149]. Investigation of apoptosis induction via the death-receptor pathway may lead to the development of a distinct group of antineoplastic agents.

9.5. *c*-myc *antisense oligonucleotides*

Analysis of c-*myc* mRNA relative to normal thyroid tissue in seven human thyroid carcinoma cell lines and in 50 thyroid tumor specimens revealed a higher level of c-*myc* expression in all the cell lines and in several thyroid tumor specimens [150]. Inhibition of c-Myc protein synthesis using *c-myc*-specific antisense oligonucleotides inhibited growth of the thyroid cancer cell lines [150]. These results suggest that c-*myc* may contribute significantly to the growth of some thyroid cancers and that further investigation of c-*myc* antisense oligonucleotides as an antineoplastic agent for thyroid cancer is indicated [150].

10. Conclusion

Although there have been moderate advances over the past decade in preclinical studies of chemotherapeutics for undifferentiated and anaplastic thyroid cancers, progress in the treatment of this disease is lagging and compared to other types of cancer. Much translational work needs to be done to bring promising agents to actual clinical use to benefit patients with aggressive thyroid cancers.

References

[1] K.B. Ain, Anaplastic thyroid carcinoma: behavior, biology, and therapeutic approaches, Thyroid 8 (1998) 715–726.
[2] D. Giuffrida, H. Gharib, Anaplastic thyroid carcinoma: current diagnosis and treatment, Ann. Oncol. 11 (2000) 1083–1089.

[3] H. Asakawa, T. Kobayashi, Y. Komoike, H. Maruyama, Y. Nakano, Y. Tamaki, Y. Matsuzawa, M. Monden, Chemosensitivity of anaplastic thyroid carcinoma and poorly differentiated thyroid carcinoma, Anticancer Res. 17 (1997) 2757–2762.

[4] H. Asakawa, T. Kobayashi, Y. Komoike, T. Yanagawa, M. Takahashi, E. Wakasugi, H. Maruyama, Y. Tamaki, Y. Matsuzawa, M. Monden, Establishment of anaplastic thyroid carcinoma cell lines useful for analysis of chemosensitivity and carcinogenesis, J. Clin. Endocrinol. Metab. 81 (1996) 3547–3552.

[5] D.A. Gewirtz, A critical evaluation of the mechanisms of action proposed for the antitumor effects of the anthracycline antibiotics adriamycin and daunorubicin, Biochem. Pharmacol. 57 (1999) 727–741.

[6] L.S. Lessin, M. Min, Chemotherapy of anaplastic thyroid cancer, in: L. Wartofsky (Ed.), Thyroid Cancer: a comprehensive guide to clinical management, Humana Press, Totowa, New Jersey, 2000, pp. 337–340.

[7] J.H. Kim, R.D. Leeper, Treatment of anaplastic giant and spindle cell carcinoma of the thyroid gland with combination Adriamycin and radiation therapy. A new approach, Cancer 52 (1983) 954–957.

[8] J.H. Kim, R.D. Leeper, Treatment of locally advanced thyroid carcinoma with combination doxorubicin and radiation therapy, Cancer 60 (1987) 2372–2375.

[9] J. Tennvall, E. Tallroth, A. el Hassan, G. Lundell, M. Akerman, A. Biorklund, H. Blomgren, T. Lowhagen, G. Wallin, Anaplastic thyroid carcinoma. Doxorubicin, hyperfractionated radiotherapy and surgery, Acta Oncologica 29 (1990) 1025–1028.

[10] J. Tennvall, G. Lundell, A. Hallquist, P. Wahlberg, G. Wallin, S. Tibblin, Combined doxorubicin, hyperfractionated radiotherapy, and surgery in anaplastic thyroid carcinoma. Report on two protocols. The Swedish Anaplastic Thyroid Cancer Group, Cancer 74 (1994) 1348–1354.

[11] J. Tennvall, G. Lundell, P. Wahlberg, A. Bergenfelz, L. Grimelius, M. Akerman, A.L. Hjelm Skog, G. Wallin, Anaplastic thyroid carcinoma: three protocols combining doxorubicin, hyperfractionated radiotherapy and surgery, Br. J. Cancer 86 (2002) 1848–1853.

[12] M. Schlumberger, C. Parmentier, M.J. Delisle, J.E. Couette, J.P. Droz, D. Sarrazin, Combination therapy for anaplastic giant cell thyroid carcinoma, Cancer 67 (1991) 564–566.

[13] B.R. Haugen, Management of the patient with progressive radioiodine non-responsive disease, Semin. Surg. Oncol. 16 (1999) 34–41.

[14] L.S. Fincman, T.A. Hamilton, A. de Gortari, P. Bonney, Cisplatin chemotherapy for treatment of thyroid carcinoma in dogs: 13 cases, J. Amer. Animal Hosp. Assoc. 34 (1998) 109–112.

[15] J.C. Morris, C.K. Kim, M.L. Padilla, J.I. Mechanick, Conversion of non-iodine-concentrating differentiated thyroid carcinoma metastases into iodine-concentrating foci after anticancer chemotherapy, Thyroid 7 (1997) 63–66.

[16] K.L. Seley, Tezacitabine, Curr. Opin. Investig. Drugs 1 (2000) 135–140.

[17] Y. Zhou, G. Achanta, H. Pelicano, V. Gandhi, W. Plunkett, P. Huang, Action of (E)-2'-deoxy-2'-(fluoromethylene)cytidine on DNA metabolism: incorporation, excision, and cellular response, Mol. Pharmacol. 61 (2002) 222–229.

[18] R. Kotchetkov, A.A. Krivtchik, J. Cinatl, B. Kornhuber, J. Cinatl Jr., Selective cytotoxic activity of a novel ribonucleoside diphosphate reductase inhibitor MDL-101,731 against thyroid cancer *in vitro*, Folia Biol. (Praha) 45 (1999) 185–191.

[19] L.Q. Sun, Y.X. Li, L. Guillou, P.A. Coucke, (E)-2'-deoxy-2'-(fluoromethylene) cytidine potentiates radioresponse of two human solid tumor xenografts, Cancer Res. 58 (1998) 5411–5417.

[20] G. Qu, E.A. Perez, Gemcitabine and targeted therapy in metastatic breast cancer, Semin. Oncol. 29 (2002) 44–52.

[21] A. Depierre, V. Westeel, P. Jacoulet, Gemcitabine induction chemotherapy in non-small cell lung cancer, Semin. Oncol. 29 (2002) 55–60.

[22] S. Culine, The present and future of combination chemotherapy in bladder cancer, Semin. Oncol. 29 (2002) 32–39.

[23] V. Heinemann, Present and future treatment of pancreatic cancer, Semin. Oncol. 29 (2002) 23–31.

[24] M.D. Ringel, M. Greenberg, X. Chen, N. Hayre, K. Suzuki, D. Priebat, M. Saji, K.D. Burman, Cytotoxic activity of 2′,2′-difluorodeoxycytidine (gemcitabine) in poorly differentiated thyroid carcinoma cells, Thyroid 10 (2000) 865–869.

[25] W. Voigt, A. Bulankin, T. Muller, C. Schoeber, A. Grothey, C. Hoang-Vu, H.J. Schmoll, Schedule-dependent antagonism of gemcitabine and cisplatin in human anaplastic thyroid cancer cell lines, Clin. Cancer Res. 6 (2000) 2087–2093.

[26] R. Kotchetkov, B. Groschel, W.H. Gmeiner, A.A. Krivtchik, E. Trump, M. Bitoova, J. Cinatl, B. Kornhuber, Antineoplastic activity of a novel multimeric gemcitabine-monophosphate prodrug against thyroid cancer cells *in vitro*, Anticancer Res. 20 (2000) 2915–2922.

[27] M.V. Blagosklonny, T. Fojo, Molecular effects of paclitaxel: myths and reality (a critical review), Int. J. Cancer 83 (1999) 151–156.

[28] P.J. Moos, F.A. Fitzpatrick, Taxanes propagate apoptosis via two cell populations with distinctive cytological and molecular traits, Cell Growth Diff. 9 (1998) 687–697.

[29] R. Danesi, W.D. Figg, E. Reed, C.E. Myers, Paclitaxel (taxol) inhibits protein isoprenylation and induces apoptosis in PC-3 human prostate cancer cells, Molec. Pharmacol. 47 (1995) 1106–1111.

[30] D. Debernardis, E.G. Sire, P. De Feudis, F. Vikhanskaya, M. Valenti, P. Russo, S. Parodi, M. D'Incalci, M. Broggini, p53 status does not affect sensitivity of human ovarian cancer cell lines to paclitaxel, Cancer Res. 57 (1997) 870–874.

[31] J.S. Lanni, S.W. Lowe, E.J. Licitra, J.O. Liu, T. Jacks, p53-independent apoptosis induced by paclitaxel through an indirect mechanism, Proc. Natl. Acad. Sci. U.S.A. 94 (1997) 9679–9683.

[32] H. Safran, T. King, H. Choy, A. Gollerkeri, H. Kwakwa, F. Lopez, B. Cole, J. Myers, J. Tarpey, A. Rosmarin, p53 Mutations do not predict response to paclitaxel/radiation for nonsmall cell lung carcinoma, Cancer 78 (1996) 1203–1210.

[33] S.S. Bacus, A.V. Gudkov, M. Lowe, L. Lyass, Y. Yung, A.P. Komarov, K. Keyomarsi, Y. Yarden, R. Seger, Taxol-induced apoptosis depends on MAP kinase pathways (ERK and p38) and is independent of p53, Oncogene 20 (2001) 147–155.

[34] J. Okano, A.K. Rustgi, Paclitaxel induces prolonged activation of the Ras/MEK/ERK pathway independently of activating the programmed cell death machinery, J. Biol. Chem. 276 (2001) 19555–19564.

[35] A.A. Stone, T.C. Chambers, Microtubule inhibitors elicit differential effects on MAP kinase (JNK, ERK, and p38) signaling pathways in human KB-3 carcinoma cells, Exper. Cell Res. 254 (2000) 110–119.

[36] L.G. Wang, X.M. Liu, W. Kreis, D.R. Budman, The effect of antimicrotubule agents on signal transduction pathways of apoptosis: a review, Cancer Chemother. Pharmacol. 44 (1999) 355–361.

[37] R.K. Srivastava, A.R. Srivastava, S.J. Korsmeyer, M. Nesterova, Y.S. Cho-Chung, D.L. Longo, Involvement of microtubules in the regulation of Bcl2 phosphorylation and apoptosis through cyclic AMP-dependent protein kinase, Molec. Cellular Biol. 18 (1998) 3509–3517.

[38] K.B. Ain, S. Tofiq, K.D. Taylor, Antineoplastic activity of taxol against human anaplastic thyroid carcinoma cell lines *in vitro* and *in vivo*, J. Clin. Endo. Metab. 81 (1996) 3650–3653.

[39] K.B. Ain, M.J. Egorin, P.A. DeSimone, Treatment of anaplastic thyroid carcinoma with paclitaxel: phase 2 trial using ninety-six-hour infusion. Collaborative Anaplastic Thyroid Cancer Health Intervention Trials (CATCHIT) Group, Thyroid 10 (2000) 587–594.

[40] S.C. Yeung, G. Xu, J. Pan, M. Christgen, A. Bamiagis, Manumycin enhances the cytotoxic effect of paclitaxel on anaplastic thyroid carcinoma cells, Cancer Res. 60 (2000) 650–656.

[41] M.M. Moasser, L. Sepp-Lorenzino, N.E. Kohl, A. Oliff, A. Balog, D.S. Su, S.J. Danishefsky, N. Rosen, Farnesyl transferase inhibitors cause enhanced mitotic sensitivity to taxol and epothilones, Proc. Natl. Acad. Sci. U.S.A. 95 (1998) 1369–1374.

[42] L.L. Nielsen, B. Shi, G. Hajian, B. Yaremko, P. Lipari, E. Ferrari, M. Gurnani, M. Malkowski, J. Chen, W.R. Bishop, M. Liu, Combination therapy with the farnesyl protein transferase inhibitor SCH66336 and SCH58500 (p53 adenovirus) in preclinical cancer models, Cancer Res. 59 (1999) 5896–5901.

[43] G. Xu, J. Pan, C. Martin, S.C. Yeung, Angiogenesis inhibition in the *in vivo* antineoplastic effect of manumycin and paclitaxel against anaplastic thyroid carcinoma, J. Clin. Endo. Metab. 86 (2001) 1769–1777.

[44] M. Karbowski, J.H. Spodnik, M. Teranishi, M. Wozniak, Y. Nishizawa, J. Usukura, T. Waka-bayashi, Opposite effects of microtubule-stabilizing and microtubule-destabilizing drugs on biogenesis of mitochondria in mammalian cells, J. Cell. Sci. 114 (2001) 281–291.

[45] P. Roswall, S. Bu, K. Rubin, M. Landstrom, N.E. Heldin, 2-Methoxyestradiol (2-ME) induces apoptosis in anaplastic thyroid carcinoma cells. In: 74th Annual Meeting of the American Thyroid Association, Los Angeles, 2002, Abstract 149, 184pp.

[46] V.K. Ngan, K. Bellman, B.T. Hill, L. Wilson, M.A. Jordan, Mechanism of mitotic block and inhibition of cell proliferation by the semisynthetic Vinca alkaloids vinorelbine and its newer derivative vinflunine, Mol. Pharmacol. 60 (2001) 225–232.

[47] K. Fukuoka, H. Arioka, Y. Iwamoto, H. Fukumoto, H. Kurokawa, T. Ishida, A. Tomonari, T. Suzuki, J. Usuda, F. Kanzawa, N. Saijo, K. Nishio, Mechanism of the radiosensitization induced by vinorelbine in human non-small cell lung cancer cells, Lung Cancer 34 (2001) 451–460.

[48] L. Zelek, S. Barthier, M. Riofrio, K. Fizazi, O. Rixe, J.P. Delord, A. Le Cesne, M. Spielmann, Weekly vinorelbine is an effective palliative regimen after failure with anthracyclines and taxanes in metastatic breast carcinoma, Cancer 92 (2001) 2267–2272.

[49] P.E. Goretzki, C. Dotzenrath, K.M. schulte, D. Simon, H.D. Roher, Oncogenes and tumor suppressor genes in differentiated thyroid cancer, in: O.H. Clark, S. Noguchi (Eds.), Thyroid Cancer: Diagnosis and Treatment, Quality Medical Publishing, St. Louis, Missouri, 2000, pp. 365–378.

[50] E. Zwick, J. Bange, A. Ullrich, Receptor tyrosine kinase signalling as a target for cancer intervention strategies, Endocrine-Related Cancer 8 (2001) 161–173.

[51] D. Hao, E.K. Rowinsky, Inhibiting signal transduction: recent advances in the development of receptor tyrosine kinase and Ras inhibitors, Cancer Invest. 20 (2002) 387–404.

[52] M.J. Morin, From oncogene to drug: development of small molecule tyrosine kinase inhibitors as anti-tumor and anti-angiogenic agents, Oncogene 19 (2000) 6574–6583.

[53] J.D. Bergstrom, A. Hermansson, T. Diaz de Stahl, N.E. Heldin, Non-autocrine, constitutive activation of Met in human anaplastic thyroid carcinoma cells in culture, Brit. J. Cancer 80 (1999) 650–656.

[54] J.D. Bergstrom, B. Westermark, N.E. Heldin, Epidermal growth factor receptor signaling activates met in human anaplastic thyroid carcinoma cells, Exp. Cell Res. 259 (2000) 293–299.

[55] E. Buchdunger, U. Trinks, H. Mett, U. Regenass, M. Muller, T. Meyer, E. McGlynn, L.A. Pinna, P. Traxler, N.B. Lydon, 4,5-Dianilinophthalimide: a protein-tyrosine kinase inhibitor with selectivity for the epidermal growth factor receptor signal transduction pathway and potent *in vivo* antitumor activity, Proc. Natl.Acad. Sci. U.S.A. 91 (1994) 2334–2338.

[56] E. Buchdunger, H. Mett, U. Trinks, U. Regenass, M. Muller, T. Meyer, P. Beilstein, B. Wirz, P. Schneider, P. Traxler, 4,5-bis(4-fluoroanilino)phthalimide: A selective inhibitor of the epidermal growth factor receptor signal transduction pathway with potent *in vivo* antitumor activity, Clin. Cancer Res. 1 (1995) 813–821.

[57] P. Furet, G. Caravatti, N. Lydon, J.P. Priestle, J.M. Sowadski, U. Trinks, P. Traxler, Modelling study of protein kinase inhibitors: binding mode of staurosporine and origin of the selectivity of CGP 52411, J. Computer-Aided Molec. Design 9 (1995) 465–472.

[58] C.P. Dinney, C. Parker, Z. Dong, D. Fan, B.Y. Eve, C. Bucana, R. Radinsky, Therapy of human transitional cell carcinoma of the bladder by oral administration of the epidermal growth factor receptor protein tyrosine kinase inhibitor 4,5-dianilinophthalimide, Clin. Cancer Res. 3 (1997) 161–168.

[59] T. Schindler, F. Sicheri, A. Pico, A. Gazit, A. Levitzki, J. Kuriyan, Crystal structure of Hck in complex with a Src family selective tyrosine kinase inhibitor, Mol. Cell 3 (1999) 639–648.

[60] F. Carlomagno, D. Vitagliano, T. Guida, M. Napolitano, G. Vecchio, A. Fusco, A. Gazit, A. Levitzki, M. Santoro, The kinase inhibitor PP1 blocks tumorigenesis induced by RET oncogenes, Cancer Res. 62 (2002) 1077–1082.

[61] M. Hara, K. Akasaka, S. Akinaga, M. Okabe, H. Nakano, R. Gomez, D. Wood, M. Uh, F. Tamanoi, Identification of Ras farnesyltransferase inhibitors by microbial screening, Proc. Natl. Acad. Sci. U.S.A. 90 (1993) 2281–2285.

[62] F. Tamanoi, Inhibitors of Ras farnesyltransferases, Trends Biochem Sci. 18 (1993) 349–353.

[63] J.B. Gibbs, N.E. Kohl, K.S. Koblan, C.A. Omer, L. Sepp-Lorenzino, N. Rosen, N.J. Anthony, M.W. Conner, S.J. deSolms, T.M. Williams, S.L. Graham, G.D. Hartman, A. Oliff, Farnesyl-ransferase inhibitors and anti-Ras therapy, Breast. Cancer Res. Treat. 38 (1996) 75–83.

[64] J.B. Gibbs, A. Oliff, The potential of farnesyltransferase inhibitors as cancer chemotherapeutics, Ann. Rev. Pharmacol. Toxicol. 37 (1997) 143–166.

[65] E.C. Lerner, A.D. Hamilton, S.M. Sebti, Inhibition of Ras prenylation: a signaling target for novel anti-cancer drug design, Anti-Cancer Drug Design 12 (1997) 229–238.

[66] C.A. Omer, N.E. Kohl, CA1A2X-competitive inhibitors of farnesyltransferase as anti-cancer agents, Trends Pharmacol. Sci. 18 (1997) 437–444.

[67] S. Sebti, A.D. Hamilton, Inhibitors of prenyl transferases, Curr. Opin. Oncol. 9 (1997) 557–561.

[68] D.B. Whyte, P. Kirschmeier, T.N. Hockenberry, I. Nunez-Oliva, L. James, J.J. Catino, W.R. Bish-op, J.K. Pai, K- and N-Ras are geranylgeranylated in cells treated with farnesyl protein transferase inhibitors, J. Biol. Chem. 272 (1997) 14459–14464.

[69] C.A. Rowell, J.J. Kowalczyk, M.D. Lewis, A.M. Garcia, Direct demonstration of geranylgeranylat-ion and farnesylation of Ki-Ras *in vivo*, J. Biol. Chem. 272 (1997) 14093–14097.

[70] P.F. Lebowitz, D. Sakamuro, G.C. Prendergast, Farnesyl transferase inhibitors induce apoptosis of Ras-transformed cells denied substratum attachment, Cancer Res. 57 (1997) 708–713.

[71] H. Ura, T. Obara, R. Shudo, A. Itoh, S. Tanno, T. Fujii, N. Nishino, Y. Kohgo, Selective cyto-toxicity of farnesylamine to pancreatic carcinoma cells and Ki-ras-transformed fibroblasts, Molec. Carcinogenesis. 21 (1998) 93–99.

[72] W. Wang, R.J. Macaulay, Apoptosis of medulloblastoma cells *in vitro* follows inhibition of far-nesylation using manumycin A, Int. J. Cancer 82 (1999) 430–434.

[73] P. Norgaard, B. Law, H. Joseph, D.L. Page, Y. Shyr, D. Mays, J.A. Pietenpol, N.E. Kohl, A. Oliff, R.J. Coffey Jr., H.S. Poulsen, H.L. Moses, Treatment with farnesyl-protein transferase inhibitor induces regression of mammary tumors in transforming growth factor (TGF) alpha and TGF alpha/neu transgenic mice by inhibition of mitogenic activity and induction of apoptosis, Clin. Cancer Res. 5 (1999) 35–42.

[74] M. Liu, M.S. Bryant, J. Chen, S. Lee, B. Yaremko, P. Lipari, M. Malkowski, E. Ferrari, L. Nielsen, N. Prioli, J. Dell, D. Sinha, J. Syed, W.A. Korfmacher, A.A. Nomeir, C.C. Lin, L. Wang, A.G. Taveras, R.J. Doll, F.G. Njoroge, A.K. Mallams, S. Remiszewski, J.J. Catino, V.M. Girijavallab-han, W.R. Bishop, et al., Antitumor activity of SCH 66336, an orally bioavailable tricyclic inhibitor of farnesyl protein transferase, in human tumor xenograft models and wap-ras transgenic mice, Cancer Res. 58 (1998) 4947–4956.

[75] L. Sepp-Lorenzino, Z. Ma, E. Rands, N.E. Kohl, J.B. Gibbs, A. Oliff, N. Rosen, A Peptidomimetic inhibitor of farnesyl: protein transferase blocks the anchorage-dependent and -independent growth of human tumor cell lines, Cancer Res. 55 (1995) 5302–5309.

[76] P. Servais, B. Gulbis, D. Fokan, P. Galand, Effects of the farnesyltransferase inhibitor UCF-1C/manumycin on growth and p21-ras post-translational processing in NIH3T3 cells, Int. J. Cancer 76 (1998) 601–608.

[77] W. Yang, K. Del Villar, J. Urano, H. Mitsuzawa, F. Tamanoi, Advances in the development of farnesyltransferase inhibitors: substrate recognition by protein farnesyltransferase, J. Cell Biochem. Suppl. 27 (1997) 12–19.

[78] T. Nagase, S. Kawata, S. Tamura, Y. Matsuda, Y. Inui, E. Yamasaki, H. Ishiguro, T. Ito, Y. Matsuzawa, Inhibition of cell growth of human hepatoma cell line (Hep G2) by a farnesyl protein transferase inhibitor: a preferential suppression of ras farnesylation, Int. J. Cancer 65 (1996) 620–626.

[79] T. Nagase, S. Kawata, S. Tamura, Y. Matsuda, Y. Inui, E. Yamasaki, H. Ishiguro, T. Ito, J. Miyagawa, H. Mitsui, K. Yamamoto, M. Kinoshita, Y. Matsuzawa, Manumycin and gliotoxin derivative KT7595 block Ras farnesylation and cell growth but do not disturb lamin farnesylation and localization in human tumour cells, Brit. J. Cancer 76 (1997) 1001–1010.

[80] T. Ito, S. Kawata, S. Tamura, T. Igura, T. Nagase, J.I. Miyagawa, E. Yamazaki, H. Ishiguro, Y. Matasuzawa, Suppression of human pancreatic cancer growth in BALB/c nude mice by man-umycin, a farnesyl: protein transferase inhibitor, Jap. J. Cancer Res. 87 (1996) 113–116.

[81] O. Kainuma, T. Asano, M. Hasegawa, T. Kenmochi, T. Nakagohri, Y. Tokoro, K. Isono, Inhibition of growth and invasive activity of human pancreatic cancer cells by a farnesyltransferase inhibitor, manumycin, Pancreas 15 (1997) 379–383.

[82] J. Pan, G. Xu, A.E. Bamiagis, S.C. Yeung, Cytochrome c and caspase-3, caspase-8 and caspase-9 are involved in the enhanced apoptosis of anaplastic thyroid cancer cells induced by the combination of manumycin and paclitaxel, J. Clin. Endo. Metab. 86 (2001) 4731–4740.

[83] C.L. Strickland, P.C. Weber, W.T. Windsor, Z. Wu, H.V. Le, M.M. Albanese, C.S. Alvarez, D. Cesarz, J. del Rosario, J. Deskus, A.K. Mallams, F.G. Njoroge, J.J. Piwinski, S. Remiszewski, R.R. Rossman, A.G. Taveras, B. Vibulbhan, R.J. Doll, V.M. Girijavallabhan, A.K. Ganguly, Tricyclic farnesyl protein transferase inhibitors: crystallographic and calorimetric studies of structure-activity relationships, J. Med. Chem. 42 (1999) 2125–2135.

[84] T. Petit, E. Izbicka, R.A. Lawrence, W.R. Bishop, S. Weitman, D.D. Von Hoff, Activity of SCH 66336, a tricyclic farnesyltransferase inhibitor, against human tumor colony-forming units, Ann. Oncol. 10 (1999) 449–453.

[85] J. Pan, G. Xu, S.C. Yeung, Cytochrome c release is upstream to activation of caspase-9, caspase-8, and caspase-3 in the enhanced apoptosis of anaplastic thyroid cancer cells induced by manumycin and paclitaxel, J. Clin. Endo. Metab. 86 (2001) 4731–4740.

[86] V.W. van Hinsbergh, A. Collen, P. Koolwijk, Angiogenesis and anti-angiogenesis: perspectives for the treatment of solid tumors, Ann. Oncol. 10 (1999) 60–63.

[87] W. Wynendaele, A.T. van Oosterom, A. Pawinski, E.A. de Bruijn, R.A. Maes, Angiogenesis: possibilities for therapeutic interventions, Pharm. World Sci. 20 (1998) 225–235.

[88] B.A. Teicher, S.A. Holden, G. Ara, D. Northey, Response of the FSaII fibrosarcoma to anti-angiogenic modulators plus cytotoxic agents, Anticancer Res. 13 (1993) 2101–2106.

[89] B.A. Teicher, S.A. Holden, G. Ara, E.A. Sotomayor, Z.D. Huang, Y.N. Chen, H. Brem, Potentiation of cytotoxic cancer therapies by TNP-470 alone and with other anti-angiogenic agents, Int. J. Cancer 57 (1994) 920–925.

[90] Y. Hama, T. Shimizu, S. Hosaka, A. Sugenoya, N. Usuda, Therapeutic efficacy of the angiogenesis inhibitor O-(chloroacetyl-carbamoyl) fumagillol (TNP-470; AGM-1470) for human anaplastic thyroid carcinoma in nude mice, Exp. Toxicol. Pathol. 49 (1997) 239–247.

[91] G.M. Tozer, C. Kanthou, C.S. Parkins, S.A. Hill, The biology of the combretastatins as tumour vascular targeting agents, Int. J. Exp. Pathol. 83 (2002) 21–38.

[92] A. Dowlati, K. Robertson, M. Cooney, W.P. Petros, M. Stratford, J. Jesberger, N. Rafie, B. Overmoyer, V. Makkar, B. Stambler, A. Taylor, J. Waas, J.S. Lewin, K.R. McCrae, S.C. Remick, A phase I pharmacokinetic and translational study of the novel vascular targeting agent combretastatin a-4 phosphate on a single-dose intravenous schedule in patients with advanced cancer, Cancer Res. 62 (2002) 3408–3416.

[93] J. Dziba, G. Marcinek, G.M. Venkataraman, J. Robinson, K. Ain, Combretastatin A4 phosphate has primary antineoplastic activity against human anaplastic thyroid carcinoma cell lines and xenograft tumors, in: 74th Annual Meeting of the American Thyroid Association, Los Angeles, Abstract 179, 199pp., 2002.

[94] R. Bicknell, A.L. Harris, Mechanisms and therapeutic implications of angiogenesis, Curr. Opin. Oncol. 8 (1996) 60–65.

[95] C. de Vries, J.A. Escobedo, H. Ueno, K. Houck, N. Ferrara, L.T. Williams, The fms-like tyrosine kinase, a receptor for vascular endothelial growth factor, Science 255 (1992) 989–991.

[96] B.I. Terman, M. Dougher-Vermazen, M.E. Carrion, D. Dimitrov, D.C. Armellino, D. Gospodarowicz, P. Bohlen, Identification of the KDR tyrosine kinase as a receptor for vascular endothelial cell growth factor, Biochem. Biophys. Res. Comm. 187 (1992) 1579–1586.

[97] F.C. White, A. Benehacene, J.S. Scheele, M. Kamps, VEGF mRNA is stabilized by ras and tyrosine kinase oncogenes, as well as by UV radiation-evidence for divergent stabilization pathways, Growth Factors 14 (1997) 199–212.

[98] S. Charvat, M. Duchesne, P. Parvaz, M.C. Chignol, D. Schmitt, M. Serres, The up-regulation of vascular endothelial growth factor in mutated Ha-ras HaCaT cell lines is reduced by a farnesyl transferase inhibitor, Anticancer Res. 19 (1999) 557–561.

[99] M.M. Feldkamp, N. Lau, J. Rak, R.S. Kerbel, A. Guha, Normoxic and hypoxic regulation of vascular endothelial growth factor (VEGF) by astrocytoma cells is mediated by Ras. Int. J. Cancer 81 (1999) 118–124.

[100] W.Z. Gu, S.K. Tahir, Y.C. Wang, H.C. Zhang, S.P. Cherian, S. O'Connor, J.A. Leal, S.H. Rosenberg, S.C. Ng, Effect of novel CAAX peptidomimetic farnesyltransferase inhibitor on angiogenesis *in vitro* and *in vivo*, Euro. J. Cancer 35 (1999) 1394–1401.

[101] E. Buchdunger, C.L. Cioffi, N. Law, D. Stover, S. Ohno-Jones, B.J. Druker, N.B. Lydon, Abl protein-tyrosine kinase inhibitor STI571 inhibits *in vitro* signal transduction mediated by c-kit and platelet-derived growth factor receptors, J. Pharmacol. Exp. Ther. 295 (2000) 139–145.

[102] D. George, Platelet-derived growth factor receptors: a therapeutic target in solid tumors, Semin. Oncol. 28 (2001) 27–33.

[103] K. Pietras, A. Ostman, M. Sjoquist, E. Buchdunger, R.K. Reed, C.H. Heldin, K. Rubin, Inhibition of platelet-derived growth factor receptors reduces interstitial hypertension and increases transcapillary transport in tumors, Cancer Res. 61 (2001) 2929–2934.

[104] K. Pietras, K. Rubin, T. Sjoblom, E. Buchdunger, M. Sjoquist, C.-H. Heldin, A. Ostman, Inhibition of PDGF receptor signaling in tumor stroma enhances antitumor affect of chemotherapy, Cancer Res. 62 (2002) 5476–5484.

[105] B. Shahedian, Y. Shi, M. Zou, N.R. Farid, Thyroid carcinoma is characterized by genomic instability: evidence from p53 mutations, Mol. Genet. Metab. 72 (2001) 155–163.

[106] Y. Nagayama, H. Yokoi, K. Takeda, M. Hasegawa, E. Nishihara, H. Namba, S. Yamashita, M. Niwa, Adenovirus-mediated tumor suppressor p53 gene therapy for anaplastic thyroid carcinoma *in vitro* and *in vivo*, J. Clin. Endo. Metab. 85 (2000) 4081–4086.

[107] M.V. Blagosklonny, P. Giannakakou, M. Wojtowicz, L.Y. Romanova, K.B. Ain, S.E. Bates, T. Fojo, Effects of p53-expressing adenovirus on the chemosensitivity and differentiation of anaplastic thyroid cancer cells, J. Clin. Endo. Metab. 83 (1998) 2516–2522.

[108] H. Shimura, H. Suzuki, A. Miyazaki, F. Furuya, K. Ohta, K. Haraguchi, T. Endo, T. Onaya, Transcriptional activation of the thyroglobulin promoter directing suicide gene expression by thyroid transcription factor-1 in thyroid cancer cells, Cancer Res. 61 (2001) 3640–3646.

[109] M. Kitazono, Y. Chuman, T. Aikou, T. Fojo, Construction of gene therapy vectors targeting thyroid cells: enhancement of activity and specificity with histone deacetylase inhibitors and agents modulating the cyclic adenosine 3′,5′-monophosphate pathway and demonstration of activity in follicular and anaplastic thyroid carcinoma cells, J. Clin. Endo. Metab. 86 (2001) 834–840.

[110] G. Portella, S. Scala, D. Vitagliano, G. Vecchio, A. Fusco, ONYX-015, an E1B gene-defective adenovirus, induces cell death in human anaplastic thyroid carcinoma cell lines, J. Clin. Endo. Metab. 87 (2002) 2525–2531.

[111] R. Brown, G. Strathdee, Epigenomics and epigenetic therapy of cancer, Trends Molec. Med. 8 (2002) S43–S48.

[112] A.R. Karpf, D.A. Jones, Reactivating the expression of methylation silenced genes in human cancer, Oncogene 21 (2002) 5496–5503.

[113] G.M. Venkataraman, M. Yatin, R. Marcinek, K.B. Ain, Restoration of iodide uptake in dedifferentiated thyroid carcinoma: relationship to human Na + /I-symporter gene methylation status, J. Clin. Endo. Metab. 84 (1999) 2449–2457.

[114] T. Kogai, J.M. Hershman, K. Motomura, T. Endo, T. Onaya, G.A. Brent, Differential regulation of the human sodium/iodide symporter gene promoter in papillary thyroid carcinoma cell lines and normal thyroid cells, Endocrinology 142 (2001) 3369–3379.

[115] S.G. Gray, B.T. Teh, Histone acetylation/deacetylation and cancer: an "open" and "shut" case?, Current Molec. Med. 1 (2001) 401–429.

[116] C. Wang, M. Fu, S. Mani, S. Wadler, A.M. Senderowicz, R.G. Pestell, Histone acetylation and the cell-cycle in cancer, Front Bioscience 6 (2001) D610–629.

[117] M. Yoshida, R. Furumai, M. Nishiyama, Y. Komatsu, N. Nishino, S. Horinouchi, Histone deacetylase as a new target for cancer chemotherapy, Cancer Chemother. Pharmacol. 48 (2001) S20–S26.

[118] W.G. Zhu, R.R. Lakshmanan, M.D. Beal, G.A. Otterson, DNA methyltransferase inhibition enhances apoptosis induced by histone deacetylase inhibitors, Cancer Res. 61 (2001) 1327–1333.

[119] V.L. Greenberg, J.M. Williams, J.P. Cogswell, M. Mendenhall, S.G. Zimmer, Histone deacetylase inhibitors promote apoptosis and differential cell cycle arrest in anaplastic thyroid cancer cells, Thyroid 11 (2001) 315–325.

[120] P. Garcia-Villalba, A.M. Jimenez-Lara, A.I. Castillo, A. Aranda, Histone acetylation influences thyroid hormone and retinoic acid-mediated gene expression, DNA Cell Biol. 16 (1997) 421–431.

[121] M.S. Eigelberger, M.G. Wong, Q.Y. Duh, O.H. Clark, Phenylacetate enhances the antiproliferative effect of retinoic acid in follicular thyroid cancer, Surgery 130 (2001) 931–935.

[122] C. Schmutzler, J. Kohrle, Retinoic acid redifferentiation therapy for thyroid cancer, Thyroid 10 (2000) 393–406.

[123] D. Simon, J. Kohrle, C. Schmutzler, K. Mainz, C. Reiners, H.D. Roher, Redifferentiation therapy of differentiated thyroid carcinoma with retinoic acid: basics and first clinical results, Exp. Clin. Endocrinol. Diabetes 104 (1996) 13–15.

[124] F. Grunwald, E. Pakos, H. Bender, C. Menzel, R. Otte, H. Palmedo, U. Pfeifer, H.J. Biersack, Redifferentiation therapy with retinoic acid in follicular thyroid cancer, J. Nucl. Med. 39 (1998) 1555–1558.

[125] D. Simon, J. Koehrle, C. Reiners, A.R. Boerner, C. Schmutzler, K. Mainz, P.E. Goretzki, H.D. Roeher, Redifferentiation therapy with retinoids: therapeutic option for advanced follicular and papillary thyroid carcinoma, World J. Surg. 22 (1998) 569–574.

[126] T. Matsumoto, Y. Sowa, N. Ohtani-Fujita, T. Tamaki, T. Takenaka, K. Kuribayashi, T. Sakai, p53-independent induction of WAF1/Cip1 is correlated with osteoblastic differentiation by vitamin D3, Cancer Lett. 129 (1998) 61–68.

[127] A. Muto, M. Kizaki, K. Yamato, Y. Kawai, M. Kamata-Matsushita, H. Ueno, M. Ohguchi, T. Nishihara, H.P. Koeffler, Y. Ikeda, 1,25-Dihydroxyvitamin D3 induces differentiation of a retinoic acid-resistant acute promyelocytic leukemia cell line (UF-1) associated with expression of p21(WAF1/CIP1) and p27(KIP1), Blood 93 (1999) 2225–2233.

[128] W. Liu, S.L. Asa, I.G. Fantus, P.G. Walfish, S. Ezzat, Vitamin D arrests thyroid carcinoma cell growth and induces p27 dephosphorylation and accumulation through PTEN/akt-dependent and -independent pathways, Am. J. Pathol. 160 (2002) 511–519.

[129] J. Matousek, Ribonucleases and their antitumor activity, Comp. Biochem. Physiol. Toxicol. Pharmacol. Chp 129 (2001) 175–191.

[130] A. Bracale, D. Spalletti-Cernia, M. Mastronicola, F. Castaldi, R. Mannucci, L. Nitsch, G. D'Alessio, Essential stations in the intracellular pathway of cytotoxic bovine seminal ribonuclease, Biochemical. J. 362 (2002) 553–560.

[131] Y. Wu, S.K. Saxena, W. Ardelt, M. Gadina, S.M. Mikulski, C. De Lorenzo, G. D'Alessio, R.J. Youle, A study of the intracellular routing of cytotoxic ribonucleases, J. Biol. Chem. 270 (1995) 17476–17481.

[132] A. Antignani, M. Naddeo, M.V. Cubellis, A. Russo, G. D'Alessio, Antitumor action of seminal ribonuclease, its dimeric structure, and its resistance to the cytosolic ribonuclease inhibitor, Biochemistry 40 (2001) 3492–3496.

[133] P. Pouckova, J. Soucek, J. Jelinek, M. Zadinova, D. Hlouskova, J. Polivkova, L. Navratil, J. Cinatl, J. Matousek, Antitumor action of bovine seminal ribonuclease. Cytostatic effect on human melanoma and mouse seminoma, Neoplasma 45 (1998) 30–34.

[134] J. Cinatl Jr., J. Cinatl, R. Kotchetkov, J.U. Vogel, B.G. Woodcock, J. Matousek, P. Pouckova, B. Kornhuber, Bovine seminal ribonuclease selectively kills human multidrug-resistant neuroblastoma cells via induction of apoptosis, Int. J. Oncol. 15 (1999) 1001–1009.

[135] I. Marinov, J. Soucek, Bovine seminal ribonuclease induces *in vitro* concentration dependent apoptosis in stimulated human lymphocytes and cells from human tumor cell lines, Neoplasma 47 (2000) 294–298.

[136] R. Kotchetkov, J. Cinatl, A.A. Krivtchik, J.U. Vogel, J. Matousek, P. Pouckova, B. Kornhuber, D. Schwabe, J. Cinatl Jr., Selective activity of BS-RNase against anaplastic thyroid cancer, Anticancer Res. 21 (2001) 1035–1042.

[137] J. Soucek, P. Pouckova, M. Zadinova, D. Hlouskova, D. Plocova, J. Strohalm, Z. Hrkal, T. Olear, K. Ulbrich, Polymer conjugated bovine seminal ribonuclease inhibits growth of solid tumors and development of metastases in mice, Neoplasma 48 (2001) 127–132.

[138] M. Michaelis, J. Cinatl, P. Pouckova, K. Langer, J. Kreuter, J. Matousek, Coupling of the antitumoral enzyme bovine seminal ribonuclease to polyethylene glycol chains increases its systemic efficacy in mice, Anti-Cancer Drugs 13 (2002) 149–154.

[139] F. Yin, A.E. Giuliano, A.J. Van Herle, Signal pathways involved in apigenin inhibition of growth and induction of apoptosis of human anaplastic thyroid cancer cells (ARO), Anticancer Res. 19 (1999) 4297–4303.

[140] J.K. Lin, Y.C. Chen, Y.T. Huang, S.Y. Lin-Shiau, Suppression of protein kinase C and nuclear oncogene expression as possible molecular mechanisms of cancer chemoprevention by apigenin and curcumin, J. Cell. Biochem. -Suppl. 28–29 (1997) 39–48.

[141] F. Boege, T. Straub, A. Kehr, C. Boesenberg, K. Christiansen, A. Andersen, F. Jakob, J. Kohrle, Selected novel flavones inhibit the DNA binding or the DNA religation step of eukaryotic topoisomerase I, J. Biol. Chem. 271 (1996) 2262–2270.

[142] S. Gupta, F. Afaq, H. Mukhtar, Involvement of nuclear factor-kappa B, Bax and Bcl-2 in induction of cell cycle arrest and apoptosis by apigenin in human prostate carcinoma cells, Oncogene 21 (2002) 3727–3738.

[143] J.P. Vanden Heuvel, Peroxisome proliferator-activated receptors (PPARS) and carcinogenesis, Toxicol. Sci. 47 (1999) 1–8.

[144] W.L. Yang, H. Frucht, Activation of the PPAR pathway induces apoptosis and COX-2 inhibition in HT-29 human colon cancer cells, Carcinogenesis 22 (2001) 1379–1383.

[145] G. Eibl, M.N. Wente, H.A. Reber, O.J. Hines, Peroxisome proliferator-activated receptor gamma induces pancreatic cancer cell apoptosis, Biochem. Biophys. Res. Comm. 287 (2001) 522–529.

[146] Y. Tsubouchi, H. Sano, Y. Kawahito, S. Mukai, R. Yamada, M. Kohno, K. Inoue, T. Hla, M. Kondo, Inhibition of human lung cancer cell growth by the peroxisome proliferator-activated receptor-gamma agonists through induction of apoptosis, Biochem. Biophys. Res. Comm. 270 (2000) 400–405.

[147] T. Shimada, K. Kojima, K. Yoshiura, H. Hiraishi, A. Terano, Characteristics of the peroxisome proliferator activated receptor gamma (PPARgamma) ligand induced apoptosis in colon cancer cells, Gut 50 (2002) 658–664.

[148] K. Ohta, T. Endo, K. Haraguchi, J.M. Hershman, T. Onaya, Ligands for peroxisome proliferator-activated receptor gamma inhibit growth and induce apoptosis of human papillary thyroid carcinoma cells, J. Clin. Endo. Metab. 86 (2001) 2170–2177.

[149] M. Ahmad, Y. Shi, TRAIL-induced apoptosis of thyroid cancer cells: potential for therapeutic intervention, Oncogene 19 (2000) 3363–3371.

[150] J. Cerutti, F. Trapasso, C. Battaglia, L. Zhang, M.L. Martelli, R. Visconti, M.T. Berlingieri, J.A. Fagin, M. Santoro, A. Fusco, Block of c-myc expression by antisense oligonucleotides inhibits proliferation of human thyroid carcinoma cell lines, Clin. Cancer Res. 2 (1996) 119–126.

Chapter 8

Medullary thyroid carcinoma

Jeffrey F. Moley

Siteman Cancer Center, Washington University School of Medicine, Box 8109, 660 South Euclid, St. Louis, MO, USA

1. Introduction

Medullary thyroid carcinoma (MTC) is a type of thyroid cancer that arises from the neuroendocrine C cells. These parafollicular cells are neural crest derivatives and are considered to be part of the amine precursor uptake and decarboxylation (APUD) group of neuroendocrine cells. The C cells comprise only 1% of the total thyroid mass and are dispersed throughout the gland, with the highest concentration in the upper poles. The C cells are named so because of their unique ability to secrete the hormone calcitonin. Calcitonin may be involved in the hormonal control of post-prandial hypercalcemia, but its exact physiologic role remains to be illuminated and pathologic changes related to hypocalcitoninemia after thyroidectomy are still under investigation [1]. C cells are capable of secreting other hormones, including carcino-embryonic antigen (CEA), histaminase, neuron-specific enolase, calcitonin gene-related peptide, somatostatin, thyroglobulin, thyrotropin-stimulating hormone, adrenocortical-stimulating hormone (ACTH), gastrin-related peptide, serotonin, chromogranin, and substance P [2,3]. MTC comprises 3–9% of all thyroid cancers.

MTC tumors are usually well demarcated, firm, gray-white, and gritty [4–6]. Microscopically, there are uniform polygonal cells with finely granular eosinophilic cytoplasm with central nuclei. Varying numbers of spindle cells are present in nearly all tumors. The presence of amyloid is considered to be a distinctive feature of MTC, although it may not be found in all cases. The amyloid differs from that of other tumors in that it is formed from calcitonin or procalcitonin molecules. In sporadic tumors, approximately 68% are solitary and 32% are bilateral or multifocal. In familial forms, 94% are bilateral or multifocal and 6% are solitary. C cell hyperplasia is associated with MTC, particularly in the familial forms. It has been suggested that C cell hyperplasia is a precursor in the malignant transformation to MTC [7–9].

Spreading of MTC may occur locally, into adjacent structures, to regional lymph nodes, and to distant sites. In a recent report, we analyzed the distribution of nodal

ADVANCES IN MOLECULAR AND CELLULAR ENDOCRINOLOGY
VOLUME   4 ISSN 1569-2566/DOI 10.1016/S1569-2566(04)04008-6

metastases in patients with MTC that presented as a palpable neck mass, and in whom central and bilateral cervical nodes were removed and examined histologically. We found that the incidence of central (levels VI and VII) node involvement was extremely high (79% for unilateral and bilateral tumors combined), regardless of the size of the primary tumor. Involvement of ipsilateral (75%) and contralateral (47%) level II, III, and IV nodes was also frequent, which supports our recommendation that these nodes be removed routinely in patients with palpable MTC [58].

It is not uncommon for primary or metastatic MTC to involve adjacent structures by direct invasion or compression. Structures that are most commonly affected include the trachea, recurrent laryngeal nerve, jugular veins, and carotid arteries. Invasion of such structures may result in stridor, upper-airway obstruction, hoarseness, dysphagia, and bleeding or arterial stenosis or occlusion.

Hematogenous MTC metastases often occur in the liver, lungs, and bone; occasionally they are found in the brain, soft tissues outside the neck, and bone marrow. In a study from a Swedish registry, it was noted that MTC patients with a palpable mass in the neck had distant metastatic disease in 20% of cases, regardless of heritability [10]. Furthermore, occult remote micrometastases are most likely the cause of persistent hypercalcitoninemia in most the cases after extensive lymph node dissection [11–13].

2. Genetics of MTC – the men 2 syndromes

MTC occurs in sporadic (75%) and hereditary (25%) clinical settings. Hereditary MTC is a component of inherited syndromes known as multiple endocrine neoplasia type 2 (MEN 2A and 2B) and non-MEN familial medullary thyroid carcinoma (FMTC). All patients with MTC should be enquired regarding the family history of thyroid, parathyroid, and adrenal disorders. The MEN 2 syndromes are inherited in Mendelian autosomal dominant fashion. There is nearly a complete penetrance but variable expression of the syndromes; essentially *all* persons who inherit the disease allele develop MTC, but other features of the disease may not necessarily be present. In MEN 2A, approximately 42% of affected patients develop pheochromocytomas, and hyperparathyroidism occurs in about 35% [14]. In MEN 2B, about half develop pheochromocytomas, and all patients develop neural ganglioneuromas, particularly in the mucosa of the digestive tract and conjunctiva. Although MEN 2B is inherited as an autosomal dominant trait, in about half the patients the disease arises [15,16] de novo. FMTC is characterized by the development of MTC without any other endocrinopathies [17].

The presentation of MTC varies in sporadic MTC, MEN 2A, MEN 2B, and FMTC (Table 1). Sporadic MTC is unilateral in the majority of cases, whereas MTC in the MEN 2 syndromes is usually bilateral and multifocal. MTC tumors in FMTC are usually indolent and appear later in life [18]. Many patients with FMTC are cured by thyroidectomy alone, and those with persistent elevation of calcitonin levels do well for many years. Death from MTC is rare in patients with FMTC [19]. MTC in MEN 2B, however, is extremely aggressive, with gross evidence of cancer present

Table 1
Clinical features of sporadic MTC, MEN 2A, MEN 2B, and FMTC

Clinical setting	Features of MTC	Inheritance pattern	Associated abnormalities	Genetic defect
Sporadic MTC	Unifocal	None	None	Somatic RET mutations in >20% of tumors
MEN 2A	Multifocal, bilateral	Autosomal dominant	Pheochromocytomas, hyperparathyroidism	Germ-line missense mutations in extracellular cysteine codons of RET
MEN 2B	Multifocal, bilateral	Autosomal dominant	Pheochromocytomas, mucosal neuromas, megacolon, skeletal abnormalities	Germ-line missense mutation in tyrosine kinase domain of RET
FMTC	Multifocal, bilateral	Autosomal dominant	None	Germ-line missense mutations in extracellular or intracellular cysteine codons of RET

Reproduced with permission from J.F. Moley, T.C. Lairmore, J.E. Phay. Curr. Problems Surg. 36 (1999) 653–764.

in children as young as 6 months of age. These patients may develop widespread metastatic MTC at an early age, underscoring the importance of early diagnosis and treatment in this particular population [20,21]. The virulence of sporadic MTC can vary and the disease can present in any age group, although the peak incidence is in the sixth decade of life [6].

In 1987, the predisposition gene for MEN 2A was localized to the pericentromeric region of chromosome 10 (10q11.2) [22]. The RET proto-oncogene is included within this critical region, and in 1993, RET was found to be the predisposition gene for these syndromes [23,24]. The RET proto-oncogene is a member of the receptor tyrosine kinase gene family and was originally found to be a dominant transforming gene activated by the replacement 5' region with a portion of a zinc finger-like gene in human lymphoma cells [25]. This transmembrane protein consists of three domains: a cysteine-rich extracellular receptor domain, a hydrophobic transmembrane domain, and an intracellular tyrosine kinase catalytic domain. RET consists of at least 20 exons [26], and is expressed as five major RNA species [27,28].

Point mutations associated with MEN 2A and FMTC were first identified in exons 10 and 11 of RET, which encode the juxtamembrane portion of the extracellular receptor domain [23,24]. These mutations result in a non-conservative substitution of one of five cysteine residue (codons 609, 611, 618, 620, and 634). Mutations associated with FMTC have also been described at codons 768 (Glu to Asp) in exons 13 and 804 (Val to Leu or Met) in exon 14 in the intracellular domain [29,30]. Over 30

Table 2
RET mutations in hereditary MTC

Syndrome	Missense Germ-line mutations in the RET proto-oncogene	
	Exon	Codon
MEN 2A, FMTC	10	609
		611
		618
		620
	11	631[a]
		634
	13	790
		791
FMTC	11	630
	13	768
	14	804
		844[a]
	15	891
MEN 2B	16	918
		883

[a]Clinical features not yet characterized. Reprinted with permission from Moley and Albinson [19].

missense mutations have been described in patients affected by these syndromes (Table 2). The mutations have been proposed to result in 'gain-of-function' in the MEN 2 syndromes with increased intrinsic tyrosine kinase activity or alterations of substrate recognition, and hence, transforming capability [31]. FMTC with non-cysteine RET mutations are not infrequent and are overrepresented in presumed sporadic MTC, suggesting that RET analysis should routinely be extended to exons 13–15 [32].

The RET proto-oncogene mutation associated with MEN 2B is characterized by allelic homogeneity with nearly all individuals sharing the identical mutation in exon 16 [33]. In these cases, a methionine is changed to threonine (ATG to ACG) at codon 918. This codon is positioned within the tyrosine kinase catalytic core of the intra-cellular domain and probably participates in the formation of the putative substrate recognition region [33]. Other mutations have been described in MEN 2B (codons 883 and 922), but these are very rare.

Mutations in the RET proto-oncogene have been associated with sporadic MTC [23,29,30,34,35]. Most commonly, these mutations involve codon 918, the codon mutated in MEN 2B. Mutations have also been found in other regions of the extra-cellular and intracellular domains. Missense, deletions, and insertion mutations have been described.

Although the exact role of the RET gene product is unclear, evidence suggests that it is important in the embryonic development of the enteric nervous system and the kidneys [36]. Glial-derived neurotrophic factor (GDNF) has been implicated as a ligand to the receptor domain of the RET gene product [37–39]. GDNF is a 32 kDa protein dimer that was first purified from glial cell lines and is a potent neurotrophic survival factor for motor neurons. There is compelling evidence that GDNF transduces a signal in RET [40–43]. A glycophosphatidylinositol (GPI)-linked protein, called glial-derived neurotrophic factor receptor-alpha (GDNFRα), is a cofactor in the signaling heterodimeric complex with RET. Current evidence suggests that GDNF binds directly to GDNFRα and directly with RET. Furthermore, it has been shown that nuclear factor (NF)-κB is activated in RET-associated C-cell carcinoma specimens [44].

In contrast to other types of cancer in which multiple genetic abnormalities are found (e.g. lung, colon, and breast), hereditary and sporadic MTC exhibit very few abnormalities apart from RET mutations on genetic analysis. Absence of amplification of N-myc, c-myc, and erb B-2 has been reported in MTCs and pheochromocytomas [45]. We also reported an absence of abnormalities in the H-ras, N-ras, K-ras, nerve growth factor receptor, and p53 genes in a series of pheochromocytomas and MTCs [45–47]. A possible mechanism for MTC formation in patients with germline RET mutations has been suggested by recent reports that describe overexpression of mutant RET in hereditary MTC, that results from duplication of the mutant RET allele or loss of the wild-type RET allele [123,124].

Germline RET mutations are found in all familial forms of MTC, and somatic RET mutations are often detected in sporadic MTC. In sporadic MTCs, the RET gene is often mutated at codon 918, where a methionine is substituted to a threonine (M918 T). In a study by Frisk et al. [48], 24 MTCs were analyzed by comparative genomic hybridization (CGH) for chromosomal imbalances. Overall, alterations were detected in approximately 60% of the samples. The most common aberrations were gains on chromosome 19q (29%), 19p (21%), 11c-q12 (12.5%), and 22q (12.5%), and losses on 13q21 (21%) and 3q23-qter (12.5%). The results indicate that MTC is a comparatively genetically stable tumor and chromosomal regions 19q, 19p, 13q, and 11q may be involved in MTC carcinogenesis [48].

3. Diagnosis

The prognosis of MTC is associated with disease state at the time of diagnosis. Nodal involvement and tumor stage are also associated with the outcome [6,49,50]. In a report from the Mayo Clinic, two-thirds of hereditary MTC patients with positive nodes died, and no patient with positive nodes had normal calcitonin levels after a median follow-up of 15.7 years [51]. Numerous studies of patients with MEN 2A treated for MTC have demonstrated a direct correlation between early diagnosis and the cure of the disease [52–57]. Clearly, early diagnosis and treatment are of significant importance.

3.1. *History and physical examination*

All patients with sporadic MTC and most index cases of MEN 2A and FMTC have a thyroid nodule. Over 75% of patients with palpable MTC have associated nodal metastases, which are often not apparent to the surgeon [58]. Respiratory complaints, hoarseness, and dysphagia are seen in approximately 13% of patients. Approximately 10–15% of patients with palpable MTC present with evidence of distant metastatic disease.

More than 50% of patients with MEN 2B have unaffected parents, and the diagnosis is not usually made until a mass is discovered in the patient's neck. Occasionally, the diagnosis is made earlier by an astute clinician, who notes the characteristic phenotype. MEN 2B patients have a 'marfanoid' habitus with long axial features, soft-tissue hypergnathism of the mid-face, and hyperflexible joints. They also typically have neuromata of the lips, conjunctiva, and gastrointestinal tract. Additionally, there is characteristic 'notching' of the tongue secondary to the presence of neuromas. (Fig. 1). Patients with MEN 2A and FMTC have a completely normal outward appearance. In these patients, the diagnosis of MTC has been made through screening efforts (genetic testing or elevated plasma calcitonin levels), because of other affected family members or by detection of a thyroid nodule on physical examination. Signs and symptoms of pheochromocytoma may be present in patients with MEN 2A and 2B.

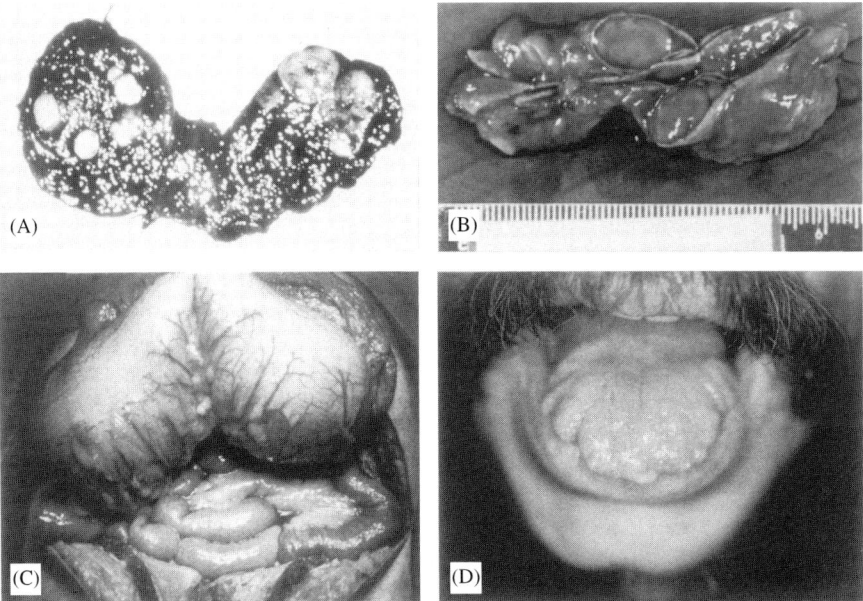

Fig. 1. Features of patients with hereditary MTC. (A) Bisected thyroid gland from a patient with MEN 2A showing multicentric, bilateral foci of MTC. (B) Adrenalectomy specimen from patient with MEN 2B demonstrating pheochromocytoma. (C) Megacolon in patient with MEN 2B. (D) Midface and tongue of patient with MEN 2B showing characteristic tongue notching secondary to plexiform neuromas. (Photograph A, courtesy of Dr. S.A. Wells; photographs B, C and D, courtesy of Dr. R. Thompson) (reprinted with permission from J.F. Moley, In: O.H. Clark, Q.-Y. Duh, (Eds.), Textbook of Endocrine Surgery, WB Saunders Co., Philadelphia, 1997).

MTC does not concentrate iodine and appears as a cold nodule on thyroid scintigraphy scans. Plain films may show areas of calcifications in the neck. Fine-needle aspirates are a sensitive means for establishing the diagnosis of MTC, especially if immunocytochemical stains for calcitonin are performed.

3.2. *Serum calcitonin screening*

Thyroid C cells and MTC cells secrete calcitonin, which has been a valuable marker for the presence of disease in screening and follow-up settings. Peripheral serum levels of this hormone are measured by radio-immunoassay. In patients with MTC, a correlation exists between basal plasma calcitonin levels and tumor mass [59]. Some patients with MTC, however, have normal basal levels of calcitonin. Provocative calcitonin stimulation tests may be performed. After an intravenous infusion of calcium gluconate ($2 \, mg \, kg^{-1}$ over 1 min) followed by pentagastrin ($0.5 \, \mu g \, kg^{-1}$ over 5 sec), blood samples are obtained before and at 1, 2, 3, and 5 min after the infusion. Peak plasma calcitonin values generally occur at 1–2 min [60]. Measurement of plasma calcitonin after the administration of calcium and pentagastrin is the most sensitive clinical test for the presence of MTC [60]. The development of immuno-radiometric assays (detection limit, $<3 \, pg^{-1} \, mL$) improves the sensitivity and specificity of the plasma calcitonin test significantly [61,62].

Routine genetic testing identifies RET mutation carriers earlier and more reliably than biochemical testing, and it obviates the need for continued testing in persons found to be unaffected. Calcitonin testing remains important, however, in follow-up of patients treated for MTC.

4. Treatment

4.1. *Surgical treatment of palpable disease*

The surgical treatment of MTC is influenced by several factors. (1) The clinical course of MTC is usually more aggressive than that of differentiated thyroid cancer (DTC), with higher rates of recurrence and mortality. (2) MTC cells do not take up radioactive iodine, and radiation therapy and chemotherapy are ineffective. (3) MTC is multicentric in 90% of patients with hereditary forms of the disease and in 20% of patients with the sporadic form. (4) Nodal metastases are present in more than 70% of patients with palpable disease. (Tables 3 and 4) (5) The ability to measure postoperative calcitonin levels has allowed the adequacy of surgical extirpation to be assessed. Total thyroidectomy is the appropriate treatment of the primary tumor, accompanied by a central node dissection in patients with a palpable thyroid tumor. In this operation, all thyroid and nodal tissues from the level of the hyoid bone to the innominate vessels, is removed. After the parathyroid glands are identified, central nodal tissue on the anterior surface of the trachea is removed, exposing the superior surface of the innominate vein behind the sternal notch. Fatty and nodal tissue between the carotid sheaths and the trachea is removed, including paratracheal

Table 3
Unilateral intrathyroid tumors-frequency and distribution of nodal metastases

Tumor size	No. patients	Central node metastases	Ipsilateral Level II–V metastases	Contralateral Level II–V metastases
0–0.9 cm	4	3/4	3/4	1/4
1–1.9 cm	9	8/9	8/9	3/9
2–2.9 cm	5	4/5	3/5	3/5
3–3.9 cm	5	2/5	4/5	3/5
4 cm or larger	9	9/9	8/9	4/9
Total	32	26/32 (81%)	26/32 (81%)	14/32 (44%)

Note: Central nodes refer to right left level VI and VII nodes. Reprinted with permission from Moley and DeBenedetti [60].

Table 4
Bilateral intrathyroid tumors—frequency and distribution of nodal metastases

Size of largest tumor (cm)	No. patients	Central node metastases	Ipsilateral level II–V metastases	Contralateral level II–V metastases
0–0.9	12	8/12	9/12	4/12
1–1.9	7	5/7	6/7	4/7
2–2.9	8	7/8	4/8	5/8
3–3.9	7	7/7	6/7	5/7
4 or larger	7	5/7	4/7	2/7
Total	41	32/41 (78%)	29/41 (71%)	20/41 (49%)

Note: Central nodes refer to right and left level VI and VII nodes. Reprinted with permission from Moley and DeBenedetti [58].

nodes along the recurrent nerves. On the right, the junction of the innominate and right carotid arteries is exposed, and on the left, nodal tissue is removed to a comparable level behind the head of the left clavicle. A systematic approach to the removal of all nodal tissue in the central neck has been reported to improve recurrence and survival rates when compared retrospectively with procedures in which only grossly involved nodes were removed [49].

4.2. *Management of the parathyroids*

Controversy exists over the optimal management of the parathyroid glands in operations for MTC. Some surgeons prefer to leave the parathyroid glands *in situ*, ensuring that the vascular pedicle is preserved [49,51,53,63–65]. At our institution, we have found that adequate total thyroidectomy and central node clearance is difficult to achieve unless the parathyroids are removed. This is especially important in patients with palpable disease. Adequate central node dissection is extremely difficult if the parathyroids are left in place with an adequate blood supply; there are nodes that are closely associated with the parathyroids and their blood supply. Attempts to leave the parathyroids in place result in either leaving central nodes in the neck or leaving devascularized parathyroids. Furthermore, if the need for re-operation in the central compartment arises, the risk of subsequent hypoparathy-roidism is negligible if the patient has a functioning autograft. Finding and preserving parathyroids in a scarred, previously operated neck is difficult and the risk of hypoparathyroidism following such procedures is significant. Therefore, we advocate parathyroidectomy with autotransplantation as part of total thyroidectomy for palpable MTC. Parathyroid glands are removed and placed in cold saline. The glands are sliced into 1 to 3 mm fragments and autotransplanted into individual muscle pockets in the sternocleidomastoid muscle in patients with sporadic MTC, FMTC, and MEN 2B, or into the nondominant forearm in patients with MEN 2A (since they have a 30% chance of developing hyperparathyroidism, even from autografts; localization of the source of hyperparathyroidism and surgical removal of the hyperfunctional tissue is greatly simplified if the grafts are placed in the forearm) [66]. If the patient becomes hyperparathyroid, operation to reduce parathyroid tissue may be carried out under local anesthesia on an outpatient basis, without the risk of a repeat neck exploration. In patients with MEN 2A, who have hyperparathyroidism at the time of operation, at least 100 mg of parathyroid tissue should be transplanted, and residual tissue should be viably frozen [67]. The autografts generally function well within 4 to 6 weeks, by which time patients can be taken off from calcium supplementation.

4.3. *Management of regional nodes*

The recommended surgical procedure for primary palpable MTC has not been well established. In the recently distributed Practice Guidelines for Major Cancer Sites, developed by the Society of Surgical Oncology, total thyroidectomy was recommended, but node dissections were recommended only for clinically palpable nodes [68]. This may be an effective strategy for DTC, where suppression with thyroxine and radioactive iodine ablation are extremely effective adjuncts to surgery, but MTC cells do not respond to these nonsurgical treatments.

In a recent report, we evaluated the incidence and pattern of nodal metastatic spread in patients with palpable MTC [58]. In this series, 73 patients with palpable MTC underwent thyroidectomy, with concurrent or delayed central and bilateral cervical node dissection. The number and location of lymph node metastases in the central (levels VI and VII) and bilateral (levels II–V) nodal groups were noted and were correlated with size and location of the primary thyroid tumor. Results of intraoperative assessment of nodal status by palpation and inspection by the operating surgeon were correlated with results of histologic examination.

Among the patients with unilateral intrathyroidal tumors, nodal metastases were present in 81% in central, 81% in ipsilateral levels II–V, and in 44% of contralateral levels II–V nodal groups. Among the patients with bilateral intrathyroidal tumors, nodal metastases were present in 78% of central nodal groups, 71% of levels II–V nodes ipsilateral to the largest intrathyroidal tumor, and 49% of levels II–V nodes contralateral to the largest intrathyroidal tumor. This is an alarmingly high incidence of nodal involvement.

Intraoperative palpation of nodes was not an accurate predictor of the presence or absence of metastases [58]. The sensitivity of intraoperative assessment by an experienced surgeon was only 64%, and the specificity was 71%. Therefore, relying on intraoperative assessment would miss involved nodes 36% of the time. The strategy or resecting only 'clinically involved nodes' is effective in differentiated thyroid cancer for which effective adjuvant therapy is available. No effective adjuvant treatments for MTC are available.

Based on the results, our recommendation for patients who present with palpable MTC is total thyroidectomy, parathyroidectomy with autotransplantation, central neck dissection (right and left levels VI and VII nodes), and unilateral or bilateral dissection of levels II–V nodes. (Fig. 2).

Alternatively, total thyroidectomy, parathyroidectomy, and central neck dissection may be performed as the initial procedure, with unilateral or bilateral dissection of levels II–V nodes (functional or modified radical neck dissection) performed as a second procedure in patients with persistent elevations of calcitonin and no evidence of distant metastatic disease.

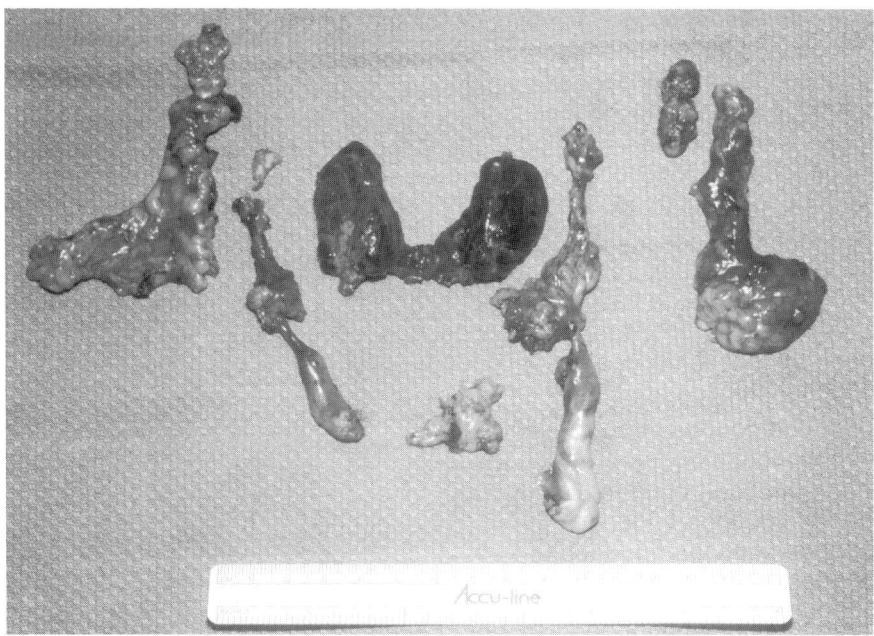

Fig. 2. Total thyroidectomy and central (levels VI and VII) and bilateral levels II–V node dissections from a thin young male with MEN 2B and a bilateral palpable thyroid masses (parathyroids not shown). Microscopic metastases were present in all nodal groups. Reprinted with permission from Moley and Albinson [19].

As with any specialized procedure undertaken for an unusual clinical problem, these operations should be performed by surgeons familiar with the disease and with expertise in the techniques described. If the surgeon is unfamiliar with these techniques, we recommend that the patient undergo a diagnostic thyroid lobectomy, with the parathyroids left undisturbed, and then be subsequently referred to an appropriate surgical specialist.

4.4. *Surgical treatment—preventative thyroidectomy in RET mutation carriers*

Discovery of RET proto-oncogene mutations associated with the MEN 2 syndromes has allowed the detection of disease gene carriers before their stimulated calcitonin levels become elevated. In principle, genetic testing, which requires the drawing of blood for extractions of lymphocyte DNA, needs to be performed only once in an at-risk individual's lifetime. Stimulated calcitonin testing remains an important modality in following patients for recurrent or residual disease after thyroidectomy.

Genetic testing should be carried out only after consultation with a geneticist or genetic counselor, and informed consent must be obtained. To test a patient for the presence of a mutation in the RET gene, DNA is extracted from peripheral white blood cells. Regions of the RET proto-oncogene are amplified by polymerase chain reaction, and mutations are detected by direct DNA sequencing, analysis of restriction sites introduced or deleted by a mutation, or gel shift analysis (denaturing gradient gel electrophoresis or single-strand conformation polymorphism analysis) [23,69,70]. Recently, a study conducted by Ruiz et al. [122] indicates that the simultaneous scanning of multiple mutations is possible via the fluorescence resonance energy transfer (FRET) system. This method allows rapid characterization of germline mutations at codon 634 in MTC patients.

Although genetic testing can be performed at birth, the age at which thyroidectomy should be performed is controversial. Presently, in children with MEN 2A and FMTC, we advocate total thyroidectomy at the age of 5 years. In patients with MEN 2B, surgery should be performed during infancy, because of the early onset and the biologic aggressiveness of MTC in these patients. We have performed total thyroidectomies with central lymph node dissection in MEN 2B children as young as 5 months [71]. Management of parathyroids in these children is controversial; we often perform parathyroidectomy with autotransplantation, because the thyroidectomy performed must be thorough, and if central nodes are removed, there is significant risk of injury to the parathyroid blood supply. Our results with parathyroid autotransplantation have been excellent [58,67,72,73]. Other surgeons routinely leave the parathyroids in place. It is important that the surgeon performing this operation be skilled in management of parathyroids. Central neck dissection has been discussed previously in this chapter.

MTC is virtually certain to develop in persons with MEN 2A or FMTC at some point in their lives (usually before 30 years of age). Therefore, at-risk family members who are found to have inherited a RET gene mutation are candidates for thyroidectomy, regardless of their stimulated plasma calcitonin levels. It has been shown in several series that RET mutation carriers often harbor foci of MTC in the thyroid gland even when stimulated calcitonin levels are normal. This indicates that the operation in these cases was therapeutic and not prophylactic. It is necessary, therefore, to apply this genetic test to other persons at risk and offer thyroidectomy to those with positive results. Patient follow-up during the next decades will determine whether the rate of recurrence is significant after preventative thyroidectomy. At present, it is advisable to follow these patients with stimulated plasma calcitonin levels every 1 to 2 years. They must also be followed for the development of pheochromocytomas and hyperparathyroidism.

Although longer follow-up of reported series is needed, prophylactic thyroidectomy with central node dissection in all probability is curative in most children who are gene carriers of MEN 2A and FMTC [72]. In contrast, 50% of patients in whom the diagnosis of hereditary MTC is made at an older age, when tumor is already present and calcitonin levels are elevated, have residual disease after total thyroidectomy [51]. Encouragingly, the number of MEN 2A and FMTC cases with synchronous metastatic disease has decreased because of the growing awareness of the hereditary variant of this cancer and the extensive screening of families at risk [10].

The discovery that mutations in the RET proto-oncogene are associated with MEN 2 syndromes was highly significant in that it demonstrated a clear correlation between genotype and phenotype; and most importantly it provided a mechanism whereby family members at risk could be identified by direct DNA analysis. Virtually all patients with MEN 2A, MEN 2B, and FMTC develop MTC; therefore, there is a clear rationale for performing thyroidectomy as soon as a RET mutation has been identified [74].

4.5. *Post-surgical follow-up*

All patients should be followed postoperatively with calcitonin and CEA levels to detect persistent or recurrent disease. Although elevated basal calcitonin levels may indicate residual disease after thyroidectomy for MTC, normal levels do not rule out residual disease [75] and are therefore not sufficient to identify early tumor progression in the postoperative follow-up of MTC patients. For this reason, provocative calcitonin stimulation testing is routinely performed. The development of immunoradiometric assays (detection limit, $<3\,\mathrm{pg\,mL}^{-1}$) improves the sensitivity and specificity of the plasma calcitonin test significantly [61,62,76]. A significant increase in calcitonin serum concentrations after calcium–pentagastrin administration is a strong indicator of tumor persistence and progression after primary surgery for MTC. However, interpretation of borderline elevated, but stable, stimulated calcitonin levels remains unclear. In more than 50% of patients with MTC, the CEA levels are elevated. This analysis has been found to be useful in following these patients postoperatively [2,77]. One study found that a rising CEA level in MTC patients with a stable or falling calcitonin level corresponded to dissemination of a virulent dedifferentiated tumor [78].

Yearly screening for pheochromocytoma (MEN 2A and MEN 2B) and hyperparathyroidism (MEN 2A) should be done. Hyperparathyroidism is monitored by serum calcium measurements. Testing for pheochromocytoma may be accomplished by measurement of 24 h urine catecholamines and metabolites. However, a recent study by Eisenhofer et al. [79] showed that the sensitivity of measurements of plasma normetanephrine and metanephrine for the detection of pheochromocytomas was 97%, whereas other biochemical tests had a sensitivity of only 47–74%. Measurements of plasma-free metanephrines appear to provide a superior test compared with other available tests for the diagnosis of pheochromocytoma.

Genetic testing for mutations in the RET gene should be done in all patients with MTC.

4.6. *Persistent or recurrent MTC*

Elevated calcitonin levels are frequently observed following primary surgery for MTC, indicating residual or recurrent MTC. In one study of patients who presented with palpable tumors, 15/18 (83%) of patients with hereditary disease and 11/20 (55%) of patients with sporadic tumors had persistent disease as indicated by elevated calcitonin levels postoperatively [7]. Many patients with persistently high levels of calcitonin following thyroidectomy and node dissection continue to do well without other evidence of the disease for many years [50,80–82]. The variable outcome of patients with positive lymph nodes is explained by differences in the biologic virulence of the tumor, the extent of spread at the time of treatment, and the adequacy of surgical extirpation.

In a recent series of reoperations for recurrent or residual MTC, the authors judged that >80% of referred patients had an inadequate primary operation [61]. Overall, persistent disease, evidenced by elevated calcitonin levels, is present in >50% of patients after surgery for MTC [7,82].

In 1986, Tisell et al. [13] described a novel surgical approach to persistent and recurrent hypercalcitoninemia. He termed this operation *microdissection*, which entails removal of all lymphatic, fatty, and connective tissue in anatomically defined compartments of the neck and mediastinum, which contain the lymphatic drainage of the thyroid. Several studies have subsequently demonstrated that this approach results in biochemical cure in 20–30% of patients and may prolong survival time in others [13,83–87].

The indications, strategies, and goals of reoperation for MTC must take into account the individual clinical setting. These considerations include the type of MTC, adequacy of primary tumor extirpation according to prior operative reports, pathology findings, and results of the preoperative staging. Careful patient evaluation is imperative for the success of a reoperation with curative or palliative intent.

Conventional imaging studies for MTC localization include computerised tomography (CT) scans, MR images, and ultrasound. Small metastases (<1.5 cm) may not be detected by these methods. *Selective venous catheterization*, with measurement of stimulated calcitonin levels from cervical, hepatic, and mediastinal veins, may localize disease to a general region such as the neck or chest, and may detect liver metastases [88,89]. This procedure is difficult and requires cooperation of interventional radiology and surgical staff. Catheters are placed into the internal and external jugular veins, innominate veins, hepatic veins, and mediastinal veins, and stimulated calcitonin levels are measured and compared with peripheral levels. Metastatic disease is localized to regions of the neck drained by veins in which a step-up is noted [90]. Although the test is extremely sensitive, not all metastatic foci are detected by SVC sampling. Cervical venous drainage may have been altered by previous surgery, and the general areas drained by these veins is large.

A number of different radiopharmaceuticals have been described to localize metastatic MTC. Thallium chloride-201 (^{201}Tl) and technetium-99 m dimercaptosuccinic acid (^{99m}Tc DMSA) have been shown to be useful in evaluating hypercalcitoninemic patients [91–94]. ^{131}I-*m*-Iodobenzyguanidine (MIBG) scintigraphy can be used to image MTC, but is not consistent. Octreotide scans with indium-111 (^{111}In) have been used to localize metastatic disease, but only have a sensitivity of approximately 57–67% [95]. Higher serum calcitonin levels are associated with greater sensitivity [96]. A study conducted by Adams et al. reported that the combination of metabolic (^{99m}Tc DMSA) and receptor (^{111}In-DTPA-d-Phe1-pentetreotide) imaging is more sensitive for tumour localization in patients with recurrent MTC than the use of only one radiopharmaceutical.

Monoclonal anti-CEA antibodies labeled with iodine-131 (^{131}I) or iodine-123 (^{123}I), ^{111}In, and ^{99m}Tc have been evaluated for localization of MTC [97]. Juweid et al. reported the largest series with 26 patients, but only 9 were identified as patients with occult disease. SPECT with labeled monoclonal anti-CEA antibodies was compared with ultrasonographic examination and CT scan, and in 4 of 9 patients, imaged metastatic foci were confirmed by operative results. Concerning the number of patients examined, the value of monoclonal antibodies in localization of occult MTC remains to be proved. Anticalcitonin monoclonal antibodies have also been evaluated in a small number of cases but have never gained broad attention [98]. Additionally, recent studies have examined the imaging of cholecystokin (CCK)-B receptors, which have been demonstrated in a high percentage of MTCs *in vitro*, in patients with MTC [99,100].

Radioimmunoguided surgery is a recently described technique designed to facilitate the intraoperative detection of metastases. After systemic administration of tumor-specific radiolabeled monoclonal antibodies, a hand-held gamma counter is used to scan the operative field. Areas of increased activity are explored, and soft tissue and nodes from these areas are resected. In five patients in whom immunoscintigraphy using an anti-CEA monoclonal antibody was applied, all previously identified metastases could be visualized. According to the authors, the technique detected tumor foci missed by intraoperative inspection and palpation in 3 of 5 patients. Radioimmunoguided surgery did not identify two small (10 mm × 10 mm) lesions that were resected and found to contain microscopic cancer [97]. In a case report, intraoperative scanning after ^{111}In pentetreotide administration was used to localize metastatic sites. Plasma calcitonin levels fell remarkably after surgery but were not reduced to normal values [101]. Although these results are promising, this method is cumbersome and can be applied effectively only if the gross location of the remaining malignant tissue is already known at the time of operation [87].

Fluorodeoxy glucose positron emission tomography (FDG-PET) has been evaluated by our group in the staging of MTC. From January 1996 to December 1996,

10 consecutively treated patients (seven men and three women) with elevated serum calcitonin levels after primary operative treatment for MTC were included in the study. FDG-PET images were compared with CT and MRI images, and suspected metastatic foci were assessed by correlation with intraoperative and histopathologic findings [102]. FDG-PET imaging proved to be more sensitive but less specific in detecting cervicomediastinal metastatic lesions compared with CT or MRI. Two patients with liver metastases detected by laparoscopy only, however, had no evidence of abnormal liver FDG uptake on PET imaging [102].

At our institution, we have found diagnostic laparoscopy to be invaluable in the evaluation of liver involvement by MTC. (Fig. 3) Metastatic MTC to the liver frequently appears as small nodules between 1 and 5 mm in size, easily seen as bright and whitish under laparoscopic magnification. Lesions of this size are generally beyond the resolution of conventional CT, nuclear scans, and ultrasonograms. The ability of laparoscopy to detect small lesions that CT scans and ultrasonograms have missed has been confirmed previously in studies of hepatic and pancreatic malignancies [103,104]. Warshaw et al. [104] noted that laparoscopic examination occasionally revealed metastatic nodules, which open examination did not. In our series of 44 patients, metastatic MTC lesions were demonstrated in 10 patients, nine of whom had negative CT or MR imaging [61,89]. In a study by Tung et al. [89], eight patients with calcitonin elevations in hepatic veins were not found to have liver metastases by laparoscopic examination. Abdelmoumene et al. [90] studied 19 patients, of whom five showed evidence of distant metastases (in the liver in four) by SVC. All five had clinical evidence of distant metastases within a mean follow-up of 3.5 years. It is possible that laparoscopy is more specific than SVC or, conversely, that the hepatic vein calcitonin gradients reflect small, relatively slow growing, and as yet otherwise undetectable foci of MTC. The long-term outcome of these patients has to be determined to address this issue adequately.

5. Treatment of patients with persistent or recurrent medullary thyroid carcinoma

5.1. *Radiation therapy*

Radioactive iodine (^{131}I) has not been found to be helpful in the treatment of patients with metastatic MTC because the C cells do not take up iodine. Nonetheless, several authors have used ^{131}I to treat MTC on the assumption that uptake by the follicular cells would expose the MTC cells to high doses of radiation based on proximity. There are, however, no data to support this use of ^{131}I in the treatment of MTC [6].

The idea of a 'targeted' radiotherapy is intriguing, and has been applied using anti-CEA monoclonal antibodies (anti-CEA Mab). In an exploratory trial of 11 patients treated with ^{131}I-labeled anti-CEA Mab in nonmyeloablative doses, Juweid et al. [105] demonstrated a 'limited antitumor effect', i.e., minor regression or stabilization of the metastatic foci in some patients lasting up to 26 months, judged by close follow-up including measurement of tumor markers (CEA, calcitonin), CT scan, and anti-CEA Mab scans.

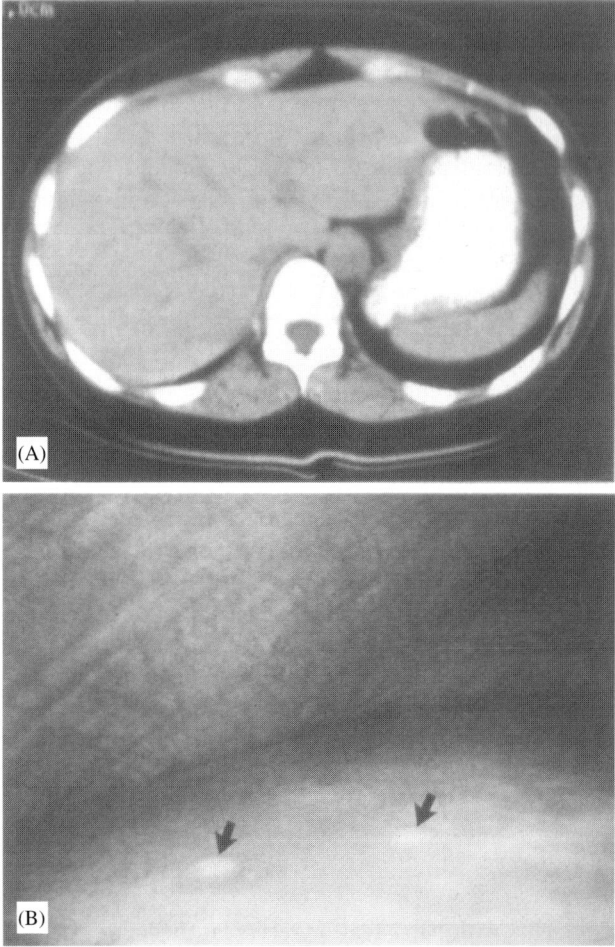

Fig. 3. (A) Computed tomography (CT) of liver from patient with MEN 2A, recurrent MTC and elevated calcitonin levels—there is no evidence of liver metastases on the scan. (B) Laparoscopic view of liver from the same patient showing multiple small raised whitish lesions on and just beneath the surface of the liver, confirmed to be metastatic MTC by biopsy. These small, multiple metastases are often not seen on routine CT scanning or other imaging modalities, including nuclear scanning. Reprinted with permission from Tung et al. [89].

The use of external beam radiation has been reported with variable results. Although several authors have advocated the use of external beam radiation therapy, these studies were retrospective and were done on small numbers of patients [106–108]. Other studies have not supported the use of radiation therapy in MTC. In one retrospective study of 202 patients, patients who underwent external beam radiation were found to have worse outcomes than those who did not [109]. The high mortality rate in patients undergoing radiotherapy was explained by recurrence of disease outside the irradiated field and by limitation of the surgical reintervention because of radiation-induced scarring, fibrosis, and vasculitis [109]. In a retrospective study from a French cooperative group, the investigators studied the effects of external beam radiation postoperatively to patients who were treated for MTC. Of the 59 patients who were followed (mean 5.4 years), 18 developed clinically evident recurrent disease and many developed local complications, primarily invasion into the aerodigestive tract [110]. Overall, the usefulness of external beam radiation in the treatment for MTC is not established, and many surgeons oppose this therapeutic option because of the severe impairment of reoperating in the irradiated field.

5.2. *Chemotherapy*

Experience with chemotherapeutic regimens as a therapeutic alternative is limited in advanced or disseminated MTC. Studies with small series of patients treated with several single agent or combination chemotherapies have failed to demonstrate substantial benefit to the MTC patient, possibly because of an intrinsic multidrug resistance of the cancer [111]. Single-agent treatment with doxorubicin was shown to provide complete response in three of the five patients in an early trial [112], but subsequent studies have failed to confirm these results. Combination chemotherapy with doxorubicin, cisplatin, and vindesine resulted in one partial remission and three minor responses out of 10 patients treated. Other combinations of chemotherapeutic regimens reported in the literature include dacarbazine and 5-fluorouracil (5-FU) cyclophosphamide, vincristine, and dacarbazine, 5-FU and streoptozocin. None of these combinations has been shown to be of significant benefit [113–116]. A phase I/II study conducted by Juweid et al. [117] indicated that therapy with (131)i-MN-14 F(ab)2 is well tolerated and shows evidence of biochemical and radiologic antitumor activity. Further dose escalation, by itself or in combination with other therapy modalities, is indicated for future trials.

On the basis of promising reports using interferon therapy in other neuroendocrine tumors, Lupoli et al. [118] used low-dose interferon-α (rIFN-α-2b) and octreotide (a somatostatin analoge) in eight cases of advanced MTC. Tumor-related clinical symptoms improved in five of six patients, who tolerated the therapy, and transient disease stabilization was demonstrated in all cases. Interestingly, although plasma calcitonin levels started to rise again after 6 months, CEA levels were still declining after 12 months of treatment.

In summary, MTC seems to be refractory to chemotherapy, and treatment strategies involving chemotherapeutic regimens have been disappointing. Recent studies with tyrosine kinase inhibitors have shown excellent *in vitro* activity, and clinical trials to test these agents are underway [125–127].

5.3. *Cervical reoperation*

Reoperation for persistent or recurrent MTC in the neck has been reported by several groups [13,80,83,85,86,119,120]. A significant reduction in stimulated calcitonin levels following reoperation was reported in many patients, and normalization of calcitonin levels was noted in some. We reported two series of cervical reoperations for medullary thyroid carcinoma: from 1990 to 1993 [86] and from 1993 to 1996 [85].

In our first reported series of such reoperations, we described experience with 37 operations in 32 patients [86]. The patients had previously undergone total thyroidectomy and most of them also had previous lymph node dissections. All patients had elevated stimulated calcitonin levels. Localization studies, including selected venous catheterization, CT scanning, and physical examination were successful in localizing tumor in half the cases.

Operative morbidity was low and there were no deaths. In 28 of the 35 operations, discharge from the hospital occurred 2 to 5 days postoperatively. In nine cases (group 1), calcitonin was reduced to undetectable levels following reoperation. In 13 cases (group 2), postoperative calcitonin levels decreased by 40% or more. In 10 cases (group 3), postoperative calcitonin levels were not improved. Patient's sex, disease, number of nodes previously resected, preoperative calcitonin levels, and preoperative localization study results were not significantly different between the three groups and therefore unlikely to predict outcome for reoperation. Previously resected tumors from patients in group 3, however, were more likely to have demonstrated invasive features (invasion of adjacent structures, extranodal, or extracapsular spread) than tumors from patients in groups 1 and 2 ($P < 0.05$, Fisher's exact test).

We concluded that reoperation with meticulous removal of residual nodal and tumor tissues in patients with persistent postoperative hypercalcitoninemia, resulted in normalization of calcitonin levels in 28% of patients, and a decrease in calcitonin levels by 40% or more in another 42% of patients. The results also suggested that determination of the degree of invasiveness of the primary tumor may help in selecting patients likely to benefit from reoperative surgery for recurrent medullary thyroid cancer.

We sought to improve our results by a more careful selection of patients, likely to benefit from reoperation [85]. We achieved this by applying systematic metastatic work-up including routing CT or MR imaging of the neck, chest, and abdomen, selective venous catheterization in selected patients, and by institution of routine staging laparoscopy, described earlier.

One hundred and fifteen patients with persistent elevation of calcitonin after primary surgery for MTC were evaluated. After metastatic work-up, which revealed distant disease in 25% of these patients, and discussion of the options (including observation), 52 patients underwent cervical reoperation. 45 patients had cervical re-exploration with curative intent. In seven patients who had palliative cervical operations, one patient had persistent postoperative hypocalcemia. There were no other complications in that group. In the 45 patients who underwent reoperation with curative intent, there were no postoperative deaths and no transfusions were required. Complications included thoracic duct leak in four patients (8.9%), and hypocalcemia (2 patients (4%) at follow-up of 3 months and 2 years). Careful identification and exposure of the RLN was done through a previously undissected area via the lateral, backdoor, or anterior approaches. This resulted in no permanent recurrent nerve injures [121]. Postoperative hoarseness was minimal, and voice returned to its preoperative state in all the patients whose nerves were preserved.

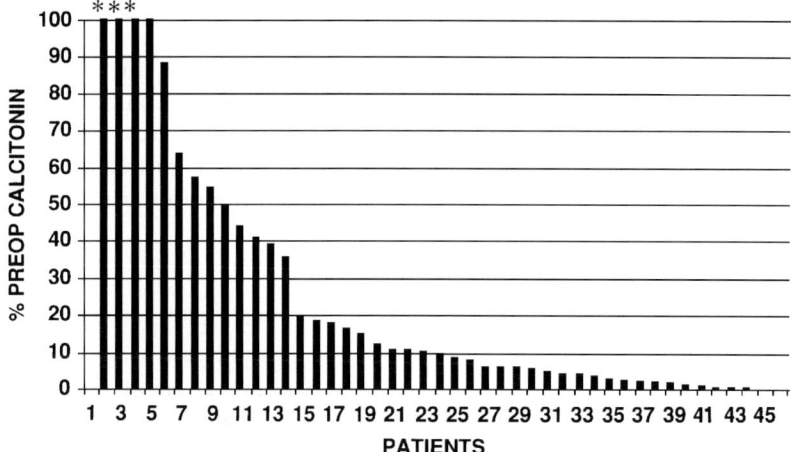

Fig. 4. Postoperative change in peak stimulated calcitonin levels in patients with MEN 2A and MEN 2B, who had reoperations for persistent or recurrent hypercalcitoninemia. The shaded bars indicate the postoperative stimulated calcitonin levels of patients who underwent cervical reexploration and dissection with curative intent. The postoperative calcitonin level is expressed as a percentage of the preoperative calcitonin level: 100% indicates no change in calcitonin level, 10% indicates that the stimulated calcitonin level decreased by 90%. Reprinted with permission from Moley et al. [85].

Of the 45 patients who underwent reoperation with curative intent, the mean decrease in postoperative stimulated calcitonin level was 73.1% (Fig. 4). In 22 of the 45 patients (48%), the postoperative stimulated calcitonin level dropped more than 90% compared with the preoperative value. Of these 45 patients, 17 (38%) had postoperative stimulated calcitonin levels that were within the normal range (group 1), and six (13%) had no significant decrease in stimulated calcitonin levels (group 3). The remaining patients had a >35% reduction in stimulated calcitonin levels (group 2). As in our earlier series, tumor invasiveness was the only parameter that correlated with failure to reduce postoperative calcitonin levels to the normal range ($P < 0.05$, Fisher's exact test). In group 1 patients, review of pathology from the primary operation did not reveal invasiveness in any case (0/17). In group 2 and 3 patients, invasiveness was identified in 8/28 cases.

These results indicate an improvement in outcome following reoperation for persistent or recurrent MTC. In the second series (1992–1996), 38% (17/45) of patients had normal postoperative stimulated calcitonin levels, compared with 28% (9/32) in the first series. Only 13% (6/45) of patients had no decrease in calcitonin levels following reoperation, compared with 31% (10/32) in the first series ($P = 0.07$, Fisher's exact test). This improvement occurred through better preoperative selection of patients and the institution of routine laparoscopic liver examination preoperatively, which identified metastases in 10 patients, nine of whom had normal CT or MR imaging of the liver and who would have otherwise undergone neck reoperation with curative intent.

In this series of 115 patients, 24 decided not to undergo further evaluation or surgical intervention for this problem [85]. If a patient with elevated calcitonin levels has had an adequate previous operation and results of imaging studies are negative, an expectant approach with routine yearly screening is appropriate in many cases. We do, however, feel that it is important to follow these patients closely with routine CT or MRI of the neck and chest. Surveillance should be carried out because if central recurrence develops, resection is possible and will prevent death from airway or great vessel invasion in some patients.

6. Conclusion

Recent advances in the understanding of MTC at the clinical, cellular, and molecular levels have led to dramatic changes in the management of the disease.

The identification of mutations in the RET proto-oncogene associated with MEN 2A, MEN 2B, FMTC, and some cases of sporadic MTC has become the cornerstone of management of patients with hereditary forms of MTC. Prophylactic thyroidectomy based on direct mutation analysis seems to be curative in MEN 2A and FMTC patients when they are screened at a young age.

Refined surgical strategies, and systemic therapies that use drugs that target the molecular basis of MTC will hopefully result in improved outcomes.

References

[1] H.G. Bone III, L.J. Deftos, W.H. Snyder, C.Y. Pak, Mineral metabolic effects of thyroidectomy and long-term outcomes in a family with MEN 2A, Henry Ford Hosp. Med. J. 40 (1992) 258–260.

[2] K.L. Becker, O.L. Liva, R.H. Snider, et al., The surgical implications of hypercalcitoninemia, Surg. Gynecology and Obstetrics 154 (1982) 897.

[3] A. Grauer, F. Raue, R.F. Gagel., Changing concepts in the management of hereditary and sporadic medullary thyroid carcinoma, Endocrinol. Metab. Clin. N. Am. 19 (1990) 613.

[4] J.B. Hazard, W.A. Hawk, G. Crile, Medullary (solid) carcinoma of the thyroid: a clinicopathologic entity, J. Clin. Endocrinol. Metab. 19 (1959) 152.

[5] A.J. Jaquet, Ein Fall von metastasierenden Amyloidtumoren (Lymphosarcoma), Virchows Archiv. [Pathol. Anat.] 185 (1906) 251.

[6] M.F. Saad, N.G. Ordonez, R.K. Rashid, et al., Medullary carcinoma of the thyroid. A study of clinical features and prognostic factors in 161 patients, Medicine 63 (1984) 319.

[7] M.A. Block, C.E. Jackson, K.A. Greenwald, et al., Clinical characteristics distinguishing hereditary from sporadic medullary thyroid carcinoma: treatment implications, Arch. Surg. 115 (1980) 142.

[8] K. Graze, I.J. Spiler, A.H. Tashjian, et al., Natural history of familial medullary thyroid carcinoma. Effect of a program for early diagnosis, N. Engl. J. Med. 299 (1978) 980.

[9] H.J. Wolfe, K.E. Melvin, S.J. Cervi-Skinner, et al., C-cell hyperplasia preceding medullary thyroid carcinoma, N. Engl. J. Med. 289 (1973) 437.

[10] U. Bergholm, H.O. Adami, R. Bergstrom, et al., Clinical characteristics in sporadic and familial medullary thyroid carcinoma: a nationwide study of 249 patients in Sweden from 1959 through 1981, Cancer 63 (1989) 1196.

[11] H. Dralle, G.F.W. Scheumann, C. Proye, et al., The value of lymph node dissection in hereditary medullary thyroid carcinoma: a retrospective, European, multicentre study, J. Intern. Med. 238 (1995) 3685–3693.

[12] T.J. Musholt, G.F.W. Scheumann, H. Dralle, Distant micrometastases-the clue to post-surgical hypercalcitoninemia in MTC (abstract), Eur. J. Surg. Oncol. 20 (1994) 287.

[13] L.E. Tisell, G. Hansson, S. Jansson, et al., Reoperation in the treatment of asymptomatic metastasizing medullary thyroid carcinoma, Surgery 99 (1986) 60.

[14] J.R. Howe, J.A. Norton, S.A. Wells Jr., Prevalence of pheochromocytoma and hyperparathyroidism in multiple endocrine neoplasia type 2A: results of long-term follow-up, Surgery 114 (1993) 1070.

[15] J.A. Carney, V.L.W. Go, G.W. Sizemore, et al., Alimentary tract ganglioneuromatosis: a major component of the syndrome of multiple endocrine neoplasia type 2b, N. Engl. J. Med. 295 (1976) 1287.

[16] M.R. Khairi, R.N. Dexter, N.J. Burzynski, et al., Mucosal neuroma, pheochromocytoma and medullary thyroid carcinoma: multiple endocrine neoplasia type 3, Medicine 54 (1975) 89.

[17] J.R. Farndon, W.G. Dilley, S.B. Baylin, et al., Familial medullary thyroid carcinoma without associated endocrinopathies: A distinct clinical entity, Br. J. Surg. 73 (1986) 278.

[18] I. Libroa, Familial medullary thyroid carcinoma: clinical management, in: Proceedings of the Seventh International Workshop on Multiple Endocrine Neoplasia, Gubbio, Italy, pp. 113–118, 1999.

[19] J.F. Moley, C. Albinson, Medullary thyroid carcinoma and the multiple endocrine neoplasia type 2 syndromes, In: G.M. Doherty, B. Skogseid, Surgical Endocrinology, Lippincott Williams and Wilkins, Philadelphia, 2001.

[20] J.A. Norton, L.C. Froome, R.E. Farrell, et al., Multiple endocrine neoplasia type 2b. The most aggressive form of medullary thyroid carcinoma, Surg. Clin. N. Am. 59 (1979) 109.

[21] R.L. Telander, D. Zimmerman, G.W. Sizemore, et al., Medullary carcinoma in children. Results of early detection and surgery, Arch. Surg. 124 (1989) 841.

[22] N.E. Simpson, K.K. Kidd, P.J. Goodfellow, et al., Assignment of multiple endocrine neoplasia type 2A to chromosome 10 by linkage, Nature 328 (1987) 528.

[23] H. Donis-Keller, S. Dou, D. Chi, et al., Mutations in the RET protooncogene associated with MEN 2A and FMTC, Hum. Mol. Genet. 2 (1993) 851.

[24] L.M. Mulligan, J.B.J. Kwok, C.S. Healey, et al., Germ-line mutations of the RET proto-oncogene in multiple endocrine neoplasia type 2A, Nature 363 (1993) 458.

[25] M. Takahashi, J. Ritz, G.M. Cooper, Activation of a novel human transforming gene, ret, by DNA arrangement, Cell 42 (1985) 581.

[26] J.B. Kwok, E. Gardner, J.P. Warner, et al., Structural analysis of the human ret proto-oncogene using exon trapping, Oncogene 8 (1993) 2575.

[27] T. Tahira, Y. Ishizaka, F. Itoh, et al., Characterization of ret proto-oncogene mRNAs encoding two isoforms of the protein product in a human neuroblastoma cell line, Oncogene 5 (1990) 97.

[28] T. Tahira, Y. Ishizaka, T. Sugimura, et al., Expression of proto-ret mRNA in embryonic and adult rat tissues, Biochem. Biophys. Res. Commun. 153 (1988) 1290.

[29] A. Bolino, L. Schuffenecker, Y. Luo, et al., RET mutations in exons 13 and 14 of FMTC patients, Oncogene 10 (1995) 2415.

[30] C. Eng, D.P. Smith, L.M. Mulligan, et al., A novel point mutation in the tyrosine kinase domain of the RET proto-oncogene in sporadic medullary thyroid carcinoma and in a family with FMTC, Oncogene 10 (1995) 509.

[31] D.J. Marsh, L.M. Mulligan, C. Eng, RET proto-oncogene mutations in multiple endocrine neoplasia type 2 and medullary thyroid carcinoma, Horm. Res. 47 (1997) 168.

[32] P. Niccoli-Sire, A. Murat, V. Rohmver, S. Franc, et al., Familial medullary thyroid carcinoma with noncysteine ret mutations: phenotype–genotype relationship in a large series of patients. J. Clin. Endocrinol. Metab. 86 (2001) 3746–3753.

[33] K.M. Carlson, S. Dou, D. Chi, et al., Single missense mutation in the tyrosine kinase catalytic domain of the RET protooncogene is associated with multiple endocrine neoplasia type 2B, Proc. Natl. Acad. Sci. U.S.A. 91 (1994) 1579.

[34] S.M. Jhiang, L. Fithian, C.M. Weghorst, et al., RET mutation screening in MEN 2 patients and discovery of a novel mutation in a sporadic medullary thyroid carcinoma, Thyroid 6 (1996) 115.

[35] K.J. Marsh, D.L. Learoyd, S.D. Andrew, et al., Somatic mutations in the RET proto-oncogene in sporadic medullary thyroid carcinoma, Clin. Endocrinol. 44 (1996) 249.

[36] A. Schuchardt, V. D'Agati, L. Larsson-Blomberg, et al., Defects in the kidney and enteric nervous system of mice lacking the tyrosine kinase receptor ret, Nature 367 (1994) 377.

[37] M.W. Moore, R.D. Klein, I. Farinas, et al., Renal and neuronal abnormalities in mice lacking GDNF, Nature 382 (1996) 76.

[38] J.G. Pichel, L. Shen, H.Z. Sheng, et al., Defects in enteric innervation and kidney development in mice lacking GDNF, Nature 386 (1996) 73.

[39] M.P. Sanchez, I. Silos-Santiago, J.F. Frisen, et al., Renal agenesis and the absence of enteric neurons in mice lacking GDNE, Nature 382 (1996) 70.

[40] P. Durbec, C.V. Marcos-Gutierrez, C. Kilkenny, et al., GDNF signalling through the RET receptor tyrosine kinase, Nature 381 (1996) 789.

[41] S. Jing, D. Wen, Y. Yu, et al., GDNF-induced activation of the Ret protein tyrosine kinase is mediated by GDNFR-a, a novel receptor for GDNF, Cell 85 (1996) 1113.

[42] J.J.S. Treanor, L. Goodman, F. de Sauvage, et al., Characterisation of a multicomponent receptor for GDNE, Nature 382 (1996) 80.

[43] M. Trupp, E. Areans, M. Fainzilber, et al., Functional receptor for GDNF encoded by the c-ret proto-oncogene, Nature 381 (1996) 785.

[44] L. Ludwig, H. Kessler, M. Wagner, C. Hoang-Vu, et al., Nuclear factor-kappaB is constitutively active in C-cell carcinoma and required for RET-induced transformation, Cancer Res. 61 (2001) 4526–4535.

[45] J. Moley, G. Wallin, M. Brother, et al., Oncogene and growth factor expression in MEN-related tumors, Henry Ford Hosp. Med. J. 40 (1992) 284–288.

[46] K. Herfarth, M. Wick, H. Marshall, et al., Absence of TP53 alternation in pheochromocytomas and medullary thyroid carcinomas, Genes Chromosome Cancer 20 (1997) 24–29.

[47] J.F. Moley, M.B. Brother, S.A. Wells, et al., Low frequency of ras gene mutation in neuroblastomas, pheochromocytomas, and medullary thyroid cancers, Cancer Res. 51 (1991) 1596–1599.

[48] T. Frisk, J. Zedenius, J. Lundberg, G. Wallin, S. Kytola, C. Larsson, CGH alterations in medullary thyroid carcinomas in relation to the RET M918T mutation and clinical outcome, Int. J. Oncol. 18 (2001) 1219–1225.

[49] H. Dralle, L. Damm, G.F.W. Scheumann, et al., Compartment-oriented microdissection of regional lymph nodes in medullary thyroid carcinoma, Surg. Today 24 (1994) 112.

[50] T. Normann, K.M. Gautvik, J.V. Johannessen, et al., Medullary carcinoma of the thyroid in Norway, Acta Endocrinol. 83 (1976) 71–85.

[51] D.S. O'Riordain, T. O'Brien, A.L. Weaver, et al., Medullary thyroid carcinoma in multiple endocrine neoplasia types 2A and 2B, Surgery 116 (1994) 1017–1023.

[52] L.L. Leape, H.H. Miller, K. Graze, et al., Total thyroidectomy for occult familial medullary carcinoma of the thyroid in children, J. Pediatr. Surg. 11 (1976) 831.

[53] C.F. Russell, J.A. van Heerden, G.W. Sizemore, et al., The surgical management of medullary thyroid carcinoma, Ann. Surg. 197 (1983) 42.

[54] R.L. Telander, D. Zimmerman, J.A. van Heerden, et al., Results of early thyroidectomy for medullary thyroid carcinoma in children with multiple endocrine neoplasia type 2, J. Pediatr. Surg. 21 (1986) 1190.

[55] S.A. Wells Jr., S.B. Baylin, G.S. Leight, et al., The importance of early diagnosis in patients with hereditary medullary thyroid carcinoma, Ann. Surg. 195 (1982) 595.

[56] S.A. Wells Jr., W.G. Dilley, J.A. Farndon, et al., Early diagnosis and treatment of medullary thyroid carcinoma, Arch. Intern. Med. 145 (1985) 1248.

[57] S.A. Wells Jr., D.A. Ontjes, C.W. Cooper, et al., The early diagnosis of medullary thyroid carcinoma of the thyroid gland in patients with multiple endocrine neoplasia type 2, Ann. Surg. 182 (1975) 362.

[58] J.F. Moley, M.K. DeBenedetti, Patterns of nodal metastases in palpable medullary thyroid carcinoma: recommendations for extent of node dissection, Ann. Surg. 229 (1999) 880–888.

[59] S.A. Wells Jr., S.B. Baylin, D.S. Gann, et al., Medullary thyroid carcinoma: relationship of method of diagnosis to pathologic staging, Ann. Surg. 188 (1978) 377.

[60] S.A. Wells Jr., S.B. Baylin, W.M. Linehan, R.E. Farrell, E.B. Cox, C.W. Cooper, Provocative agents and the diagnosis of medullary carcinoma of the thyroid gland, Ann. Surg. 188 (1978) 139–141.

[61] P. Motte, M. Ait-Abdellah, P. Vauzelle, P. Gardet, C. Bohuon, D. Bellet, A two-site immunora-diometric assay for serum calcitonin using monoclonal anti-peptide antibodies, Henry Ford Hosp. Med. J. 35 (1987) 129–132.

[62] S.J. Wimalawansa, F. Bailey, Validation, role in perioperative assessment, and clinical applications of an immunoradiometric assay for human calcitonin, Peptides 16 (1995) 307–312.

[63] R.A. Decker, J.D. Geiger, C.E. Cox, et al., Prophylactic surgery for multiple endocrine neoplasia type lia after genetic diagnosis: is parathyroid transplantation indicated?, World J. Surg. 20 (1996) 814–820 (discussion 820–821).

[64] A. Frilling, H. Dralle, C. Eng, et al., Presymptomatic DNA screening in families with multiple endocrine neoplasia type 2 and familial medullary thyroid carcinoma, Surgery 118 (1995) 1099–1104.

[65] C.J.M. Lips, R.M. Landsvater, J.W.M. Hoppener, et al., Clinical screening as compared with DNA analysis in families with multiple endocrine neoplasia type 2A, N. Engl. J. Med. 331 (1994) 828–835.

[66] J.A. Olson Jr., M.K. DeBenedetti, D.S. Baumann, et al., Parathyroid autotransplantation during thyroidectomy. Results of long-term follow-up, Ann. Surg. 223 (1996) 472.

[67] S.A. Wells Jr., A.J. Ross, J.K. Dale, et al., Transplantation of the parathyroid glands: current status, Surg. Clin. N. Am. 59 (1979) 167–177.

[68] A.R. Shaha, R.M. Byers, J.J. Terz, Thyroid cancer surgical practice guidelines in practice guidelines for major cancer sites. Arlington Heights IL: Society of Surgical Oncology, 1997.

[69] P. Musholt, T. Musholt, P. Goodfellow, et al., "Cold" SSCV for mutation analysis of the RET proto-oncogene, Surgery 122 (1997) 363–371.

[70] M.L. Peacock, M.J. Borst, J.D. Sweet, et al., Detection of RET mutations in multiple endocrine neoplasia type 2a and familial medullary thyroid carcinoma by denaturing gradient gel electrophoresis, Hum. Mutat. 7 (1996) 100–104.

[71] M.A. Skinner, M.K. DeBenedetti, J.F. Moley, et al., Medullary thyroid carcinoma in children with multiple endocrine neoplasia types 2A and 2B, J. Pediatr. Surg. 31 (1996) 177.

[72] S.A. Wells Jr., D.D. Chi, K. Toshima, et al., Predictive DNA testing and prophylactic thyroidectomy in patients at risk for multiple endocrine neoplasia type 2A, Ann. Surg. 220 (1994) 237.

[73] S.A. Wells Jr., M.A. Skinner, Prophylactic thyroidectomy, based on direct genetic testing, in patients at risk for the multiple endocrine neoplasia type 2 syndromes, Exp. Clin. Endocrinol. Diabetes 106 (1998) 29–34.

[74] S.A. Wells, C. Franz, Medullary carcinoma of the thyroid gland, World J. Surg. 24 (2000) 952–956.

[75] L.E. Tisell, W.G. Dilley, S.A. Wells Jr., Progression of postoperative residual medullary thyroid carcinoma as monitored by plasma calcitonin levels, Surgery 119 (1996) 34.

[76] D. Guilloteau, R. Perdristo, C. Calmettes, et al., Diagnosis of medullary carcinoma of the thyroid (MCT) by calcitonin assay using monoclonal antibodies: criteria for the pentagastrin stimulation test in hereditary MCT, J. Clin. Endocrinol. Metab. 71 (1990) 1064–1067.

[77] S.A. Wells, D. Haagensen, W. Linehan, et al., The detection of elevated plasma levels of carcinoembryonic antigen in patients with suspected or established medullary thyroid carcinoma, Cancer 42 (1978) 1498.

[78] B. Busnardo, M.E. Girelli, N. Simioni, et al., Nonparallel patterns of calcitonin and carcinoembryonic antigen levels in the follow-up of medullary thyroid carcinoma, Cancer 53 (1984) 278.

[79] G. Eisenhofer, J.W. Lenders, W.M. Linehan, et al., Plasma normetanephrine and metanephrine for detecting pheochromocytoma in von Hippel-Lindau disease and multiple endocrine neoplasia 2, N. Engl. J. Med. 340 (1999) 1872–1879.

[80] M.A. Block, C.E. Jackson, A.H. Tshjian Jr., Management of occult medullary thyroid carcinoma: evidenced only by serum calcitonin level elevations after apparently adequate neck operations, Arch. Surg. 113 (1978) 368.

[81] A.V. Stepanas, N.A. Samaan, C.S. Hill Jr., et al., Medullary thyroid carcinoma: importance of serial serum calcitonin measurement, Cancer 43 (1979) 825.

[82] J.A. van Heerden, C.S. Grant, H. Gharib, et al., Long-term course of patients with persistent hypercalcitoninemia after apparent curative primary surgery for medullary thyroid carcinoma, Ann. Surg. 212 (1990) 395.

[83] H.J. Buhr, F. Kallinowski, F. Raue, et al., Microsurgical neck dissection for occultly metastasizing medullary thyroid carcinoma. Three-year results, Cancer 72 (1993) 3685.

[84] G.C. Chong, O.H. Beahrs, G.W. Sizemore, et al., Medullary carcinoma of the thyroid gland, Cancer 35 (1975) 695.

[85] J.F. Moley, W.G. Dilley, M.K. DeBenedetti, Improved results of cervical reoperation for medullary thyroid carcinoma, Ann. Surg. 225 (1997) 734–743.

[86] J.F. Moley, S.A. Wells Jr., W.G. Dilley, et al., Reoperation for recurrent or persistent medullary thyroid cancer, Surgery 114 (1993) 1090–1096.

[87] T.J. Musholt, J.F. Moley, Management of recurrent medullary thyroid carcinoma after total thyroidectomy, Prob. Gen. Surg. 14 (1997) 89–110.

[88] K.M. Gautvik, K. Talle, B. Hager, et al., Early liver metastases in patients with medullary carcinoma of the thyroid gland, Cancer 63 (1989) 175.

[89] W.S. Tung, T.M. Vesely, J.F. Moley, Laparoscopic detection of hepatic metastases in patients with residual or recurrent medullary thyroid cancer, Surgery 118 (1995) 1024–1030.

[90] N. Abdelmoumene, M. Schlumberger, P. Gardet, et al., Selective venous sampling catheterisation for localization of persisting medullary thyroid carcinoma, Br. J. Cancer 69 (1994) 1141–1144.

[91] R.J. Bigsby, E.K. Lepp, D.E. Litwin, et al., Technetium 99 m pentavalent dimercaptosuccinic acid and thallium 201 in detecting recurrent medullary carcinoma of the thyroid, Can. J. Surg. 35 (1992) 388–392.

[92] M. Koizumi, H. Taguchi, M. Goto, et al., Thallium-201 scintigraphy in the evaluation of thyroid nodules A retrospective study of 246 cases, Ann. Nucl. Med. 7 (1993) 147–152.

[93] T. Ohnishi, S. Noguchi, N. Murakami, et al., Detection of recurrent thyroid cancer: MR versus thallium-201 scintigraphy, Am. J. Neuroradiol. 14 (1993) 1051–1057.

[94] P.S. Sinha, D.I. Beeby, P. Ryan, An evaluation of thallium imaging for detection of carcinoma in clinically palpable solitary, nonfunctioning thyroid nodules, Thyroid 11 (2001) 85–89.

[95] K. Frank-Raue, H. Bihl, U. Dorr, et al., Somatostatin receptor imaging in persistent medullary thyroid carcinoma, Clin. Endocrinol. (Oxf.) 42 (1995) 31–37.

[96] L. Berna, A. Chico, X. Matias-Guiu, E. Mato, et al., Use of somatostatin analogue scintigraphy in the localization of recurrent medullary thyroid carcinoma, Eur. J. Nucl. Med. 25 (1998) 1482–1488.

[97] P. Peltier, C. Curtet, J.F. Chatal, et al., Radioimmunodetection of medullary thyroid cancer using a bispecific anti-CEA/anti-indium-DTPA antibody and an indium-111-labeled DTPA dimer, J. Nucl. Med. 34 (1993) 1267–1273.

[98] L. Manil, F. Boudet, P. Motte, et al., Positive anticalcitonin immunoscintigraphy in patients with medullary thyroid carcinoma, Cancer Res. 49 (1989) 5480–5485.

[99] T.M. Behr, N. Jenner, M. Behe, et al., Radiolabeled peptides for targeting cholecystokinin-B/gastrin receptor-expressing tumors, J. Nucl. Med. 40 (1999) 1029–1044.

[100] D.J. Kwekkeboom, W.H. Bakker, P.P. Kooij, et al., Cholecystokin receptor imaging using octapeptide DTPA-CCK analogue in patients with medullary thyroid carcinoma, Eur. J. Nucl. Med. 27 (2000) 1312–1317.

[101] W.A. Waddington, A.G. Kettle, R.M. Heddle, A.J. Coakley, Intraoperative localization of recurrent medullary carcinoma of the thyroid using indium-111 pentetreotide and a nuclear surgical probe, Eur. J. Nucl. Med. 21 (1994) 363–364.

[102] T.J. Musholt, P.B. Musholt, F. Dehdashti, J.F. Moley, Evaluation of fluorodeoxyglucose positron emission tomographic scanning and its association with glucose transporter expression in medullary thyroid carcinoma and pheochromocytoma: a clinical and molecular study, Surgery 122 (1997) 1049–1061.

[103] T.J. Babineau, W.D. Lewis, R.L. Jenkins, R. Bleday, G.J. Steele, R.A. Forse, Role of staging laparoscopy in the treatment of hepatic malignancy, Am. J. surg. 167 (1994) 151–154.

[104] A.L. Warshaw, J.E. Tepper, W.U. Shipley, Laparoscopy in the staging and planning of therapy for pancreatic cancer, Am. J. Surg. 51 (1986) 76–80.

[105] M. Juweid, R.M. Sharkey, T. Behr, et al., Targeting and initial radioimmunotherapy of medullary thyroid carcinoma with 131I-labeled monoclonal antibodies to carcinoembryonic antigen, Cancer Res. 55 (suppl) (1995) 5946S–5951S.

[106] P. Rougier, C. Parmnetier, A. Laplanche, et al., Medullary thyroid carcinoma: prognostic factors and treatment, Int. J. Radiat. Oncol. Biol. Phys. 9 (1983) 161.

[107] W.J. Simpson, Radiotherapy in thyroid cancer, Can. Med. Assoc. J. 113 (1975) 115–118.

[108] A.D. Steinfeld, The role of radiation therapy in medullary carcinoma of the thyroid, Radiology 123 (1977) 745–746.

[109] N.A. Samaan, P.N. Schultz, R.C. Hickey, Medullary thyroid carcinoma: prognosis of familial versus sporadic disease and the role of radiotherapy, J. Clin. Endocrinol. Metab. 67 (1988) 801–805.

[110] T.D. Nguyen, J.L. Chassard, P. Lagarde, et al., Results of postoperative radiation therapy in medullary carcinoma of the thyroid: a retrospective study by the French Federation of Cancer Institutes-the Radiotherapy Cooperative Group, Radiother. Oncol. 23 (1992) 1–5.

[111] K.P. Yang, Y.P. Liang, N.A. Samaan, Intrinsic drug resistance in a human medullary thyroid carcinoma cell line: association with overexpression of mdrl gene and low proliferation fraction, Anticancer Res. 11 (1991) 1065–1068.

[112] J.A. Gottlib, D.S. Hill Jr., Chemotherapy of thyroid cancer with Adriamycin. Experience with 30 patients, N. Engl. J. Med. 290 (1974) 193–197.

[113] F. Orlandi, P. Caraci, A. Berruti, et al., Chemotherapy with dacarbazine and 5-fluorouracil in advanced medullary thyroid cancer, Ann. Oncol. 5 (1994) 763–765.

[114] S.R. Petursson, Metastatic medullary thyroid carcinoma. Complete response to combination chemotherapy with dacarbazine and 5-fluorouracil, Cancer 62 (1988) 1899–1903.

[115] M. Schlumberger, N. Abdelmoumene, M.J. Deiisle, et al., Treatment of advanced medullary thyroid cancer with an alternating combination of 5 FU-streptozocin and 5 Fudacarbazine. The Groupe D'Etudedes Tumeurs a Calcitonine (GETC), Br. J. Cancer 71 (1995) 363–365.

[116] L.T. Wu, S.D. Averbuch, D.W. Ball, et al., Treatment of advanced medullary thyroid carcinoma with a combination of cyclophosphamide, vincristine, and dacarbazine, Cancer 73 (1994) 432–436.

[117] M.E. Juweid, G. Hajjar, L.C. Swayne, et al., Phase I/II trial of (131)I-MN-14F(ab)2 anti-carcinoembryonic antigen monoclonal antibody in the treatment of patients with metastatic medullary thyroid carcinoma, Cancer 85 (1999) 1828–1842.

[118] G. Lupoli, E. Cascone, F. Arlotta, G. Vitale, L. Celentano, M. Salvatore, G. Lombardi, Treatment of advanced medullary thyroid carcinoma with a combination of recombinant interferon α-2b octreotide, Cancer 78 (1996) 1114–1118.

[119] J.D. Ellenhorn, J.P. Shah, M.F. Brennan, Impact of therapeutic regional lymph node dissection for medullary carcinoma of the thyroid gland, Surgery 114 (1993) 1078.

[120] J.A. Norton, J.L. Doppman, M.F. Brennan, Localization and resection of clinically inapparent medullary carcinoma of the thyroid, Surgery 87 (1980) 616–622.

[121] J.F. Moley, T.C. Lairmore, G.M. Doherty, M. Brunt, M.K. DeBenedetti, Preservation of the recurrent laryngeal nerves in thyroid and parathyroid reoperations, Surgery 125 (1999) 673–679.

[122] A. Ruiz, G. Antinolo, I. Marcos, S. Borrego, Novel technique for scanning of codon 634 of the RET protooncogene with fluorescence resonance energy transfer and real-time PCR in patients with medullary thyroid carcinoma, Clin. Chem. 47 (2001) 1939–1944.

[123] C.A. Koch, S.C. Huang, J.F. Moley, N. Azumi, G.P. Chrousos, R.F. Gagel, Z. Zhuang, K. Pacak, A.O. Vortmeyer, Allelic imbalance of the mutant and wild-type RET allele in MEN 2A-associated medullary thyroid carcinoma, Oncogene 20 (2001) 7809–7811.

[124] S.C. Huang, J. Torres-Cruz, S.D. Pack, C.A. Koch, A.O. Vortmeyer, P. Mannan, I.A. Lubensky, R.F. Gagel, Z.J. Zhuang, Amplification and overexpression of mutant RET in multiple endocrine neoplasia type 2-associated medullary thyroid carcinoma, Clin. Endocrinol. Metab. 88 (2003) 459–463.

[125] M.S. Cohen, H.B. Hussain, J.F. Moley, Inhibition of medullary thyroid carcinoma cell proliferation and RET phosphorylation by tyrosine kinase inhibitors, Surgery 132 (2002) 960–966.

[126] F. Carlomagno, et al., ZD6474, an orally available inhibitor of KDR tyrosine kinase activity, efficiently blocks oncogenic RET kinases, Cancer Res. 62 (2002) 7284–7290.

[127] F. Carlomagno, et al., The kinase inhibitor PP1 blocks tumorigenesis induced by RET oncogenes, Cancer Res. 62 (2002) 1077–1082.

Chapter 9

Thyroid neoplasms in children and adolescents

Wellington Hung

*Division of Pediatric Endocrinology and Metabolism, Department of Pediatrics,
Georgetown University Medical Center, Washington, DC*

Occurence of thyroid carcinomas in the pediatric age group is rare. Well-differentiated thyroid carcinoma (WDTC), papillary, and follicular carcinomas comprised only 1.3% of all the newly diagnosed childhood carcinomas in the United States reported from 1973 to 1987, as determined from data collected by the National Cancer Institute of the National Institutes of Health [1]. Two-thirds of WDTC occur in females, with a peak incidence between 7 and 12 years of age [2]. WDTC in children and adolescents have a relatively favorable prognosis in contrast to other malignancies. Most pediatric studies group papillary and follicular thyroid neoplasma as WDTC and this convention will be followed in this chapter.

1. Epidemiology

1.1. *Well-differentiated thyroid carcinoma*

The epidemiology of WDTC is not well understood, and the relative proportion of papillary and follicular carcinomas varies geographically, perhaps as a function of the iodine content of the diet [3]. Recent studies indicate that iodine deficiency alters the pathology of thyroid carcinoma by increasing the relative incidence of follicular and anaplastic carcinomas, while sufficient iodine increases the percentage of papillary thyroid carcinomas [4].

From 1920 to 1960, radiotherapy was widely used in children for treating benign conditions of the head, neck, and upper chest such as tinea capitis, acne and thymic enlargement. In 1949, Quimby and Werner [5] suggested the possibility of a relationship between neck radiation and subsequent development of thyroid cancer. The thyroid gland during childhood is highly sensitive to irradiation. Numerous investigations have verified the relationship suggested by Quimby and Werner. After 1950, radiotherapy for benign conditions gradually stopped. Investigational techniques,

ADVANCES IN MOLECULAR AND CELLULAR ENDOCRINOLOGY
VOLUME 4   ISSN 1569-2566/DOI 10.1016/S1569-2566(04)04009-8

especially fluoroscopy, can involve radiation exposure in the range implicated in the pathogenesis of thyroid tumors [6].

Exposure to γ radiation as well as higher energy β emitters such as radioiodines following atomic fallout are associated with development of thyroid carcinoma [7]. The accident at the nuclear power plant in Chernobyl, Ukraine on April 26, 1986, released into the atmosphere $\sim$1800 PBq (49MCi) of ^{131}I, 2500 PBq (68MCi) of ^{133}I and 1000 PBq (27MCi) of ^{132}Tel, which decays to ^{132}I [8,9]. As early as 4 years after the accident, the incidence of papillary thyroid carcinoma in pediatric patients in the most contaminated region, the province of Gomel, Belarus, increased dramatically [10,11]. These findings provide evidence that the marked increase in thyroid carcinoma was a direct consequence of exposure to radioactive iodine fallout [12]. The short latency period of 4 years for thyroid carcinoma to be detected is in contrast to 18 years observed in other radiation-associated thyroid papillary carcinomas [13].

Cytogenetic studies on papillary and follicular carcinomas from pediatric patients exposed to radiation in Belarus have been performed to study the pathogenetic mechanism(s) of carcinogenic induction by ionizing radiation. Proto-oncogenes are protein products that regulate cell growth. When proto-oncogenes undergo activating mutations, they become oncogenes and contribute to uncontrolled proliferation and growth. The RET proto-oncogene is located on human chromosome 10q11.2 and encodes a transmembrane receptor with a tyrosine kinase domain [14]. The RET proto-oncogene is a member of a large class of protein tyrosine kinases that function as signal transduction molecules to regulate cellular function and proliferation [15]. RET activation is found in papillary thyroid carcinomas, hence the name RET/PTC. Oncogene rearrangements result from fusion of the tyrosine kinase domain of the *RET* gene and the 5′ regulatory parts of other ubiquitously expressed genes, particularly ELE1 [16]. Three main RET/PTC rearrangements have been identified in thyroid epithelial tumors: RET/PTC1, RET/PTC2, and RET/PTC3. In papillary thyroid carcinomas, which occurred in Belarus after the Chernobyl accident, RET rearrangements were detected in 60–80% of children while in adults only RET/PTC1 rearrangements were observed. However, RET/PTC1 and RET/PTC3 rearrangements were seen in children [17]. It is likely that RET/PTC1 rearrangement is correlated with radiation-induced carcinogenesis because it is observed in only 3–35% of 'spontaneous' papillary thyroid carcinomas [18,19]. Some investigators have suggested that RET/PTC3 rearrangement is preferentially formed after exposure to high radiation and is related to aggressive growth of carcinomas [20]. Point gene mutations of RAS, TP53, and GSP were not significant following the Chernobyl accident, thereby differing from sporadic cases of papillary thyroid carcinoma [21,22].

Another cytogenetic change observed in Belarussian children was receptor tyrosine kinase NTRK1 rearrangement in some of the papillary carcinomas [23]. Santoro et al. [24] suggest that activation of receptor tyrosine kinase genes played a predominant role in the carcinogenesis in these children.

Activating point mutations of the RAS genes are found in a high frequency in thyroid adenomas and follicular carcinomas, which suggested that RAS mutations may represent an early event in thyroid tumorigenesis [25,26]. There are other stimuli for thyroid growth and function, including insulin-like growth factor 1, prostaglandin, and growth hormone. Although these stimuli are thought to have a growth-promoting effect in benign thyroid disease, it is not clear that they have an effect on the growth of WDTC.

Survival rates for patients with many pediatric malignancies have improved, but therapeutic radiation and chemotherapy have been implicated in the development of secondary thyroid carcinomas in some patients [27]. Genetic factors have been suggested as etiologic factors in reports of thyroid carcinomas in familial syndromes such as Pendred syndrome, Gardner syndrome, Cowden syndrome, and Familial polyposis [28]. Pal et al. [29] have suggested that there may be familial factors that predispose children to develop thyroid carcinoma.

1.2. *Medullary thyroid carcinoma*

Medullary thyroid carcinoma (MTC) originate in calcitonin-producing cells (C-cells) of the thyroid. C-cells are of neuroectodermal origin and do not accumulate iodine. There are familial and sporadic variants of MTC. Patients with MTC or its precursor, C-cell hyperplasia, have elevated basal plasma immunoreactive plasma calcitonin (iCT) levels and responses to various stimuli. Multiple endocrine neoplasia type 2 (MEN 2) is an autosomal dominant syndrome. All variants of MEN 2 show a high penetrance for MTC and are caused by germline mutations of the RET proto-oncogene. MEN 2A is characterized by the presence of MTC, pheochromocytoma, and parathyroid adenoma [30]. MEN 2B is characterized by MTC, pheochromocytoma, mucosal ganglioneuroma, and a marfanoid habitus [31]. MEN 2B is the most aggressive of the MEN 2 variants [32]. In familial MTC (FMTC), MTC occurs without other abnormalities [33].

Specific mutations are present in each of the above forms of MTC. The inherited defects responsible for these mutations map to the pericentromere region of chromosome 10 [34,35]. The specifically mutated RET correlates with the MEN 2 variant, including the aggressiveness of MTC [32]. The mutations in the RET proto-oncogene may be responsible for the development of neoplasia in these disorders [36].

1.3. *Anaplastic thyroid carcinoma*

Anaplastic carcinomas of the thyroid gland probably represent the terminal stage in the dedifferentiation of differentiated carcinomas [37]. The cause of the dedifferentiation is not known.

RAS oncogene activation is high in anaplastic carcinomas and in differentiated thyroid tumors [26]. Activation of RAS has been thought to be an early occurrence in thyroid tumorigenesis [25]. The p53 gene is a tumor suppressor gene and is the most commonly affected gene in human cancer [38]. Inactivating point mutations of p53 are frequently present in anaplastic but not in differentiated thyroid carcinoma, suggesting that p53 mutations play an important role in progression from differentiated to undifferentiated or anaplastic carcinoma [38].

2. Pathological features

2.1. *Papillary thyroid carcinoma*

Papillary thyroid carcinoma is usually unencapsulated, welldifferentiated, and sharply circumscribed from surrounding thyroid parenchyma. The cancer may be multicentric. Papillary foci have a moderately dense fibrous stroma and tend to invade between follicles. Psammona bodies are a feature of papillary carcinoma. The tumors spread to normal surrounding thyroid parenchyma and regional lymph nodes. These carcinomas characteristically grow slowly [39].

2.2. *Follicular thyroid carcinoma*

These carcinomas are well-differentiated tumors characterized by well-developed follicles and by the absence of well-differentiated papillae. They are usually encapsulated and have a marked tendency to vascular invasion and spread to bone and lung.

2.3. *Medullary thyroid carcinoma*

MTC vary in size from barely visible to those that replace the entire thyroid gland. Most sporadic and FMTC are not encapsulated and show a solid pattern of growth. They exhibit a wide spectrum of histological patterns that mimic other types of thyroid malignancies. The presence of amyloid is diagnostic. C-cell hyperplasia is present either adjacent to the carcinoma or at a distance from it. FMTC characteristically involve both lobes. MTC initially metastasize to lymph nodes of the neck and mediastinum. The tumor may replace an entire lobe and extend into perithyroidal soft tissues. MTC metastasize to lung, bone, and liver.

2.4. *Anaplastaic thyroid carcinoma*

Anaplastic thyroid carcinomas are usually large and widely invasive. Three distinct microscopic morphological patterns exist: (1) squamoid, (2) spindle cell, and (3) giant cell. The tumor usually replaces most of the thyroid gland and spreads into the soft tissues of the neck, lungs, bone, and brain.

3. Clinical features

Most pediatric patients with thyroid carcinoma present with a solitary thyroid nodule, multinodular goiter, goiter, or cervical lymphadenopathy [28]. Single or multiple nodules of the thyroid gland are an uncommon finding in pediatric patients. The implications of a solitary thyroid nodule are different from those of multiple nodules. The risk of malignancy is supposedly lower in a thyroid gland with discrete multiple nodules than in a solitary thyroid nodule. However, Garcia et al. [40] reported 16 children and adolescents with multiple thyroid nodules and 4 of the patients had carcinoma. Three of the patients had follicular carcinomas and a history of radiation

Table 1
Differential diagnosis of solitary thyroid nodules

Adenomas	Follicular
	Colloid
	Toxic
Carcinomas	Papillary
	Follicular
	Mixed papillary-follicular
	Medullary
	Anaplastic
Chronic lymphocytic thyroiditis	Cysts
	Abscess
Developmental anomalies	Agenesis of lone lobe
	Intrathyroidal thyroglossal duct cyst

Table 2
Differential diagnosis of multinodular thyroid disease

Chronic lymphocytic thyroiditis	Prior to medical therapy
	Secondary to medical therapy
Infections	Bacterial
	Viral
Multiple follicular adenomas	
Cysts	Colloid
	Adenomatous
Carcinoma secondary to radiation therapy	Iodine deficiency
	Hyperplasia
	Goitrogen-induced
	Inborn errors of thyroid hormone synthesis

therapy to the neck and upper chest. The other patient had no history of exposure to radiation and had a papillary carcinoma.

Clinically, it is not always possible to be certain that a single thyroid nodule is indeed single. Some thyroid glands, judged on physical examination, are found by ultrasonography or surgical exploration to have more than one nodule. Table 1 lists the differential diagnosis of a solitary thyroid nodule in pediatric patients and Table 2 lists the differential diagnosis of multiple nodules of the thyroid.

4. Diagnosis

4.1. *History and physical examination*

The history is important and should include questions about external irradiation to the head, neck, and upper chest. A history of goitrogen exposure should be sought.

Information regarding the rate of growth of the mass(es), the presence of local or systemic symptoms, hoarseness, or dysphagia should be obtained. The family history should be explored for the presence of thyroid disease, hyperparathyroidism, and pheochromocytoma. Rapid painless growth of a nodule suggests the presence of carcinoma. Pain or tenderness in the thyroid gland is an unusual complaint with malignancy, but may be marked in viral or bacterial thyroiditis. A rapidly enlarging nodule with transient pain suggest hemorrhage into a cyst.

Careful palpation of a thyroid nodule helps in defining its nature. A soft compressible nodule is unlikely to be malignant and is more likely to be a cyst. However, on occasions a cyst can be quite firm on palpation. Tenderness in a nodule suggests hemorrhage into a cyst or an inflammatory process. Malignancy should be suspected if the nodule is hard, if there is fixation to surrounding structures, or if there is vocal cord paralysis. Lymphadenopathy, particularly low in the neck, increases the likelihood of malignancy. In most pediatric patients with a malignant nodule, the surrounding thyroid tissue appears normal and the gland is not enlarged.

Children with MTC generally have no clinical symptoms but are evaluated either because they have a thyroid nodule, palpable cervical lymphadenopathy, or because they are members of a kindred with MTC and have a positive RET germline mutation or have increased iCT levels of testing.

Patients with MEN 2A have a normal appearance, while those with MEN 2B have a 'marfanoid' body build and multiple neuromas of the lips, eyelids, and tongue. Slit-lamp examination of the cornea may show enlargement of the corneal nerves. Ganglioneuromas may be present throughout the gasatrointestinal tract and cause symptoms including constipation and diarrhea, often beginning in infancy.

4.2. *Blood studies*

In general, there is no blood test that is of value in diagnosing WDTC or anaplastic carcinoma. Nevertheless, serum T4, T3, and TSH determinations are helpful in determining the functional status of the thyroid gland. It should be stressed that the degree of hyperthyroidism due to a toxic nodule may not be sufficiently severe to allow diagnosis on clinical grounds. Hypothyroidism should be ruled out, which, if secondary to chronic lymphocytic thyroiditis, can be associated with solitary or multiple nodules. Serum thyroglobulin (Tg) levels are not only elevated in patients with WDTC, but also elevated in benign thyroid disorders. Thus, measurement of serum TG is not helpful initially but is of great importance in the management of patients with WDTC.

Measurement of plasma iCT, both basally and in response to pentagastrin, permits the detection of MTC in some patients before the appearance of any clinical signs or symptoms [41]. Testing with pentagastrin allows screening of families with MTC who are at risk of developing of C-cell disease. Unfortunately, this biochemical testing does not detect all patients at risk [42]. The stimulation test may be performed with infusion of the stimuli over 1 min Calcium gluconate (2 mg of Ca^{2+} kg^{-1}) and petagastrin ($0.5 \mu g \, kg^{-1}$). Plasma iCT is measured at 1–5 min [43]. Abnormal basal and stimulated plasma iCT values must be obtained from the reference laboratory performing the study.

The recent identification of mutations in the RET proto-oncogene allows diagnosis of patients who are gene carriers and are predisposed to develop C-cell hyperplasia and MTC. This knowledge allows prophylactic thyroidectomy to be performed before development of any neoplastic changes [44,45]. Molecular genetic testing is more specific than biochemical testing and should replace biochemical testing when possible.

4.3. *Radionuclide imaging*

The traditional approach to evaluating patients with nodular thyroid disease has been radioisotope scanning, aiming to classify nodules as 'cold', 'hot', or 'warm' depending on their ability to concentrate the isotope. Scanning can be done with iodine-123 (^{123}I) or technetium-99m pertechnetate (^{99m}Tc). The value of such scans is limited by poor differentiation of benign from malignant disease. However, scans allow one to rule out the presence of anomalies such as agenesis of a lobe with compensatory hypertrophy of the contralateral lobe presenting as a solitary nodule.

A solitary hot nodule can be toxic or non-toxic and may or may not be autonomous in function. Hot nodules that do not produce hyperthyroidism initially can increase their secretion of thyroid hormones gradually and insidiously until clinical hyperthyroidism results. In pediatric patients, there is a more rapid progression to hyperthyroidism and a higher incidence of carcinoma when compared with adults [46]. It has been recommended that all hot solitary thyroid nodules in pediatric patients be removed surgically [46].

Patients with solitary thyroid nodules most commonly have cold nodules on scintiscanning [47]. A study of 93 pediatric with solitary thyroid nodules revealed that 77 nodules (82.8%) were cold [47]. The most common cause of a cold solitary nodule is a follicular adenoma. It is the patient with a cold nodule who presents the greatest clinical challenge in differentiating a benign from a malignant nodule. Cold nodules can be found in carcinomas, chronic lymphocytic thyroiditis, cysts, follicular adenomas, abscesses, and embryonic defects. The highest incidence of carcinomas occur in patients with cold solitary nodules.

4.4. *Ultrasonography*

Ultrasonographic examination of the thyroid provides an accurate means of assessing thyroid size and the presence, number, and size of thyroid nodules. Sonography will differentiate solid lesions from cystic lesions and is more sensitive than radionuclide scans in detecting multiple nodules.

Cystic lesions are generally considered to be benign lesions. Most cysts result from necrosis and degeneration of nodules. Desjardin and associates [48] reported a series of 12 pediatric patients with thyroid carcinoma in whom nearly half had cystic nodules. Surgical removal of all cystic nodules for diagnosis as well as for therapy has been recommended [47].

5. Thyroid hormone suppression

It is not clear whether long-term levothyroxine (LT4) therapy to achieve partial suppression of TSH is an effective method of treating thyroid nodules. The use of high-dose LT4 to fully suppress TSH for benign thyroid disease is not beneficial or safe [49]. The rationale for LT4 suppression therapy is based on evidence that TSH is the main stimulator of thyroid growth and function [50]. LT4 suppression therapy for unknown nodular thyroid is not recommended for pediatric patients.

5.1. *Biopsy*

There has been an increase in the successful use of fine-needle aspiration biopsy (FNAB) in pediatric patients with thyroid nodules [51,52]. The use of FNAB in pediatric patients requires an experienced aspirationist working in close association with an experienced cytopathologist. FNAB is recommended if a solid solitary nodule is present and there is no suspicion of malignancy based on history or physical findings. If an experienced aspirationist and cytopathologist are not available, open surgical biopsy is recommended.

6. Treatment of thyroid carcinoma

6.1. *Well-differentiated thyroid carcinoma*

There is a continuing controversy regarding the optimal management of children and adolescents with WDTC because of various features of this malignancy. These features include: (1) its aggressive behavior compared to that in adults, (2) its tendency to metastasize early, and (3) its usual good long-term prognosis with an overall survival rate >95% [53]. There are no prospective randomized clinical trials to guide the clinician in the management of pediatric patients with WDTC. It is unlikely that any such trials will ever be conducted, given the relatively small number of patients, slow progression of the disease, and its overall good prognosis. The most controversial aspect of management is the extent and/or aggressiveness of treatment required, which mainly include surgery and [131]I.

Surgery is the primary therapy for WDTC in pediatric patients [54]. Controversy exist as to whether total (or near-total) thyroidectomy versus subtotal thyroidectomy is the procedure of choice [55]. There is very seldom an indication for radical neck dissection in pediatric patients [56]. Regardless of the surgical procedure, it should be performed by an experienced thyroid surgeon. A minority of surgeons recommend subtotal thyroidectomy because they believe that the literature has not provided enough support for the conclusion that total (or near-total) thyroidectomy leads to improved survival when compared with subtotal thyroidectomy. This group of surgeons also argue that the more complete surgical procedure may increase the incidence of serious complications such as permanent hypoparathyroidism or recurrent laryngeal nerve damage.

Most surgeons currently perform total or near-total thyroidectomy in pediatric patients with WDTC, based on favorable interpretation of the available data, that this type of surgery reduces the rate of local recurrences [57,58]. In addition, they point to the well-known frequent occurrence of multiple, bilateral foci of papillary micro-carcinoma in glands of patients with papillary thyroid carcinoma [59]. Total thyroidectomy will increase the efficiency of ^{131}I therapy as well as the sensitivity of diagnostic RAI whole body scanning (WBS) at the time of ablation therapy. This is based on the fact that normal thyroid tissue concentrates RAI much more efficiently than WDTC tissue. Also, serum Tg levels will be significantly lower after total thyroidectomy compared with the level after subtotal thyroidectomy, thereby allowing this tumor marker to be used as a sensitive indicator of residual or recurrent disease. Following thyroidectomy, patients are placed on TSH-suppressive doses of LT4 by most clinicians.

Depending on the amount of residual postoperative normal thyroid remnant, any coexisting carcinoma metastases may not be detected at the time of a diagnostic RAI WBS [60]. Additionally, without ablation of thyroid remnants, the treatment of metastases may be less effective because normal thyroid tissue accumulates ^{131}I more efficiently than WDTC. Thyroid remnant ablation has been successful in the majority of pediatric patients after a single dose of 29.9 MCi [131]I (1.1 GBq) administered as an outpatient [61]. Some clinicians recommend obtaining a WBS 5 to 7 days after the ablation dose of [131]I [54]. Usually, the scan visualizes the thyroid remnant, and may reveal previously unsuspected areas of local or disseminated spread of disease that can be treated by further ^{131}I treatment(s).

Following surgery and ^{131}I ablation of thyroid remnants, a diagnostic WBS is recommended to assess the need for further ^{131}I therapy; this should be performed within 6 months after the remnant ablation and in conjunction with measurement of serum Tg. In preparation for the WBS, patients are made hypothyroid over a period of 6 weeks. In order to increase the affinity of any thyroid tissue for ^{131}I, it has been recommended that a low-iodine diet be instituted (daily iodine content $< 50 \, \mu g$) for 2 weeks prior to scanning. Patients who take LT4 following thyroidectomy should discontinue it and start L-triiodothyronine (LT3), $1 \, \mu g^{-1} \, kg^{-1} \, day^{-1}$, divided into 2 or 3 doses for 4 weeks. LT3 is discontinued 2 weeks before ^{131}I therapy. The serum TSH level should be $> 25 \, mU \, L^{-1}$ (third generation) to optimize iodine uptake. An increasing number of adult endocrinologists administer recombinant human TSH (rhTSH), while the patients remain on LT4 therapy [62]. The use of rhTSH avoids the necessity of producing hypothyroidism. At present, the use of rhTSH in pediatric patients has not been approved by the United States Food and Drug Administration.

The diagnostic WBS can be performed using 0.5–1 mCi (18–74 MBq) of ^{131}I or 150–300 μCi (5.6–11.1 MBq) of ^{123}I as the tracer and quantitative uptakes can be measured at 24 h (as well as at 48 and 72 h when ^{131}I is used) [63]. Some clinicians prefer to use larger doses of ^{131}I but most metastatic lesions amenable to ^{131}I therapy are unlikely to be missed in an athyreotic patient using diagnostic doses of ^{131}I cited above, especially when the information obtained from the diagnostic WBS is combined with measurement of serum Tg under hypothyroid conditions. The use of larger ^{131}I scanning doses may result in thyroid 'stunning'. This phenomenon occurs when the radiation dose from ^{131}I, which has been administered for an imaging study, results in a lower uptake of ^{131}I given subsequently for remnant ablation or cancer therapy [64]. There is no well-documented evidence that ^{131}I tracer doses of 2 mCi (74 MBq) causes stunning. Therefore, following thyroidectomy, it has been recommended that imaging be done with a maximum of 2 mCi (74 MBq) of ^{131}I in children and adolescents [61]. During the first follow-up evaluation, if a negative diagnostic WBS is obtained, the necessity for repeat therapy is determined by the serum Tg level as well as clinical and radiologic findings. If the WBS shows the presence of residual neck activity or extracervical disease, repeat ^{131}I therapy is indicated. If cervical cancer lymph nodes are present, surgical removal is indicated before ^{131}I therapy. If the diagnostic WBS is negative but the serum Tg level is above 10 ng ml^{-1}, there is a high probability that carcinoma is present and further ^{131}I therapy is recommended [65].

Yeh and La Quaglia [61] have reported that most institutions treating pediatric patients use empirical fixed therapy doses of [131]I. Estimation of the therapeutic dose of ^{131}I can be based on body surface or total body weight as suggested by Reynolds [66]. Another approach to calculate the pediatric dose of ^{131}I has been proposed by Maxon [67] and involves the use of quantitative blood and whole body dosimetry. This method is more complicated than using the empirical, fixed dose method, and is not widely available.

Few reports of immediate side effects and complications in pediatric patients treated with ^{131}I have been reviewed by Yeh and LaQuaglia [61]. Early side effects include painful swelling of the remnant tissue or metastases, nausea, vomiting, acute swelling of the salivary glands, and transient loss of taste and smell. Transient bone marrow suppression may occur resulting in leucopenia and thrombocytopenia, with a blood count nadir occurring approximately 6–8 weeks after therapy. A complete blood count should be obtained during this period, and at 10–12 weeks after therapy. Pulmonary fibrosis can occur following therapy of pulmonary metastases. There is a paucity of data regarding long-term complications that may appear many years or decades after therapy. The long-term complications reported to date have been reviewed by Wiersinga [68].

Total cumulative doses of ^{131}I are generally kept below 500 mCi (18,000 MBq) in children and 800 mCi (29,600 MBq) in adolescents [69,70]. Larger doses are more likely to be associated with serious long-term complications. Cumulative ^{131}I doses greater than those reported may be administered with extreme caution and depends on the patient's clinical status.

The risk of induction of secondary solid tumors after therapy in children and adolescents is probably small, although actual data are not available. The most comprehensive study on the outcome of pregnancies in females after receiving ^{131}I for WDTC has been published by Schlumberger et al. [71]. Their data on 2,130 pregnancies did not provide evidence that such therapy affected the outcome of subsequent pregnancies, with the exception of a small increase in the frequency of miscarriages during the first year after therapy.

6.2. *LT4 therapy*

Many clinicians prescribe LT4 therapy immediately after thyroidectomy to prevent hypothyroidism and suppress TSH secretion. A minority of clinicians prefer that their patient become hypothyroid and do not start LT4 therapy in order to prepare for RAI diagnostic studies and serum Tg measurements [54]. LT4 therapy is based on the assumption that suppression of endogenous TSH deprives TSH-dependent stimulation of WDTC cell growth. The dose of LT4 is higher in patients with thyroid carcinoma than that given for hormone replacement for spontaneously occurring primary hypothyroidism [72]. The physiologic replacement dosage of LT4 during childhood and adolescence is approximately $1-3\,\mu g\,kg^{-1}\,day^{-1}$ or $100\,\mu g\,m^{-2}\,day^{-1}$, given orally once daily. The LT4 dose to fully suppress serum TSH in children and adolescents is $\sim 2.1-4.5\,\mu g\,kg^{-1}\,day^{-1}$.

6.3. *Other therapies*

External beam irradiation is rarely used in pediatric patients but may be indicated in select patients with advanced disease that are unresponsive to any modality of therapy. This can be used if the integrity of local structures is threatened. The irradiation may slow down the rapid tumor growth.

There has been very little experience with the use of chemotherapy in pediatric patients. However, combined chemotherapy might be tried in rapidly growing, widely metastatic disease.

6.4. *Follow-up*

The most important biochemical test to detect recurrence of disease in patients with WDTC is measurement of serum Tg, is an effective tumor marker after total thyroidectomy and ^{131}I ablation of thyroid remnants [73]. The presumption is that following thyroidectomy and ablation of thyroid remnants, and while under LT4 suppression therapy, the serum Tg should be undetectable. Serum Tg determinations are unreliable in the presence of serum antithyroglobulin antibodies [74]. It is essential to screen for the presence of these antibodies to avoid misinterpretation of the Tg value. Serum Tg levels should be obtained both while on LT4 suppression therapy as well as under conditions of TSH stimulation, i.e., either after LT4 therapy has been discontinued for 6 weeks or after rhTSH administration. Kirk et al. [73] have suggested that in the absence of residual, recurrent or metastatic disease, the serum Tg levels measured under hypothyroid conditions should be less than $10\,ng\,ml^{-1}$.

Patients should be evaluated every 6 months following initial thyroid surgery and ^{131}I therapy by serum Tg assay and diagnostic ^{131}I WBS for the first 12–18 months

[54]. If the serum Tg level and diagnostic WBS are 'positive' for the disease, repeat ^{131}I therapy is indicated. [131]I therapy should be repeated every 6 to 12 months until the serum Tg level and WBS indicate that carcinoma is no longer present or until a 'maximal' cumulative dose of ^{131}I has been given. Further administration of ^{131}I therapy must be decided based on the patient's clinical status.

For patients who remain with no evidence of the disease after the first 18 months, another 2 year follow-up evaluation (with diagnostic WBS and serum Tg assay), followed by another revaluation 3 years thereafter has been recommended [54]. If the patient remains disease-free, the next evaluation may be 5 years later and then on 5 year basis. Thyroid function testing and serum Tg assay while on LT4 therapy should be performed on a yearly basis for life time. It must be emphasized that lifelong follow-up is essential. It is extremely important to transfer care to an adult endocrinologist when the patient reaches adulthood.

Chest X-rays have been traditionally obtained every 6 to 12 months after the initial surgery to detect pulmonary metastases. Chest X-rays are not sensitive to detect metastases early in most patients, and may be documented only on WBS [75].

The role of neck and mediastinal magnetic resonance imaging as well as nuclear medicine scanning using radionuclides other than ^{131}I in the follow-up evaluation of pediatric patients has not been validated.

6.5. *Prognosis*

The prognosis for pediatric patients with WDTC is better than that for adults. The survival of children and adolescents up to 1970 was ~82% at 20 years [76], but in a series published in the late 1980s, survival rates of >95% at 15 to 20 years of age were reported [77,78]. The presence of distant metastases does not necessarily predict a poor prognosis. In the series of young patients reported in 1988 from the Mayo Clinic who had distant metastases, 14% died by 15 years compared with 68% of adults with distant metastases [77]. It is important to remember that recurrences can occur very late. In the Mayo Clinic series, 33% of metastases were detected 5 years after the initial therapy, and 15% were diagnosed 15 or more years later.

According to multivariate Cox regression analysis of prognostic factors in 109 children with WDTC, 6–17 years of age, disease-free survival is longer in children older than 10 years than in those younger than 10 years [79]. Disease-free survival is also longer after total thyroidectomy than after less extensive surgery, and after ^{131}I treatment than after no ^{131}I therapy. Alessandri et al. [80], in a pediatric population, identified age as the major determinant of time to recurrence in WDTC. In this study young patients (< 10 years of age) experienced recurrences more frequently and early than patients 10 to 17 years of age.

Mortality from WDTC in pediatric patients is low and in many series no neoplasm-induced deaths are reported [81]. It should be remembered that a non-negligible percentage of neoplasm-induced deaths occur years and decades after diagnosis and are therefore reported only in studies carried out over very long periods of follow-up.

7. Medullary thyroid carcinoma

Total thyroidectomy with resection of the central cervical lymph node compartment is the procedure of choice in patients with MTC [32]. Total thyroidectomy is indicated because MTC is multi-focal. In addition to regional lymph nodes, other common sites of metastases include the lung and liver. All patients with MEN 2 syndromes should be screened for the presence of pheochromocytoma. Lifelong LT4 therapy is necessary postoperatively. If pheochromocytoma(s) are present, bilateral adrenalectomy may be necessary because of multicentricity and bilaterality of these tumors.

Once a patient has been diagnosed as having one of the MEN 2 variants, RET germline mutation testing should be done on all relatives to detect gene carriers who are predisposed to develop C-cell hyperplasia and MTC [32]. Molecular genetic testing permits early identification of gene carriers before MTC is clinically apparent and allows for prophylactic total thyroidectomy and any additional surgical procedures to be performed [32,79]. Brandi et al. [32] have summarized possible surgical management strategies based on the specific RET codon mutation. RET germline mutation testing has replaced plasma iCT testing as the prime testing study for detection of gene carriers in MEN 2 families [32,86].

The ideal age at which prophylactic total thyroidectomy should be performed in children with RET germline mutations is controversial. Some clinicians recommend surgery in mutation carriers of MEN 2B in the first year of life and for those with gene mutation for MEN 2A at 5 years of age [82,83]. Heptulla et al. [44] recommend prophylactic total thyroidectomy during the first decade of life in patients with FMTC and RET mutations. Following thyroidectomy, measurement of plasma iCT basally and after stimulation should be carried out yearly for at least 5 years to detect the presence of MTC.

7.1. *Prognosis*

The prognosis in patients with MTC is poor [84,87]. There is an early tendency for metastases to occur in the lungs and bone [88]. Treatment of patients with persistent MTC is controversial. Van Heerden et al. [85] reported a study of 31 patients with MTC who had 5 and 10 year survival rates of 90% and 86%, respectively.

8. Anaplastic thyroid carcinoma

The clinical presentation of anaplastic thyroid carcinoma is typically that of a rapidly enlarging neck mass in the thyroid area. This is usually associated with compression signs such as dyspnea and dysphagia. The duration of the disease is short, ranging from a few weeks to a few months. At the time of diagnosis, at lest 50% of patients have metastases in the lungs, bone, or brain [31]. Surgical excision is the first line of therapy, although in most cases, the tumor is so widespread that total removal is impossible. Surgery may be necessary to relieve compression signs. ^{131}I, LT4 suppression, and multi-drug chemotherapy are not effective.

8.1. *Prognosis*

Anaplastic thyroid carcinoma in the pediatric population is fatal in almost all cases.

References

[1] R.W. Miller, J.L. Young Jr., B. Novakovic, Childhood cancer, Cancer 75 (1995) 395–405.
[2] H.R. Harach, E.D. Williams, Childhood thyroid cancer in England and Wales, Br. J. Cancer 72 (1995) 777–783.
[3] A. Belfiore, G.L. LaRosa, G. Padove, L. Sava, O. Ippolito, R. Vigneri, The frequency of cold thyroid nodules and thyroid malignancies in patients from an iodine deficient area, Cancer 60 (1987) 3096–3102.
[4] A. Aghini-Lombardi, L. Antonangeli, E. Martino, P. Vitti, A. Maccherini, F. Leoli, T. Rago, L. Grasso, R. Valeriano, A. Balestrieri, A. Pinchera, The spectrum of thyroid disorders in an iodine-deficient community: the Pescopagano survey, J. Clin. Endocrinol. Metab. 84 (1999) 561–566.
[5] E.H. Quimby, S.C. Werner, Late radiation effects in Roentgen therapy for hyperthyroidism, JAMA 140 (1949) 1046–1047.
[6] A. Yoshida, S. Noguchi, K. Fukuda, T. Hirohata, Low-dose irradiation to head, neck, or chest during infancy as a possible cause of thyroid carcinoma in teenagers: a match case-control study, Jpn. J. Cancer 78 (1987) 991–994.
[7] R.L. Prentice, H. Kato, M. Mason, A. Yoshimoto, Radiation Exposure and Thyroid Cancer Incidence among Hiroshima and Nagasaki Resident, National Cancer Institute Monograph 62, 1982, pp. 207–212.
[8] US Nuclear Regulatory Commission, Report on the Accident at the Chernobyl Power Station 1987 NUREG-1250, US Government Printing Office, Washington, DC.
[9] J. Robbins, Lessons from Chernobyl: the event, the after-math fallout: radioactive, political, social, Thyroid 7 (1997) 182–192.
[10] A. Antonelli, P. Miccoli, V.E. Derzhitski, G. Panasiuk, N. Solovieva, L. Baschieri, Epidemiological and clinical evaluation of thyroid cancer in children coming from the Gomel region (Belarus), World J. Surg. 20 (1996) 867–871.
[11] K. Baverstock, B. Egloff, A. Pinchera, C. Ruchti, E.D. Williams, Thyroid cancer after Chernobyl, Nature 359 (1992) 21–22.
[12] L. Leehardt, A. Aurengo, Post-Chernobyl thyroid carcinoma in children, Bailliere's Clin. Endocrinol. Metab. 14 (2000) 667–677.
[13] A. Bounacer, R. Wicker, B. Caillou, A.F. Cailleux, A. Sarasin, M. Schlumberger, H.G. Suarez, High prevalence of activating ret proto-oncogene rearrangements in thyroid tumors from patients who had received external radiation, Oncogene 15 (1997) 1263–1273.
[14] R.M. Tuttle, D.V. Becker, The Chernobyl accident and its consequences: update at the millennium, Semin. Nucl. Med. 30 (2000) 133–140.
[15] L.M. Mulligan, J.B.J. Kwok, C.S. Healy, M.J. Eldson, Germline mutations of the RET proto-oncogene in multiple endocrine neoplasia type 2A, Nature 363 (1993) 458–460.
[16] H.M. Rabes, S. Klugbauer, Molecular genetics of childhood papillary thyroid carcinomas after irradiation: high prevalence of RET rearrangement, Recent Results Cancer Res. 154 (1998) 249–265.
[17] L. Fugazzola, S. Pilotti, A. Pinchera, T.V. Vorontsova, P. Mondellini, I. Bongarzone, A. Greco, L. Astakhova, M.G. Butti, E.P. Demidchik, F. Pacini, M.S. Pierotti, Oncogenic rearrangements of the RET proto-oncogene in papillary thyroid carcinomas from children exposed to the Chernobyl nuclear accident, Cancer Res. 55 (1995) 5617–5620.

[18] M. Santoro, F. Carlomagno, I.D. Hay, M.A. Herrmann, M. Grieco, P. Melillo, M.A. Pierotti, I. Bongarzona, G.D. Porta, N. Berger, J.L. Peix, C. Paulin, N. Fabien, G. Vecchio, R.B. Jenkins, A. Fusco, RET oncogene activation in human thyroid neoplasms restricted to the papillar subtype, J. Clin. Invest. 89 (1992) 1517–1522.

[19] I. Bongarzone, L. Fugazzola, P. Vigneri, L. Mariani, P. Mondellini, F. Pacini, F. Basolo, A. Pinchera, S. Pilotti, A. Pierotti, Age-related activation of the tyrosine kinase receptor proto-oncogene RET and NTRK1 in papillary thyroid carcinoma, J. Clin. Endocrinol. Metab. 81 (1996) 2006–2009.

[20] H.M. Rabes, E.P. Demidchik, J.D. Sidorow, E. Lengfelder, C. Beimfohr, D. Hoelzel, S. Klugbauer, Pattern of radiation-induced RET and NTRK1 rearrangements in 191 post-Chernobyl papillary thyroid carcinomas: biological, phenotype, and clinical implications, Clin. Cancer Res. 6 (2000) 1093–1103.

[21] Y.E. Nikiforov, J.M. Rowland, K.E. Bove, H. Monforte-Munoz, J.A. Fagin, Distinct pattern of ret oncogene rearrangements in morphological variants of radiation-induced and sporadic thyroid papillary carcinomas in children, Cancer Res. 57 (1997) 1690–1694.

[22] J. Smida, K. Salassidis, L. Hieber, H. Zitzelsberger, A.M. Keller, E.P. Demidchik, T. Nagele, F. Spelsberg, E. Lengfelder, M. Werner, M. Bauchinger, Distinct frequency of ret rearrangements in papillary thyroid carcinomas of children and adults from Belarus, Int. J. Cancer 80 (1999) 32–38.

[23] C. Beimfohr, S. Klugbauer, E.P. Demidchik, E. Lengfelder, H.M. Rabes, NTRK1 re-arrangement in papillary thyroid carcinoma of children after the Chernobyl reactor accident, Int. J. Cancer 80 (1999) 842–847.

[24] M. Santoto, G.A. Thoas, G. Vecchio, G.H. Williams, A. Fusco, T. Chiappetta, V. Pozcharskaya, T.I. Bogdanova, E.P. Demidchik, E.D. Cherstvoy, L. Voscoboinik, N.D. Tronko, A. Carss, H. Bunnell, M. Tonnachera, J. Parma, J.E. Dumont, G. Keller, H. Hofler, E.D. Williams, Gene rearrangement and Chernobyl related thyroid cancers, Br. J. Cancer 82 (2000) 315–322.

[25] H. Namba, S.A. Rubin, J.A. Fagin, Point mutations of RAS oncogene are an early event in thyroid tumorigenesis, Mol. Endocrinol. 4 (1990) 1474–1479.

[26] N.R. Lemoine, E.S. Mayall, F.S. Wyllier, E.D. Williams, M. Goyns, B. Stringer, D. Wynford-Thomas, High frequency of RAS oncogene activation in all stages of human thyroid tumorigenesis, Oncogene 4 (1989) 159–164.

[27] J. Blatt, A. Gishan, M.J. Gula, P.S. Dickman, B. Zaranek, Second malignancies in very-long term survivors of childhood cancer, Am. J. Med. 93 (1992) 57–60.

[28] L.F.M. De Keyser, A.J. Van Herle, Differentiated thyroid cancer in children, Head Neck Surg. 8 (1985) 100–114.

[29] T. Pal, F.D. Vogl, P.O. Chappuis, R. Tsang, J. Brierley, H. Renard, K. Sanders, T. Kantemiroff, S. Bagha, D.E. Goldger, S.A. Narod, W.D. Foulkes, Increased risk for nonmedullary thyroid cancers in the first degree relatives of prevalent cases of nonmedullary thyroid cancer: a hospital-based study, J. Clin. Endocrinol. Metab. 86 (2001) 5307–5312.

[30] A.L. Steiner, A.D. Goodman, S.R. Powers, Study of a kindred with pheochromocytoma, medullary thyroid carcinoma, hyperparathyroidism and Cushing's disease: multiple endocrine neoplasia, type 2, Medicine 47 (1968) 371–409.

[31] R.N. Schimke, W.H. Hartmann, T.E. Prout, D.L. Rimon, Syndrome of bilateral pheochromocytomas, medullary thyroid carcinoma and multiple neuromas: a possible regulatory defect in differentiation of chromoffin tissue, New Engl. J. Med. 279 (1968) 1–7.

[32] M.L. Brandi, R.F. Gagel, A. Angeli, J.P. Bilezikian, P. Beck-Peccoz, C. Bordi, B. Conte-Devolx, A. Falchetti, R.G. Gheri, A. Libroia, C.J.M. Lips, G. Lombardi, M. Mannelli, F. Pacini, B.A.J. Ponder, F. Raue, B. Skogseid, G. Tamburrano, R.V. Thakker, N.W. Thompson, P. Tomassetti, F. Tonelli, S.A. Wells Jr., S.J. Marx, Guidelines for diagnosis and therapy of MEN Type 1 and Type 2, J. Clin. Endocrinol. Metab. 86 (2001) 5658–5671.

[33] J.R. Farndon, G.S. Leight, W.G. Dilley, S.B. Baylin, R.C. Smallridge, T.S. Harrison, S.A. Wells Jr., Familial medullary thyroid carcinoma without associated endocrinopathies: a distinct clinical entity, Br. J. Surg. 73 (1986) 278–281.

[34] T.C. Lairmore, J.R. Howe, J.A. Korte, W.G. Dilley, L. Aine, E. Aine, S.A. Wells Jr., H. Donis-Keller, Familial medullary thyroid carcinoma and multiple endocrine neoplasia type 2B map to the same region of chromosome 10 as multiple endocrine neoplasia type 2A, Genomics 9 (1991) 181–192.

[35] G.P. Matthew, K.S. Chin, D.F. Easton, K. Thrope, C. Carter, G.I. Liou, S.L. Fong, C.D. Bridges, C.D.B. Haak, H.N. Kruseman, A.C. Schifter, S. Hansen, H.H. Telenius, M. Telenius-Berg, B.A.J. Ponder, A linked genetic marker for multiple endocrine neoplasia type 2A on chromosome 10, Nature 328 (1987) 527–528.

[36] H. Donis-Keller, S. Dou, D. Chi, K.M. Carlson, K. Toshima, T.D. Lairmore, J.R. Howe, J.F. Moley, P. Goodfellow, S.A. Wells Jr., Mutations in the RET proto-oncogene associated with MEN 2A and FMTC, Human Mol. Genet. 2 (1993) 851–856.

[37] K.B. Ain, Anaplastic thyroid carcinoma: behavior, biology, and therapeutic approaches, Thyroid 8 (1998) 716–728.

[38] J.A. Fagin, K. Matsuo, A. Karmakar, D.L. Chen, S.H. Tang, H.P. Koeffler, High prevalence of mutations of the p53 gene in poorly differentiated human thyroid carcinomas, J. Clin. Invest. 91 (1993) 179–184.

[39] B.M. Wenig, C.S. Heffess, C.F. Adair, Atlas of Endocrine Pathology, WB Saunders Co., Philadelphia, 1997.

[40] C.J. Garcia, A. Daneman, P. Thorner, D. Daneman, Sonography of multi-nodular thyroid gland in children and adolescents, Am. J. Dis. Child. 146 (1992) 811–816.

[41] R.L. Telander, D. Zimmerman, G.W. Sizemore, J.A. Van Heerden, C.S. Grant, Medullary carcinoma in children: results of early detection and surgery, Arch. Surg. 124 (1989) 841–843.

[42] G.A. Ledger, S. Khosla, N.M. Lindor, S.N. Thibodeau, H. Gharib, Genetic testing in the diagnosis and management of multiple endocrine neoplasia type II, Ann. Int. Med. 112 (1995) 118–124.

[43] S.A. Wells Jr., H. Donis-Keller, Current Perspectives on the diagnosis and management of patients with multiple endocrine neoplasia type 2 syndromes, Endocrinol. Metab. Clin. North Am. 23 (1994) 215–228.

[44] R.A. Heptulla, R.P. Schwartz, A.E. Bale, S. Flynn, M. Genel, Familial medullary thyroid carcinoma: presymptomatic diagnosis and management in children, J. Pediatr. 135 (1999) 327–331.

[45] C.J.M. Lips, R.M. Landsvater, J.W.M. Hoppener, R.A. Geerdink, G. Blijham, J.M.J. Van Veen, A.P.G. Van Gils, M.J. de Wit, R.A. Zewald, M.J.H. Berends, F.A. Beemer, J. Brouwers-Smalbraak, R.P.M. Jansen, H.K.P. Van Amstel, T.J.M.V. Van Vroonhoven, T.M. Vroom, Clinical screening as compared with DNA analysis in families with multiple endocrine neoplasia type 2A, New Engl. J. Med. 331 (1994) 828–835.

[46] R.D. Groom III, C.G. Thomas Jr., R.L. Reddick, Autonomously functioning thyroid nodules in childhood and adolescence, Surgery 102 (1987) 1101–1108.

[47] W. Hung, Solitary thyroid nodules in 93 children and adolescents: a 35-years experience, Horm. Res. 52 (1999) 15–18.

[48] J.G. Desjardin, A.H. Khan, P. Montupet, P.P. Collin, G. Leboeuf, C. Polychronakos, P. Simard, J. Boisvert, L.J. Dube, Management of thyroid nodules in children: a 20-year experience, J. Pediatr. 22 (1987) 736–739.

[49] E.L. Mazzaferri, R.L. Young, J.E. Oertel, Papillary thyroid carcinoma: the impact of therapy in 576 patients, Medicine 56 (1977) 171–196.

[50] H. Gharib, E.L. Mazzaferri, Thyroxine suppressive therapy in patients with nodular thyroid disease, Ann. Int. Med. 128 (1998) 386–394.

[51] A. Corrias, S. Einaudi, G. Chiorboli, G. Weber, A. Crino, M. Andreo, G. Cesaretti, L. de Sanctis, M.F. Messina, F. Segni, M. Cicchetti, M. Vigone, A.M. Pasquino, S. Spera, F. de Luca, G.C. Mussa, G. Bona, Accuracy of fine-needle aspiration biopsy of thyroid nodules in detecting malignancy in childhood: comparison with conventional clinical, laboratory and imaging approaches, J. Clin. Endocrinol. Metab. 86 (2001) 4644–4648.

[52] A. Al'Shaikh, B. Ngan, A. Daneman, D. Daneman, Fine-needle aspiration biopsy in the management of thyroid nodules in children and adolescents, J. Pediatr. 138 (2001) 140–142.

[53] J.B. Gorlin, S.E. Sallen, Thyroid cancer in childhood, Endocrinol. Metab. Clin. North Am. 19 (1990) 649–662.

[54] W. Hung, N.J. Sarlis, Current controversies in the management of pediatric patients with well-differentiated nonmedullary thyroid cancer: A review, Thyroid 12 (2002) 683–702.

[55] M. Friedman, B.C. Pacella Jr., Total versus subtotal thyroidectomy: arguments, approaches, and recommendations, Otolaryngol, Clin. North Am. 23 (1990) 413–427.

[56] S.A. De Jong, J.G. Demeter, A.M. Lawrence, E. Paloyan, Necessity and safety of completion thyroidectomy for differentiated thyroid carcinoma, Surgery 112 (1992) 734–739.

[57] M.E. Dottorini, A. Vignati, L. Mazzucchelli, G. Lomuscio, L. Colombo, Differentiated thyroid carcinoma in children and adolescents: a 37-year experience in 85 patients, J. Nucl. Med. 38 (1997) 669–675.

[58] U. Hallwirth, J. Flores, K. Kaserer, B. Niederle, Differentiated thyroid cancer in children and adolescents: the importance of adequate surgery and review of the literature, Eur. J. Pediatr. Surg. 9 (1999) 359–363.

[59] R. Katoh, J. Sasaki, H. Kurihara, K. Suzuki, Y. Iida, A. Kawaoi, Multiple thyroid involvement in intraglandular metastases in papillary thyroid carcinoma, Cancer 70 (1992) 1585–1590.

[60] S.B. Paryani, R.J. Chobe, W. Scott, J. Wells, D. Johnson, A. Kuruvilla, S. Schoeppel, A. Deshukh, R. Miller, L. Dajani, C.T. Montogomery, E. Puestow, J. Purcell, M. Roura, D. Sutton, R. Mallett, J. Peer, Management of thyroid carcinoma with radioactive ^{131}I, Int. J. Rad. Oncol. Biol. Phys. 36 (1996) 583–586.

[61] S.D. Yeh, M.P. La Quaglia, 131-I therapy for pediatric thyroid cancer, Semin. Pediatr. Surg. 6 (1997) 128–133.

[62] E.L. Mazzaferri, R.T. Kloos, Using recombinant human TSH in the management of thyroid cancer: current strategies and future direction, Thyroid 10 (2000) 767–778.

[63] S.J. Mandel, L.K. Shankar, F. Benard, A. Yamamoto, A. Alavi, Superiority of iodine-123 compared with iodine-131 scanning for thyroid remnants in patients with differentiated thyroid cancer, Clin. Nucl. Med. 26 (2001) 6–9.

[64] H.M. Park, O.W. Perkins, J.W. Edmondson, R.B. Schnute, A. Manatunga, Influence of diagnostic radioiodine in the uptake of ablative dose iodine-131, Thyroid 4 (1994) 49–54.

[65] J. Robbins, Management of thyroglobulin-positive, body-scan negative thyroid cancer patients: evidence for the utility of I-131 therapy, J. Endocrinol. Invest. 22 (1999) 808–810.

[66] J.C. Reynolds, Comparison of I-131 absorbed radiation doses in children and adults: a tool for estimating therapeutic I-131 doses in children, in: J. Robbins (Ed.), Treatment of Thyroid Cancer in Childhood, Dept. of Energy: Publication DOE/EH-0406, Washington, DC, 1993, pp. 127–135.

[67] H.R. Maxon, Quantitative radioiodine therapy in the treatment of differentiated thyroid cancer, Q. J. Nucl. Med. 43 (1999) 313–323.

[68] W.M. Wiersinga, Thyroid cancer in children and adolescents consequences in later life, J. Pediatr. Endocrinol. Metab. 14 (2001) 1289–1296.

[69] C. Menzel, F. Grunwald, A. Schomburg, "High-dose" radioiodine therapy in advanced differentiated thyroid carcinoma, J. Nucl. Med. 37 (1996) 1496–1503.

[70] J.C. Sisson, Medical treatment of benign and malignant thyroid tumors, Endocrinol. Metab. Clin. North Am. 18 (1989) 359–387.

[71] M. Schlumberger, F. De Vathaire, C. Ceccarelli, Exposure to radioactive iodine-131 for scintigraphy or therapy does not preclude pregnancy in thyroid cancer patients, J. Nucl. Med. 37 (1996) 606–612.

[72] L. Burmeister, M.O. Goumaz, C.N. Mariash, J.H. Oppenheimer, Levothyroxine dose requirements for throtropin suppression in the treatment of differentiated thyroid cancer, J. Clin. Endocrinol. Metab. 75 (1992) 344–350.

[73] J.M.W. Kirk, C. Mort, D.B. Grant, R.J. Touzel, N. Plowman, The usefulness of serum thyroglobulin in the follow-up of differentiated thyroid carcinoma in children, Med. Pediatr. Oncol. 20 (1992) 201–208.

[74] C.A. Spencer, Serum thyroglobulin measurements: clinical utility and technical limitations in the management of patients with differentiated thyroid carcinoma, Endocr. Pract. 6 (2000) 481–484.

[75] A.M. Samuel, B. Rajashejharrao, D.H. Shah, Pulmonary metastases in children and adolescents with well-differentiated thyroid cancer, J. Nucl. Med. 39 (1998) 1531–1536.

[76] T. Winship, R. Rosvoll, Thyroid carcinoma in childhood: final report on a 20 year study, Clin. Proc. Child. Hosp. Wash. DC 26 (1970) 327–349.

[77] D. Zimmerman, I.D. Hay, I.R. Gough, J.R. Goellner, J.J. Ryan, C.S. Grant, W.M. McConahey, Papillary thyroid carcinoma in children and adults: long-term follow-up of 1039 patients conservatively treated at one institution during three decades, Surgery 104 (1988) 1157–1166.

[78] M.P. La Quaglia, M.T. Corbally, G. Heller, Recurrence and morbidity in differentiated thyroid carcinoma in children, Surgery 104 (1988) 1149–1156.

[79] B. Jarzab, D.H. Junak, J. Wloch, B. Kalemba, J. Roskosz, A. Kukulska, Z. Puch, Multivariate analysis of prognostic factors for differentiated thyroid carcinoma in children, Eur. J. Nucl. Med. 27 (2000) 833–841.

[80] A.J. Alessandri, K.J. Goddard, G.K. Blair, C.J.H. Fryer, K.R. Schultz, Age is the major determinant of recurrence in pediatric differentiated thyroid carcinoma, Med. Pediatr. Oncol. 35 (2000) 41–46.

[81] M.E. Dottorini, Differentiated thyroid carcinoma in childhood, RAYS 25 (2000) 245–255.

[82] M.A. Skinner, M.K. DeBendetti, J.F. Moley, J.A. Norton, S.A. Wells Jr., Medullary thyroid carcinoma in children with multiple endocrine neoplasia type 2A and 2B, J. Pediatr. Surg. 31 (1996) 177–181.

[83] M.A. Iler, D.R. King, M.E. Ginn-Pease, T.M. O'Dorisio, J.F. Soto, Multiple endocrine neoplasia type 2A: a 25 year review, J. Prediatr. Surg. 34 (1999) 92–97.

[84] T. Parlowsky, P. Bucsky, M. Hof, P. Kaatsch, Malignant endocrine tumors in childhood and adolescence - results of a retrospective analysis, Klin. Pediatr. 208 (1996) 205–209.

[85] A. van Heerden, C.S. Grant, H. Gharib, V.D. Hat, D.M. Iistrup, Long-term course of patients with persistent hypercalcitoninemia after apparent curative primary surgery for medullary thyroid carcinoma, Ann. Surg. 212 (1990) 395–400.

[86] D.J. Marsh, B.G. Robinson, S. Andrew, A.L. Richardson, R. Pojer, M. Schnitzler, L.M. Mulligan, V.J. Hyland, A rapid screening method for the detection of mutations in the RET proto-oncogene in multiple endocrine neoplasia type 2A and familial medullary thyroid carcinoma families, Genomics 23 (1994) 447–479.

[87] R.L. Telander, C.R. Moir, Medullary thyroid carcinoma in children, Semin. Pediatr. Surg. 3 (1994) 188–193.

[88] J.R. Gill, M. Reyes-Mugica, S. Lyengar, K.K. Kidd, R.J. Touloukian, C. Smith, M.S. Keller, M. Genel, Early presentation of metastatic medullary carcinoma in multiple endocrine neoplasia, type IIA: implications for therapy, J. Pediatr. 129 (1996) 456–464.

scale at 0/cm. In general, Raman bands can be easily attributed to a chemical structure. The spectra are very specific and are cleaner than infrared spectra. Raman bands are narrower and overlap, combination bands are generally weak, and chemical identifications can be performed by using search algorithms in digital databases. Raman spectroscopy can be used to measure bands of symmetric linkages that are weak in an infrared spectrum (e.g. -S·S-, -C-S-, -C=C-). Other advantages include the fact that water and CO_2 vapours are very weak scatterers – hence, purging is unnecessary and no special accessories are needed for measuring polymers dissolved in aqueous solutions. It is believed that in many cases Raman spectroscopy may be superior to infrared spectroscopy and may provide a better answer to polymer analysis problems.

2.2 Specific properties of polymers in the presence of liquid media

In liquid media, polymers can be found in three states, depending on various parameters. Full dissolution can be obtained in appropriate solvents when the concentration and molecular weight are in the proper range to allow complete solubilisation. Polymers form gels when the concentration is high, when the molecular weight is very high (e.g. after cross-linking), or when the polymer can form liquid crystals resulting from the self-organisation of the polymer chains thanks to their nature and structure. Polymers can be dispersed as tiny particles of insoluble material to form colloidal suspensions. Polymers incorporated in all these systems can confer unique properties, for instance to improve the performance of drug-delivery formulations or to provide drug-delivery formulations with specific properties. As will be discussed later in this chapter, the use of polymers formulated in solution can greatly facilitate the process of fabrication of pharmaceutical formulations.

2.2.1 Polymer solutions: preparation and properties

Polymer solutions are obtained by complete dissolution of the macromolecule into a solvent. As in any case of dissolution of a solute in a solvent, dissolution phenomena are controlled by the balance between, on the one hand, solute–solute and solvent–solvent interaction forces and, on the other hand, solute–solvent interaction forces. Thus, general thermodynamic considerations, including solubility parameters and cohesive energy density notions, can help us to predict whether or not a polymer can be soluble in a given solvent. Nevertheless, solubilisation of a polymer in a suitable solvent is a more complex phenomenon than solubilisation of a small molecule, and it generally takes a long time because it requires several steps.

As illustrated in Figure 2.9, swelling of the dried polymer powder by the solvent is the first step; this is a slow process. During swelling, mobility of the polymer chains increases, resulting in increased freedom. In a second step,

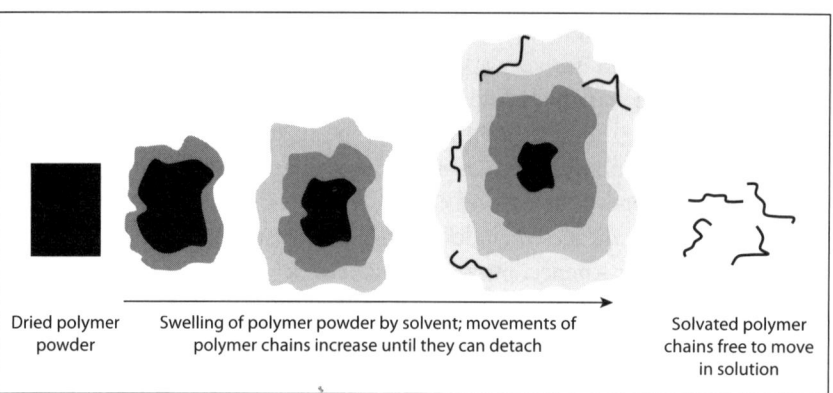

Dried polymer | Swelling of polymer powder by solvent; movements of | Solvated polymer
powder | polymer chains increase until they can detach | chains free to move in solution

Figure 2.9   Dissolution of a polymer in a suitable solvent.

polymer chains that have gained enough mobility and freedom are detached from the swollen polymer. This finally leads to complete solubilisation, which is obtained when the solvated chains are individualised in the solution.

Solubilisation is also affected by several parameters inherent to the polymer itself. For instance, the rate of the initial stage of swelling is influenced by the glass transition temperature, T_g (see Section 2.3.3), which is related to the mobility of the polymer chains in the solid state. Swelling of a polymer endowed with a T_g lower than the solubilisation temperature starts much more rapidly than swelling of polymers with a high T_g in which the chains are mainly immobile. The molecular weight of the polymer is also an important parameter that controls the rate of dissolution. Low-molecular-weight polymers dissolve faster than large macromolecular chains.

It is noteworthy that some polymers have a very narrow window of solubilisation in some solvents. Poly(ethylene glycols) and their derivatives, which are used widely in pharmaceutical formulations, are among such polymer species. In general, these are highly soluble in water but they can also dissolve in some organic solvents. In aqueous solvents, their solubilisation results in the formation of hydrogen bonds with the surrounding water molecules. Because of this solubilisation mechanism, they are only soluble below a given temperature, which can vary by the addition of small solutes such as ions or sugars in the aqueous dissolution medium. Thus, such polymers may be not soluble above 30 °C but they may be perfectly soluble at room temperature. This may be an important parameter to consider, as most preparations are performed at room temperature but the human in vivo temperature is 37 °C. When using such polymers and copolymers in formulation of a solution, it is important to check systematically whether the PEG-containing compound soluble at room temperature will become insoluble at body temperature. Conversely, such temperature-dependent behaviour can be taken advantage of, e.g. for obtaining temporary embolisation or jellifying eye drops (see Section 4.1.1). This is typically the case for aqueous solutions of poloxamer 407, which are liquid below 25 °C and form a gel at higher temperatures.

Adding polymers to a solution confers new physicochemical properties to the solution. In pharmaceutical formulations, the property that is used is the increase in viscosity. Indeed, the viscosity of a polymer solution is influenced directly by both the concentration of the polymer and its molecular weight. Relationships between the viscosity of the solution and the polymer concentration and molecular weight can be found in Section 2.1.1.

Another property of polymers in the solubilised state that may be interesting for pharmaceutical formulations is a property specific to amphiphilic copolymers (see Section 4.1.1). Such copolymers can be used to formulate stable dispersions and emulsions. In general, they are highly efficient surfactants. Their critical concentration for micelle formation (CMC) is much lower, e.g. about 0.005 wt% in water, than the CMC of low-molecular-weight surfactants, e.g. 0.2 wt% for sodium dodecylsulphate.

2.2.2 Gels and hydrogels

Gels can be formed with various polymers. The polymer forms the backbone of a cross-linked matrix including channels filled with a liquid phase, as shown in Figure 2.10. Depending on the nature of the polymer forming the

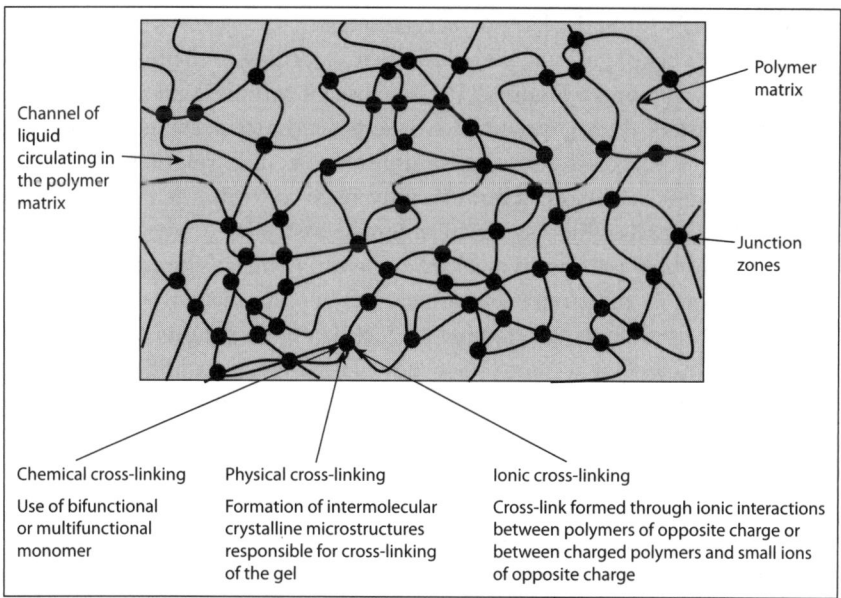

Figure 2.10 Schematic representation of the structure of a gel. The black lines show the polymer chains forming the matrix of the gel. The black dots represent the cross-linking zones that can result from different mechanisms of gel formation. The grey colour of the background represents the liquid phase filling the channels formed in the matrix of polymer.

matrix, and on its affinity for given types of solvent, gels can be obtained with either an organic or an aqueous liquid phase. In the latter case, they are named hydrogels. Swelling properties of hydrogels are linked both to the affinity of the polymeric backbone for a solvent and to the degree of cross-linking. If the polymeric network is cross-linked enough to be insoluble, but not too much to be able to swell, then the general shape of the material is kept; however, its total size increases.

In many cases, gels are mainly composed of the liquid phase, which can represent more than 90% of the total composition. However, some hydrogels contain less water, as shown in the case of poly(2-hydroxyethylmethacrylate) (PHEMA). Thanks to the presence of the polymeric network, the internal viscosity of hydrogels is high, resulting in structural strength, decreased resistance to sliding, and decreased permeability to large molecules, making their retention possible. The main characteristic of the liquid phase is that it is not able to flow, because it is trapped in the channels formed by the polymer chains. However, this liquid can be used to dissolve components in the gel, or it can be used for chemical reactions.

Many natural hydrogels are known to be constituents of the extracellular matrix, mucin, glycocalix and so on. Jelly is a well-known example of the use of hydrogels in food. Hydrogels can be obtained from many hydrophilic polymers, either natural (e.g. cellulose, dextran, alginate, hyaluronic acid, chitosan, pectin) or synthetic (e.g. poly(vinyl alcohol) (PVA), PEG, poly(vinyl pyrrolidone) (PVP), PHEMA, polyacrylamides).

Different types of gel have been described according to their mechanism of formation, as shown in Figure 2.10. The use of bifunctional or multifunctional monomers during polymer synthesis leads to permanent chemical cross-linking of polymers with almost infinite molecular weight. Cross-linked polymers cannot be dissolved but can only swell to form gels in appropriate solvents. Poly(acrylamide) gels used in biochemistry for analysis of proteins by gel electrophoresis are a typical example of chemically cross-linked gels. Polymerisation of the simple monomer, i.e. acrylamide, in water leads to formation of linear poly(acrylamide), which is highly soluble in water even at very high molecular weight (10^6 g/mol). However, by addition of a small amount of a bifunctional monomer, e.g. bis-acrylamide, in the polymerisation medium, a solid gel is formed, entrapping the water used for the polymerisation reaction.

A second method that can be used to obtain chemically cross-linked polymers is to start with a linear polymer containing free chemical groups that can be used to react with a cross-linking agent. A typical example of such a polymer, which is widely used as an excipient in the pharmaceutical industry, is poly(acrylic acid). As many carboxylic acid groups are available along the polymer chain, poly(acrylic acid) can be cross-linked by any component containing for instance at least two hydroxyl groups in their structure. In practice,

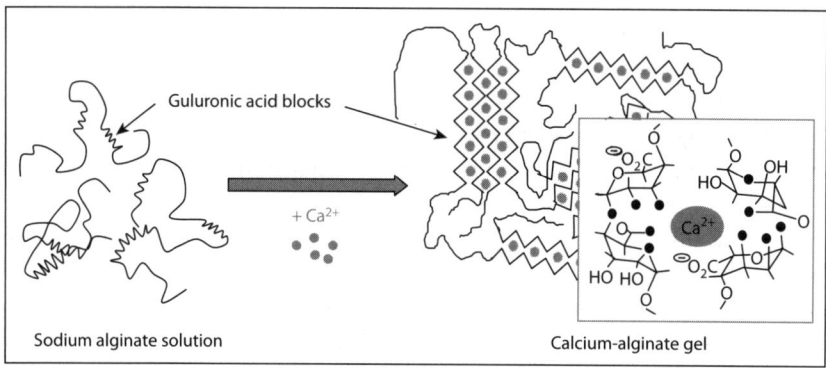

Guluronic acid blocks

+ Ca²⁺

Sodium alginate solution

Calcium-alginate gel

Figure 2.11   Ionic gel formed from alginate.

cross-linking can be achieved by using sugars or glycol derivatives. In both cases, the mesh size of the polymer matrix forming the gel is controlled by the amount of cross-linking agent. Properties of the gel are conditioned by this important parameter.

Another cross-linking method is based on the formation of ionic bonds between polymers of opposite charges or between charged polymers and small molecules of opposite charges. A very popular example of such a gel is illustrated by the polysaccharide alginate. This natural polymer extracted from brown seaweeds is composed of guluronic acid and manuronic acid units. The gelling property is due to the oligoguluronic acid segments or blocks included in the structure of the polymer, as shown in Figure 2.11. In the presence of calcium, oligoguluronic blocks can be organised in crystalline-like structures in the presence of calcium ions. The calcium ion fits in the guluronic blocks as eggs in an egg box, forming highly compact junction zones as ionic cross-linking points of the gel structure. Such hydrogels have also been proposed to encapsulate enzymes and even cells.

Several polymers are able to form gels by ionic gelation controlled by the pH of the external medium. Gels are formed by pectin, another polysaccharide, in acidic medium. In contrast with the gels obtained by covalent cross-linking methods, ionic gels are reversible. In the case of the calcium alginate gels, calcium can be displaced by using both a monovalent cation such as sodium and a complexing agent able to trap the released calcium.

Poly(methacrylic acid) and its derivatives are other polymers with pH-dependent swelling. Poly(methacrylic acid) is barely hydrophilic, whereas its sodium salts are easily dissolved in water. This property is used to prepare gastro-resistant coatings for tablets. Cross-linked poly(methacrylic acid) does not swell at low pH, but its salts swell above pH 6. Such polymers and copolymers have been used as matrices for intestinal controlled delivery of drugs. Conversely, linear polymers bearing amino groups are water-soluble at low pH, whereas cross-linked polymers are swollen. Gastro-soluble and gastro-resistant derivatives of poly(methacrylic acid) have been developed under the trade name Eudragit® (see Section 4.4.2).

There are many other physicochemical mechanisms that can result in the formation of gels from polymer solutions. Indeed, polymer gels may also be obtained by formation of hydrogen bonds, hydrophobic interactions and formation of crystallised domains. This is the case for cellulose, which is highly crystalline and swells into water without dissolving, despite the fact that it is not chemically cross-linked. On the other hand, dextrans, which are also polymers of glucose, are water-soluble when non-cross-linked. Cross-linked forms, known as Sephadex®, are well known as beads with various degrees of swelling.

The sol–gel transition can be induced by various physicochemical parameters, such as the temperature, the concentration in salt in the solution and the pH. Poly(N-isopropylacrylamide) (PNIPAm) exhibits a thermosensitive transition. Below 31 °C, the polymer is hydrophilic and swollen by water. Above this temperature, the polymer is hydrophobic and the network collapses, as shown in Figure 2.12. Such temperature-dependent behaviour can be of great interest.

Other mechanisms are based on stereo-complexation, self-assembling and host–guest interactions. In certain cases, the simple mixing of two polymers with complementary assembling functionalities is enough to obtain the formation of a gel; for instance, polymers containing cyclodextrins as a host for hydrophobic compounds are able to form gels via this mechanism. In the presence of a second polymer containing hydrophobic compounds able to form complexes with the host cavity of the cyclodextrins, gels can be readily formed.

Many polymers forming gels according to these mechanisms are tailor-made copolymers that can be designed in a very precise way in order to form

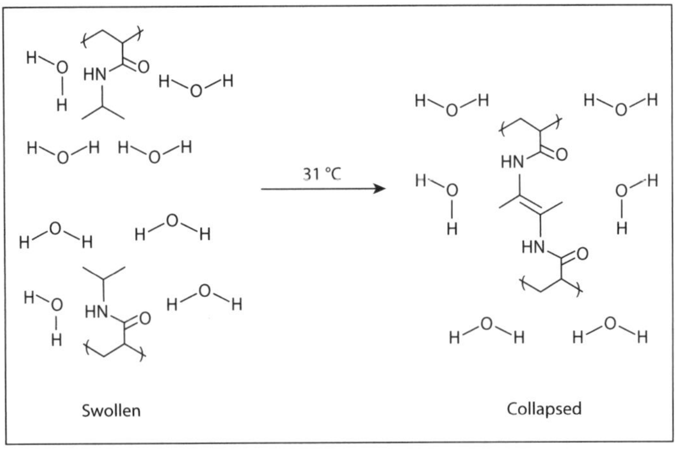

Figure 2.12   Thermal sensitive hydrogels of poly(N-isopropyl acrylamide) (PNIPAm).

gels under defined physicochemical conditions. In general, the gels formed are reversible and can be obtained with very specific properties. Because of the stringent conditions required for their formation, interest in them is growing for the development of new applications in drug-delivery formulations. For instance, many amphiphilic copolymers can form liquid crystals thanks to the supramolecular arrangements of polymer chains in an ordered orientation. Such gels behave in some ways like liquids and in some ways like solids. They include thermotropic phases that undergo phase transition at a very precise temperature and lyotropic phases that undergo phase transition at a very precise temperature and polymer concentration. Thus, they may be suitable for developing stimuli-responsive drug-delivery systems. Another interesting area is the development of formulations administrable as a liquid form but that solidify as a gel to form a solid depot at the administration site as soon as the formulation is in contact with the biological medium. A typical application is the development of eye-drop formulations in which the solution is converted into a gel in contact with the cornea, hence prolonging the residence time of the drug on the surface of the ocular mucosa. Examples of polymers capable of forming gels according to the mechanisms described above are PEG-containing copolymers, which can be used for many applications in pharmacy. Agarose and agar-agar are polysaccharides that form gels by cooling down the temperature of the solution.

Finally, gels can be formed by increasing the concentration of the polymer in such a way that the polymer chains do not have enough space in the solvent to move freely in the solution. In these gels, the polymer chains are entangled together, forming a polymer network in which a liquid phase can be entrapped. Low concentrations of polymers with high molecular weight are required to form gels by this approach compared with polymers of a lower molecular weight. By diluting the gel with a large amount of solvent, the gel structure is lost simply because enough solvent is then available to solubilise the polymer chains.

Polymer gels, and especially polymer hydrogels, show interesting properties for pharmaceutical applications. As already mentioned, polymer gels are mostly composed of a liquid entrapped in the polymer matrix. Thus, some of the properties of a gel are given by the liquid phase it contains.

The other properties are governed by the gelling polymer. For instance, it can be understood that gels obtained from a chemical cross-linked polymer contain permanent covalent bonds. These gels cannot break easily and are permanent. In contrast, gels obtained by other mechanisms are generally reversible gels under certain conditions, except for a few gels. All kinds of gels can be characterised by a swelling ratio defined as the ratio of the weight of the swollen gel to the weight of the dried gel. This ratio defines the capacity of the gel to absorb a liquid phase. The mobility of solute dissolved in the liquid phase depends on its diffusion in the liquid but also on the mesh size of the matrix formed by the polymer, which can slow down the mobility of the larger molecules due to geometry constraints. This last property makes gels very interesting in the formulation of drug-delivery systems with controlled-release properties. Indeed, gels can be used as a reservoir for a drug, which can move out of the gel matrix when the gel matrix has been placed in contact with receiver media, for instance gastrointestinal fluids or the skin surface. The driving force responsible for the drug release from the gel is the difference in concentration between the inside and the outside of the gel. The release rate of the solute depends on many parameters inherent to the properties of the gel, of the solute itself, and of the interactions of the solute with both the gel and the liquid phase entrapped in the gel. The release rate depends also on the characteristics of the releasing medium.

PHEMA is probably the most widely used hydrogel for biomedical applications. PHEMA can contain about one-third of its weight of water. In addition to the monofunctional monomer, commercial monomers usually contain a small percentage of bifunctional residues resulting from synthesis. Polymerisation leads to a material that is water-insoluble but that can be swollen by an aqueous medium. PHEMA was developed in the 1960s to make hydrophilic soft contact lenses (see Section 4.3.7). PHEMA is also used as a lubricating surface coating for catheters and, due to its capacity to incorporate drugs into its network, is used as a matrix for controlled sustained release of drugs.

As the porous structure of the network can be adjusted, and due to their high water content, hydrogels are first-choice materials to incorporate magnetic resonance imaging (MRI) markers. Colloidal superparamagnetic iron oxide stabilised by binding of dextran chains has been manufactured, e.g. Endorem®. Hydrogels containing such an MRI contrast agent have been developed to prepare labelled microparticles for embolisation (see Section 4.3.8).

2.2.4   Polymer dispersions

Another formulation of polymers in liquid media that is of great interest in pharmaceutical applications consists of tiny particles of insoluble polymer dispersed in an aqueous phase. Polymer dispersions are obtained mainly by polymerisation in heterogeneous medium (see Section 3.7.2). In such dispersed systems, polymers are present as spherical particles of diameter less than $1\,\mu m$. In general, aqueous dispersions of such polymer particles are characterised by a low viscosity, just above the viscosity of water, even at high concentration, i.e. at several 10% in the dispersed polymer particles. Polymer dispersions in aqueous-based formulations have been developed as coating material to replace the organic solutions of polymers used in the past. Coating operations are facilitated by the coating material being provided in an aqueous medium and by its having a low viscosity for a high solid content. Gastro-resistant films formed with poly(acrylic) polymers at the surface of tablets or capsules are now obtained from polymer dispersions of the corresponding polymers. Alternative methods require that the polymer is precipitated under small particles in defined conditions. The main difficulty after formation of the polymer particles with the correct size characteristics is to preserve their stability under a dispersed form. This can be achieved by using surfactants or other types of stabilising agent. Finally, in order to be used as coating agents, the polymer particles should display surface properties allowing fusion of particles when they come into contact with each other after they have been sprayed on the surface of tablets or capsules, and after the solvent has been removed during the drying process. Formulations of polymer dispersions for this purpose need to fulfil these crucial requirements in order to be used successfully as a coating material.

Another field of application of polymer dispersions is in the advanced research of drug-delivery systems that aim to design drug carriers that can target the loaded drugs to diseased cells. Dispersed polymer particles of diameter less than 1 μm were found to be suitable for this. Using polymers compatible with this application, such particles can be obtained by polymerisation in heterogeneous systems (see Section 3.7.2) or by precipitation methods directly from the polymer. These polymer dispersions need to remain stable in media that can be used for in vivo administration and to display suitable surface properties to fulfil the drug-delivery duty with the desired pharmacokinetic and biodistribution profiles. A tremendous amount of work has been spent on designing the polymer particle surface to ensure stability of the particles as dispersions and to confer the particles with the desired biopharmaceutical characteristics. It remains a challenging milestone in the battle that aims to increase the specificity of the action of drugs used in the treatment of severe diseases.

Polymer dispersions containing polymer micelles are another system of interest for pharmaceutical applications. These are obtained from amphiphilic polymers that self-aggregate as small spherical entities above a critical concentration of polymer in the solution named the critical micelle concentration (CMC). The main difference between polymer micelles and the particles described above is that the micelle-forming polymer is fully soluble in the dispersing medium below the CMC and itself aggregates to form micelles just by raising the concentration in polymer above the CMC. Micelles are reversible aggregates and can be solubilised by diluting the polymer solution to reach a concentration below the CMC. This is fundamentally different from the previously described particles that form only when applying a more or less sophisticated preparation method and that are not destroyed by simple dilution with an excess of dispersing medium. Micelles are characterised by a well-defined structure; this results from the aggregation of the amphiphilic copolymers in such a way that the surface energy at the interface between the aggregate and the dispersing medium is minimal. Thus, in aqueous medium, the lipophilic part of the copolymers assembles to form lipophilic compartments surrounded by the hydrophilic part of the copolymers, which ensures the stability of the micelle. Micelles consist of core shell particles of nanometric size in which lipophilic drugs can be solubilised.

2.3 Relationships between structure of polymers and cohesion of materials

Many polymers are used as materials. The cohesive properties of polymeric materials result from their structural characteristics and in many cases from the thermomechanical processes used to transform the crude polymer into objects (Box 2.1). The aim of this section is to examine the structural parameters of polymers capable of influencing the cohesive properties of polymeric materials.

2.3.1 Influence of molecular weight

In a molecule, the binding energy between atoms does not depend on the molecular weight of the molecule. Typically, energy of a few hundreds of kilojoules has to be spent in order to break one mole of covalent carbon–carbon bonds. However, the energy that has to be spent in order to separate two molecules, i.e. the cohesive energy, strongly depends on the molecular weight of the molecules. The interactions between molecules, due to van der Waals forces, can be broken by supplying a few tens of kilojoules per mole in the case of small molecules. The high molecular weight of polymers results in increasing cohesive properties. The resulting physical properties such as melting and boiling temperatures are also increased, as shown in Table 2.4.

The shortest hydrocarbons, i.e. methane to butane, are gaseous at room temperature. The thermal energy at this temperature is not sufficient to separate larger molecules from each other, which are more cohesive and in the condensed state, either liquid or solid. The cohesive energy between linear

---

Box 2.1

The structural characteristics resulting from synthesis provide the possibility of a regular structure. Strong interactions between chains leading to high crystallinity and high mechanical strength are strongly improved by thermomechanical treatments. See, for instance, Table 4.2 for the thermomechanical properties of some biodegradable polymers before and after processing.

Table 2.4 Increasing molecular weight of linear alkanes results in increasing melting and boiling temperatures

Molecule	CH_4	C_2H_6	C_4H_{10}	C_6H_{14}	C_8H_{18}	$C_{12}H_{26}$	$C_{20}H_{42}$
Molecular weight (g/mol)	16.04	30.07	58.12	86.18	114.23	170.34	282.54
Melting temperature (°C)	−182	−182	−138	−95	−56.5	−9.6	36.8
Boiling temperature (°C)	−161	−89	−0.5	68	125	216	343
State at room temperature	Gas	Gas	Gas	Liquid	Liquid	Liquid	Solid

hydrocarbon chains tends towards a limit. However, in the case of polymers, the cohesive energy can surpass the energy of the carbon–carbon bond, which can be broken when a sufficient amount of energy is provided to the material in a short time, e.g. during a shock.

2.3.2 Influence of crystallinity

Cohesive energy, which depends on molecular weight for all molecules, depends also on the organisation between macromolecular chains. The existence of a long-range order between chains is characterised by crystallinity. In crystalline fusion, a sharp change occurs from an ordered solid state to a more disordered liquid state with rising temperature. The phenomenon is sharp for metals and small organic molecules, but it is usually less sharp for macromolecules. This is due to the fact that polymers are usually not completely crystalline but are composed of crystalline and amorphous domains. However, highly crystalline polymers are endowed with a defined melting temperature (T_m) (see Section 2.1.2 for method of determination).

The structure of the polymer resulting from synthesis determines the possibility of the presence of crystalline domains. The possibility of the presence of stereo-regular domains can be found in linear polymers with a regular and compact chain structure. Stacking up of chains is favoured by such structural conditions. This is typically the case for high-density polyethylene (HDPE), which is highly linear, with only hydrogen atoms borne by the backbone, and also for poly(tetrafluoroethylene) (PTFE) as the fluorine atoms are small enough. In the case of low-density polyethylene (LDPE), which bears about one butyl group per 100 methylene units, crystallinity is strongly reduced. Isotactic polypropylene, but not atactic polypropylene, is also endowed with a high stereo-regularity. The possibility of the presence of crystalline domains is still increased by the presence in the chains of polar groups such as carbonyl groups (acceptors) and amino groups (donors), inducing hydrogen bonds between chains, e.g. in polyamides (Nylons) or in polyimides. Some examples are given in Figure 2.13.

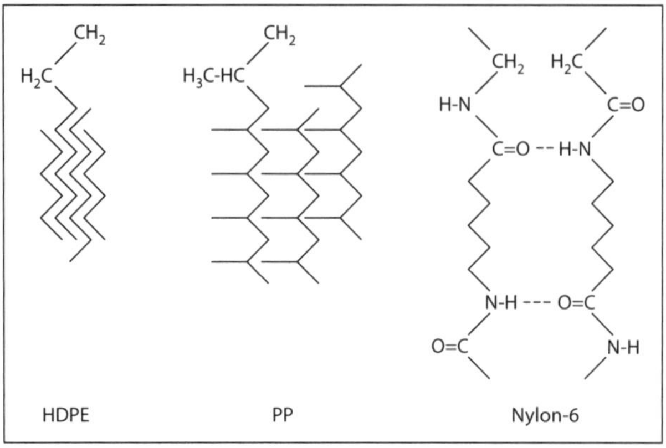

Figure 2.13 Examples of crystalline polymers: high-density polyethylene (HDPE), isotactic polypropylene (PP) and polyamide-6 (Nylon-6).

The possibility of the presence of crystalline domains is thus linked only to the structure of the polymer, but the percentage of crystallinity in the material can be increased by thermomechanical processing such as hot drawing, which makes possible an optimal alignment of all the chains and stacking up.

2.3.3   Glass transition of amorphous domains

Large crystalline domains cannot easily be generated in many polymers that remain mainly amorphous. This can be due to the presence of bulky and/or rigid substituents inducing a steric hindrance, which prevents alignment and stacking of chains. This is typically the case for polystyrene (PS) and poly (methylmethacrylate) (PMMA), shown in Figure 2.14, which are in a rigid and fragile glassy state at room temperature.

With increasing temperature (above T_g), such amorphous polymeric materials can become viscous and more flexible and the shape of the material can

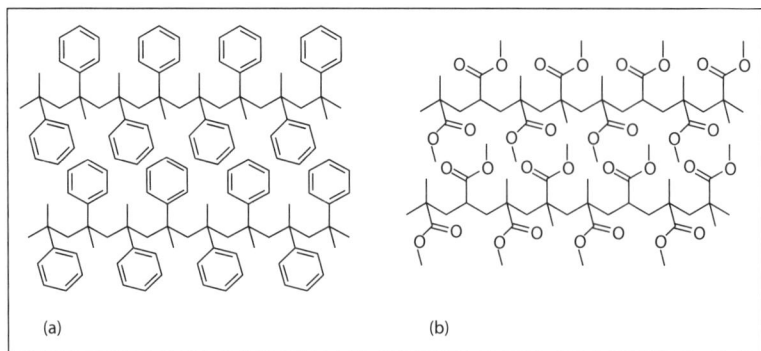

(a)   (b)

Figure 2.14 Examples of amorphous polymers. The phenyl group on polystyrene (PS) (a) and the ester group on PMMA (b) are too bulky to make possible easy crystallisation of the polymers.

be changed by various processes, e.g. extrusion and moulding. Below T_g the polymer chains in the material are immobile, while above T_g the chains can move, explaining why the material properties change. A further decrease of temperature below T_g regenerates the rigid properties and stabilises the shape of the object. In semi-crystalline polymers, only the amorphous domains are concerned by glass transition. Mechanical properties depend on T_g compared with the temperature of the surrounding medium.

When T_g is well above the surrounding temperature, the bulky side groups can hardly move and the polymer is rigid, glassy and fragile. When T_g is close to the temperature of the surrounding medium, segments of molecules can move and the polymer is viscous. When T_g is well below the temperature of the surrounding medium, the chains can move and the polymer behaves as an elastomer.

Examples of glass transition temperature of some polymers are given in Table 2.5.

The influence of the side groups is well illustrated in the case of poly (alkylacrylates) and poly(alkylmethacrylates). It is interesting to compare these polymers, since the difference lies only in the presence of a methyl group as a side chain of poly(alkylmethacrylates) instead of simple hydrogen in the poly(alkylacrylates). In the poly(alkylacrylates), the main chains are repelled from each other by the ester side chains. Increasing size of the side chain decreases T_g. In the poly(alkylmethacrylates), the methyl group hinders the movement of the main chains. For a similar ester side chain, T_g is markedly increased when compared with corresponding poly(alkylacrylates).

Table 2.5 Glass transition temperature of some polymers and their properties at room temperature

Polymer	T_g (°C)	At room temperature
Poly(dimethylsiloxane)	−127	Elastomer
Polybutadiene	−85	Elastomer
Polyisoprene 1–4 *cis* (natural rubber)	−70	Elastomer
Polystyrene	100	Rigid
Poly(methylacrylate)	0	Viscous
Poly(ethylacrylate)	−25	Rather elastic
Poly(*n*-butylacrylate)	−60	Elastomer
Poly(methylmethacrylate)	85	Rigid
Poly(ethylmethacrylate)	50	Rigid
Poly(*n*-butylmethacrylate)	20	Rather viscous

Poly(dimethylsiloxane) (PDMS) is interesting because it possesses the required structural qualities to crystallise. This can be achieved at low temperatures, but the chains are so mobile that PDMS does not remain crystalline at room temperature.

2.4   Properties of polymers as materials

Polymeric materials used in medical devices are selected in order to meet different requirements depending on the specific in vivo application. The reactions of living tissues in contact with a material are exquisitely sensitive to the material's surface properties, and so these and the mechanical properties given by the bulk of the material have to be characterised.

2.4.1   Some mechanical properties

The mechanical behaviour of polymeric materials is often characterised by their stress/strain properties. A tension stress is applied at a very slow rate to a piece of material, which usually has a standardised dumbbell shape, as illustrated in Figure 2.15. Elongation, i.e. strain, is measured until the sample breaks. The results are usually displayed as a plot of stress versus strain. The stress reported to the smallest section of the sample is expressed in newtons per square centimetre (N/cm^2). The strain is usually expressed as the percentage of the original length of the sample ($\Delta L/L \times 100$). Some typical stress/strain plots are shown in Figure 2.16.

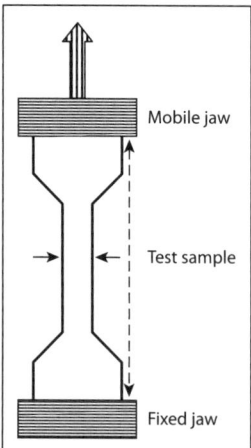

Figure 2.15   Measurement of tensile strength (stress/strain) of a sample of material. A force (in newtons, N) is applied to a dumbbell test sample of initial length L (in cm) and initial section S (in cm^2). The mobile jaw is moving at a slow speed and the relative strain ($\Delta L/L \times 100$) is measured.

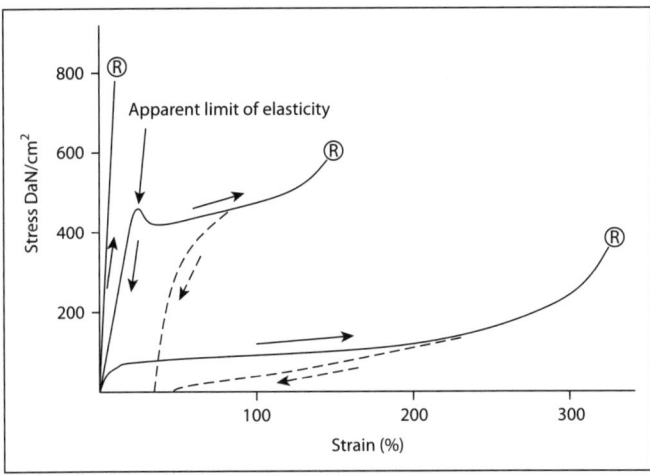

Figure 2.16 Typical stress/strain graphs. Clockwise: rigid plastic, $T_g \gg$ room temperature; flexible plastic, $T_g \cong$ room temperature; elastomer, $T_g \ll$ room temperature; ® = rupture.

Important information can be drawn from such stress/strain plots:

- The modulus of elasticity is given by the initial slope of stress versus strain. It should be determined at a given temperature in conditions of quasi-reversibility, i.e. at a very low rate of elongation, in order to be as accurate as possible. The modulus is also expressed in N/cm^2.
- Elastic elongation is determined by the extent of reversible elongation. For flexible 'plastics', it corresponds only to the first part of the plot.
- Strength and elongation at breaking are sometimes named ultimate strength and elongation. As rupture is initiated at defects of the sample, these data are usually not very accurate.

The mechanical behaviour of polymeric materials depends on several parameters such as degree of crystallinity, melting temperature, glass transition and cross-linking. Typically, elastomers are highly amorphous, with a very low T_g. Their modulus of elasticity is low and they can undergo a very large elongation. However, elongation may be not completely reversible and a slight degree of cross-linking is generally necessary in order to obtain a completely reversible behaviour. In contrast, the modulus of elasticity of highly crystalline or highly cross-linked polymers, and of polymers with a T_g well over room temperature, is high; such polymers can undergo only a very small elongation before breaking. Rigid and amorphous polymers such as PS are much more fragile than crystalline polymers such as Nylon fibres. The behaviour of flexible 'plastics' is in between, with a rather high initial modulus that depends strongly on the degree of crystallinity, and a domain of irreversible elongation that can be extended. A complete view of the mechanical behaviour of polymers can be

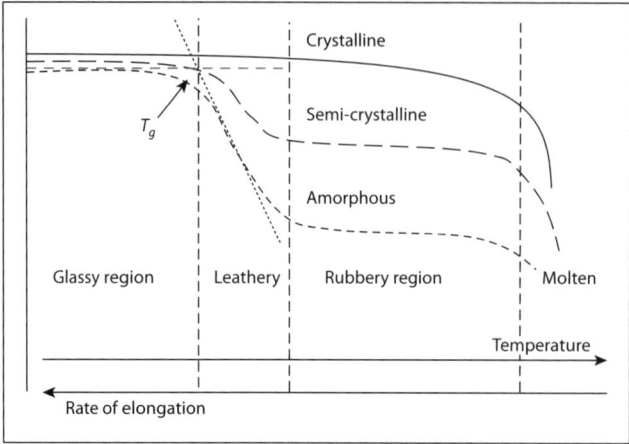

Figure 2.17 Variation of the initial modulus of elasticity with temperature increase (from left to right) or increasing rate of elongation (from right to left).

represented by the variation of the modulus of elasticity as a function of either temperature or rate of elongation, as shown in Figure 2.17.

Whatever the polymer, when the rate of elongation is very fast or the temperature is very low, the polymer behaves as a rigid and fragile material. With highly crystalline polymers, increasing temperature decreases the modulus only slightly until the melting temperature is reached. With amorphous polymers, a sharp decrease in the modulus is observed in the range of glass transition. The behaviour of semi-crystalline polymers is in between.

Other mechanical properties can be tested, depending on the specific application. Mechanical properties can be strongly affected by implantation in a living tissue, which can be very aggressive for some types of polymeric material that are otherwise usually stable in vitro.

2.4.2   Surface properties

The biocompatibility of a material strongly depends on its surface properties, as living tissues are in contact with the surface of the material (see Section 4.3.3). The surface composition of a material can be very different from the bulk composition. This is well known for metals, e.g. the surface of titanium and titanium alloys is generally covered with titanium oxide. This can also be true for polymers, depending on the history of the material and even in the absence of contamination (an example of contamination is given in Section 4.3.5).

For instance, PS has been widely used for in vitro biomedical applications. Storage boxes, Petri dishes for cell or tissue culture, and latexes for diagnosis purposes are frequently made of PS. However, although the bulk composition of these materials is similar, the surface compositions are different: the surface of storage boxes made of pure PS is hydrophobic, whereas that of Petri dishes and latexes for diagnosis purposes is more hydrophilic. Pure PS is not suitable for cell or tissue culture, as cells do not spread on it and cannot survive; Petri dishes are therefore submitted to surface treatments, for instance by glow discharge (i.e. an electrical cold gas plasma), in order to modify the surface chemistry and make the attachment and survival of cells possible. Latexes for diagnosis purposes are prepared by emulsion polymerisation in aqueous phase (see Section 3.7.2). As the initiator of polymerisation is generally a peroxodisulphate, the surface of the resulting latex is covered by covalently linked sulphate groups, which are highly hydrophilic, bear negative charges and are able to stabilise the latex.

It can be seen from these examples that cells and tissues are very sensitive to the composition of the materials surface. Several physicochemical techniques for analysing the composition of materials surface have been described. However, attention is drawn to the fact that the surface analysed by most of these methods is not the surface 'analysed' by living cells, as cells recognise only the outermost layer of a hydrated material. Analysing this ultimate hydrated layer by a physicochemical method is a real challenge. Indeed, the most surface-sensitive methods such as electron spectroscopy for chemical analysis (ESCA; also known as X-ray photoelectron spectroscopy, XPS) and secondary-ion mass spectrometry (SIMS) can analyse respectively a few layers at once or one layer after the other, but in strictly dry conditions. Performing an ESCA analysis at a very low temperature in order to keep water frozen has been described, but this is currently far from a routine method. Conversely, analysis of hydrated surfaces by ATR-IR is usual, but this method determines the composition of many layers in addition to the ultimate layer, as it analyses a depth of more than 1 μm.

Because of the restrictive possibilities of relevant physicochemical surface analysis, different strategies can be adopted. For instance, the effects of surface composition on cells or tissues can be tested on completely modified model materials in which the surface and the bulk are similar. The relevant modification can then be achieved only on the surface.

A simple experimental evidence of surface modification, for instance concerning the hydrophilic/hydrophobic balance of the surface, can be searched for. To do this, the simplest and oldest method measures the contact angle at 'equilibrium' between the clean surface of a material, a liquid and its vapour. This method permits evaluation of the surface tension of material surfaces, which can be related to the hydrophilic/hydrophobic balance. Several experimental processes have been described, but the simplest is deposition of a droplet of liquid on the surface, as shown in Figure 2.18.

The surface tension is calculated by using the Young–Dupré equation (Equation 2.10). In this equation, γ_{LV} is the surface tension between the liquid and its vapour, and θ_e is the solid/liquid contact angle measured at 'equilibrium'. The critical surface tension, which is characteristic of a material surface, corresponds to $\theta_e = 0$ (or $\cos \theta_e = 1$). As zero angles cannot be

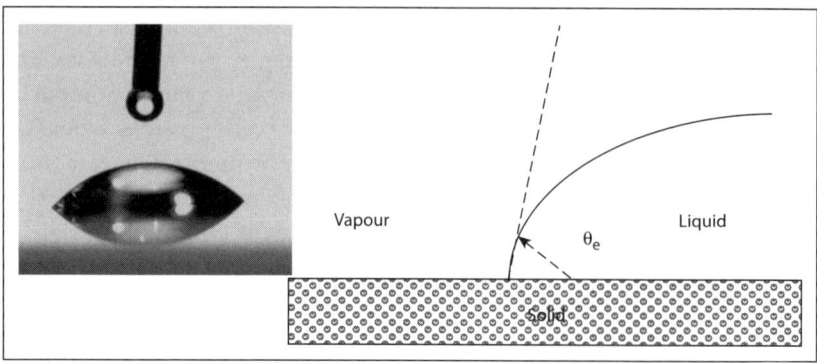

Figure 2.18   Measuring the contact angle at 'equilibrium'. A droplet of liquid is deposited on the horizontal clean surface of the material. The size of the droplet should be small enough to decrease the effects of gravity. When apparent equilibrium has been reached, the contact angle is measured.

measured, the critical surface tension can be assessed by extrapolation after measuring the contact angles between the material surface and several liquids of different γ_{LV}. The surface tension is expressed in energy unit per surface unit. As this equation is rather old, surface tensions are still expressed in some tables as dyne/cm (erg/cm^2), corresponding to mN/m (mJ/m^2) in SI units. The critical surface tension of some polymeric surfaces is given in Table 2.6.

$$\gamma = \gamma_{LV} \cdot \cos \theta_e \qquad (2.10)$$

Table 2.6 Critical surface tension of some polymers		
Polymeric material	**Abbreviation**	**Tension (mJ/m^2)**
Polytetrafluoroethylene	PTFE	19
Poly(dimethylsiloxane)	PDMS	24
Poly(vinylidene fluoride)	PVDF	25
Polyethylene	PE	31
Polystyrene	PS	33
Poly(2-hydroxyethylmethacrylate)	PHEMA	37
Poly(methylmethacrylate)	PMMA	39
Poly(vinyl chloride)	PVC	39
Poly(ε-caprolactame) (Nylon-6)	PA-6	42
Poly(ethylene terephthalate)	PET	43
Polyacrylonitrile	PAN	50

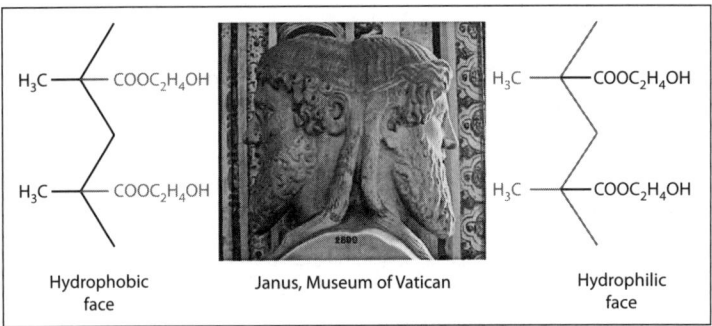

Figure 2.19 Like Janus, poly(2-hydroxyethylmethacrylate) (PHEMA) has two faces. The face presenting the carbon–carbon chain and methyl groups is hydrophobic. The face presenting the hydroxyethyl esters is hydrophilic.

These values found in several reference books require a comment. Concerning 'simple' polymers such as PTFE, polyethylene (PE) and PS, the given values are a direct reflection of their hydrophobicity and even lipophobicity for PTFE. For PHEMA, the value of the critical surface tension is questionable as this polymer is well known as the main constituent of hydrophilic soft contact lenses. This can be explained by the fact that PHEMA has two faces, one hydrophobic, the other hydrophilic, like the Roman god Janus shown in Figure 2.19.

When PHEMA is prepared, it is surrounded by a hydrophobic medium and the polymer is hydrophobic. When the medium surrounding PHEMA is replaced by a hydrophilic medium, the polymer is able to become hydrophilic. However, since dry PHEMA is rigid at room temperature, changing from the hydrophobic material to the hydrated material takes a long time. Thus, it can be assumed that the conditions in which the critical surface tension of PHEMA was measured were not at true thermodynamic equilibrium. This was clearly demonstrated by determining the advancing and receding contact angles on a partially immersed plate.

Bibliography

Determination of molecular weight of polymers, MALDI-TOF and determination of copolymer composition

Ibbeth NR, ed. (1993). *NMR Spectroscopy of Polymers*. London: Blackie Academic & Professional.

Koenig JL, ed. (1999). *Spectroscopy of Polymers*. Amsterdam, New York: Elsevier.

Pasch H, Schrepp W, eds (2003). *MALDI-TOF Mass Spectrometry of Synthetic Polymers*. Berlin, New York: Springer.

Gels and hydrogels

Steinbüchel A, Marchessault RH, eds (2005). *Biopolymers for Medical and Pharmaceutical Applications. Vol: 1: Humic Substances, Polyisoprenoids, Polyesters and Polysaccharides.* Weinheim: Wiley-VCH.

Polymer dispersions

Carraher CE, ed. (2003). *Polymer Chemistry*, 6th edn. New York: Marcel Dekker.
Ebewele RE, ed. (2000). *Polymer Science and Technology*. Boca Raton, FL: CRC Press.

Mechanical properties

Barton AFM, ed. (1983). *Handbook of Solubility Parameters and other Cohesion Parameters.* Boca Raton, FL: CRC Press.
Ferry JD (1980). *Viscoelastic Properties of Polymers*, 3rd edn. New York: John Wiley & Sons.

Surface properties

Andrade JD, ed. (1985). *Surface and Interfacial Aspects of Biomedical Polymers. Vol. 1: Surface Chemistry and Physics*; and *Vol. 2: Protein Adsorption*. New York: Plenum Press.
Ratner BD, ed. (1988). *Surface Characterization of Biomaterials*. Amsterdam: Elsevier.
Stuart B, ed. (2002). *Polymer Analysis*. Chichester: John Wiley & Sons.

3

Main methods and processes to synthesise polymers

3.1   Why there is a need to synthesise polymers

It was shown in Chapter 1 that life is supported by many natural polymers or macromolecules. Natural polymers have been used for centuries, e.g. natural rubber. Modification of natural polymers permitted new useful goods to be made, but sometimes not very well adapted to everyday life, e.g. the highly flammable celluloid.

The domain of health provides remarkable illustrations of the necessity to create new polymers. Natural materials have been used for centuries to replace missing parts of the body: parietal plates made of gold or silver have been found in mummies; silk and 'catgut' sutures have been used for many years by surgeons; and cellulose and derivatives are still used as excipients in formulations of drugs designed to be administered by the oral route. However, such materials were not always adequate and their properties were not always reproducible. Some adverse reactions have occurred, leading to failure of the material, for reasons unknown at the time. Box 3.1 describes some examples of the problems associated with 'technical-grade' polymers.

> **Box 3.1** *Examples of drawbacks encountered when using technical-grade polymers*
>
> For storage of blood, single-use plasticised poly(vinyl chloride) (PVC) bags replaced heavy, breakable glass flasks. However, migration of the plasticiser di-(2-ethylhexyl) phthalate (DEHP) into blood has been observed. Plasticised PVC is still used but is restricted to short-time contact as single-use tubing.
>
> For the joints of hip prostheses, poly(tetrafluoroethylene) (PTFE, e.g. Teflon®) was tested for its well-known low-friction properties. However, this material does not resist wear under compression, leading to failure of the prosthesis.
>
> For the main piece of hip prostheses, the use of carbon-fibre-based composites was suggested because of their lightness and excellent mechanical properties. However, debris of carbon fibres was found in the surrounding tissues, leading to the withdrawal of such types of composite for use in living tissues.

In the 1980s, the need to create materials designed for use in the body gave the impetus to biomaterials. In pharmacy, sustained controlled-release systems and later targeted drug-delivery systems led to the development of hydrogels, biodegradable polymers and nanomaterials.

In order to understand how synthetic polymers are prepared, the methods and processes of polymerisation are presented in this chapter and Chapter 4. It can be seen that some properties of polymers, especially surface properties, depend on the synthesis. The classical techniques are introduced first, but the more specific techniques needed to synthesise special polymers are emphasised.

3.2   Introducing step and chain polymerisation

Two mechanisms of polymerisation have been described: step polymerisation and chain polymerisation. The monomers that are used are completely different. Monomers used in step polymerisation bear at least two chemically reactive groups per molecule (e.g. alcohol, amine, epoxy, carboxylic acid or chloride, isocyanate). The groups may be similar (e.g. diols) or different (e.g. acid and alcohol), as shown in Figure 3.1.

The mechanisms that are implied and the composition of the reaction media versus time are completely different in step and chain polymerisation, as shown in Figure 3.2.

At each step of step polymerisation, two groups react together, e.g. alcohol and acid, whatever the length of the molecule bearing the groups. As the

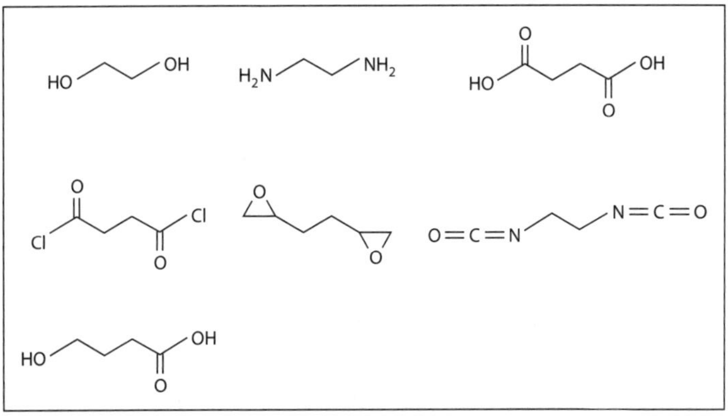

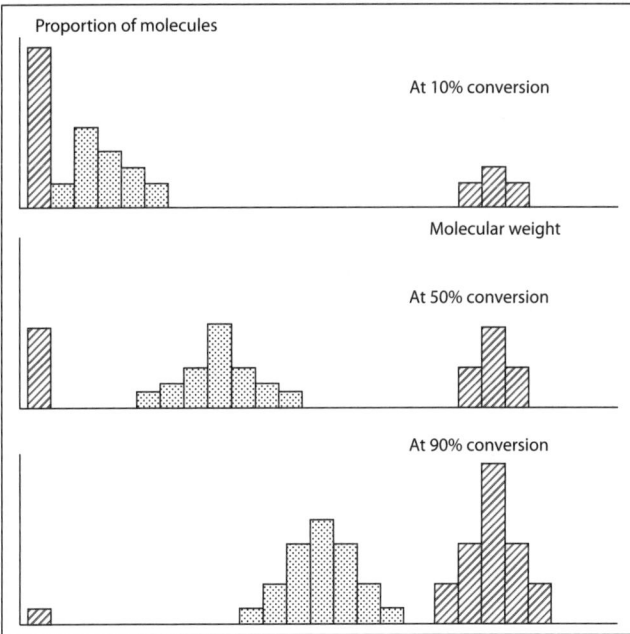

Figure 3.1 Some bifunctional monomers used in step polymerisation: diol, diamine, dicarboxylic acid, dicarboxylic acid chloride, diepoxide, diisocyanate, hydroxyacid.

reaction proceeds, elongation of the chains can occur either by reaction of oligomers with other oligomeric chains or by reaction of oligomers with remaining monomers. The molar fraction of monomers in the reactive medium decreases very rapidly, leading to fast formation of oligomers at the beginning of polymerisation. Thus, the reaction medium is composed of molecules of

Figure 3.2 Composition of reaction medium as a function of conversion. In chain polymerisation (hatched), the reaction medium contains monomers and high-molecular-weight polymer even at low conversion. Increasing conversion increases yield in polymer, not molecular weight. In step polymerisation (dotted), the reaction medium contains monomers and oligomers at low conversion. Increasing conversion increases polymer molecular weight.

slowly increasing length. Concentration of reactive groups decreases with increasing time and a long time is required to obtain high-molecular-weight polymers, at least when using small molecules as monomers.

Monomers used in chain polymerisation contain one or two double bonds, or a triple bond or a cycle. Following generation of an active site able to open the bonds or cycles, the chain grows by successive and fast additions of monomers. The molar fraction of monomers in the reactive medium decreases rather slowly, leading to formation of long polymeric chains. Thus, the reaction medium is composed of a mixture of monomer and high polymer, even at low conversion. The active sites usually have a short life and their concentration is low and almost constant with time. Increasing the reaction time increases the conversion yield of monomer into polymers but not the average chain length of the polymers.

3.3 Some examples of step polymerisation: from small reagents and from prepolymers

The first industrial success in step polymerisation was the synthesis and development by Carothers and co-workers at DuPont of the famous polyamide Nylon 6-6, starting from hexamethylene diamine and adipic acid dichloride. As shown in Equation 3.1, this reaction is favoured by elimination of hydrochloric acid.

$$\text{ClCO-}(CH_2)_4\text{-COCl} + H_2N\text{-}(CH_2)_6\text{-NH}_2$$
$$\rightarrow \text{ClCO-}[(CH_2)_4\text{-CONH-}(CH_2)_6]\text{-NH}_2 + HCl \qquad (3.1)$$

The number average degree of polymerisation (DP_n) can be calculated as a function of functionality of the monomers, i.e. the number of reactive groups per monomer, and as a function of the extent of conversion. For a functionality of 2.000, i.e. corresponding to very pure difunctional monomers, and for 99.9% conversion, it can be calculated that $DP_n = 1000$, i.e. a number-average molecular weight of about 200 000.

The following conditions are required in order to obtain high-molecular-weight linear Nylon 6-6:

* highly purified monomers, as the presence of monofunctional impurities stops the chain growing and the presence of trifunctional impurities leads to branched polymers
* good control of stoichiometry
* long reaction time.

Thus, such a synthesis is expensive and Nylon 6-6 has now been replaced by Nylon 6 produced by ring-opening polymerisation (see Section 3.6).

Some high-molecular-weight polymers can be obtained by using reagents that are already small polymers, called prepolymers. This is the case for polyurethanes and poly(urethanurea)s. For instance, a poly(ether urethane) can be obtained by reacting a poly(ethylene glycol) (PEG), which has two OH end groups, with a diisocyanate such as methylene bis-4-phenyl isocyanate, as shown in Equation 3.2. In this example, R = methylene bis-4-phenyl.

$$O=C=N-R-N=C=O + H-(-O-CH_2-CH_2-)_n-OH$$
$$\rightarrow O=C=N-R-NH-CO-(-O-CH_2-CH_2-)_n-OH \quad (3.2)$$

Addition of a diamine such as ethylene diamine leads to a poly(ether urethane urea), as shown in Equation 3.3.

$$O=C=N-R-NH-CO-(-O-CH_2-CH_2-)_n-OH$$
$$+ H_2N-CH_2-CH_2-NH_2$$
$$\rightarrow H_2N-CH_2-CH_2-NH-CO-NH-R-NH-CO-$$
$$(-O-CH_2-CH_2-)_n-OH \quad (3.3)$$

Such poly(ether urethane urea)s are well known as Lycra® and Spandex® in the textile industry and as Biomer® and Pellethane® in the biomedical field.

3.4   Free radical chain polymerisation

Free radical chain polymerisation is the method used to prepare the most common polymers. A free radical is generated and reacts with one molecule of monomer (initiation). Then monomer molecules react with this first species, leading to formation of a long chain by successive additions of monomer (propagation). Finally, chains are terminated by reaction of two chains bearing radicals (termination). As radicals are very reactive species, side reactions are likely to occur and modify the simple process (transfer).

3.4.1   Initiation: generation of radicals

Chain polymerisation can be initiated by free radicals generated through different mechanisms. Free radicals are generally very unstable and reactive species; thus, they can easily react with the π electrons of carbon=carbon double bonds, leading to the bonds opening and starting chain polymerisation.

Chemical initiation by thermal decomposition of fragile bonds

The most common process used to generate free radicals is the homolytic thermal decomposition of a molecule containing a fragile symmetrical bond, such as peroxides (R-O-O-R), hydroperoxides (R-O-O-H), azonitriles (R-N=N-R) or peroxodisulphates (see Equations 3.4–3.6).

$$C_6H_5-\underset{\underset{O}{\|}}{C}-O-O-\underset{\underset{O}{\|}}{C}-C_6H_5 \quad \rightarrow \quad 2C_6H_5-\underset{\underset{O}{\|}}{C}-O^{\bullet} \quad (3.4)$$

$$
\begin{array}{ccc}
\underset{\underset{N\equiv C}{|}}{\overset{\overset{CH_3}{|}}{CH_3-C}}-N=N-\underset{\underset{C\equiv N}{|}}{\overset{\overset{CH_3}{|}}{C}}-CH_3 & \rightarrow & 2\,CH_3-\underset{\underset{C\equiv N}{|}}{\overset{\overset{CH_3}{|}}{C^\bullet}}+N\equiv N
\end{array}
$$

$$(3.5)$$

$$
\underset{\underset{O}{\|}}{\overset{\overset{O}{\|}}{K^{+-}O-S}}-O-O-\underset{\underset{O}{\|}}{\overset{\overset{O}{\|}}{S}}-O^{-+}K \quad \rightarrow \quad 2\,K^{+-}O-\underset{\underset{O}{\|}}{\overset{\overset{O}{\|}}{S}}-O^\bullet \quad (3.6)
$$

Benzoyl peroxide (BPO) and 2,2′-azo-bis-isobutyronitrile (AIBN) are soluble in organic medium, whereas peroxodisulphates are water-soluble. The rate of decomposition is significant for AIBN over 60 °C and for peroxides over 80 °C.

Redox initiation

Redox catalysis of peroxide decomposition
To permit the generation of radicals at a sufficient rate, the temperature used in industrial processes ranges between 60 °C and 150 °C, depending mainly on the type of initiator used. Addition of reductants as catalysts of peroxide decomposition can increase the rate of radical generation, allowing the use of such initiators at lower temperatures. An example of catalysis by dimethyltoluidine is given in Equation 3.7.

$$
C_6H_5-\underset{\underset{O}{\|}}{C}-O-O-\underset{\underset{O}{\|}}{C}-C_6H_5 + C_6H_5-N(CH_3)_2
$$

$$
\rightarrow (C_6H_5-\underset{\underset{CH_3}{|}}{\overset{\overset{CH_3}{|}}{N}}-O-C-C_6H_5)^+(C_6H_5-\underset{\underset{O}{\|}}{C}-O)^-
$$

$$(3.7)$$

$$
C_6H_5-\underset{\underset{O}{\|}}{C}-O^\bullet + (C_6H_5-\underset{\underset{CH_3}{|}}{\overset{\overset{CH_3}{|}}{N}})^+(C_6H_5-\underset{\underset{O}{\|}}{C}-O)^-
$$

The rate constant (k_d) for decomposition of BPO alone at 90 °C is $k_d = 1.3 \times 10^{-4}$/s. In the presence of dimethyltoluidine the rate constant becomes $k_d = 2.3 \times 10^{-3}$ l/mol.s at 30 °C. Such a catalysed system is used to initiate polymerisation of methyl methacrylate for sealing hip or knee prostheses in vivo, as described in Section 4.3.4.

Ferrous ions can also promote peroxide decomposition, as shown in Equation 3.8; thus, peroxides should not be kept in containers made from iron.

$$R-O-O-R + Fe^{2+} \rightarrow R-O^- + R-O^{\bullet} + Fe^{3+} \qquad (3.8)$$

Organic–inorganic redox pairs
Different inorganic oxidants can react with organic molecules to generate radicals. An example of the reaction between cerium (IV) ions and an alcohol is given in Equation 3.9. Such a reaction has been used to initiate polymerisation of monomers on polysaccharides to obtain mainly graft copolymers and sometimes block copolymers (see Section 3.8).

$$R-CH_2OH + Ce^{4+} \rightarrow R-C^{\bullet}HOH + Ce^{3+} + H^+ \qquad (3.9)$$

Thermal initiation and storage of monomers

WARNING! To avoid uncontrolled polymerisation, monomers should be stored in small quantities, at a low temperature, in a dark non-reflecting flask (glass, not metal) and in the presence of 0.1–1% of polymerisation inhibitors.

Spontaneous polymerisation of some monomers such as styrene can occur in the presence of sunlight and heat, conditions in which free radicals may be generated. Such an uncontrolled initiation is a dangerous hazard. As polymerisation is an exothermic process, temperature increases in the bulk of the monomer and the process can lead to a blast.

Photochemical and radiochemical initiations

High-energy radiation such as ultraviolet (UV) radiation, X-rays, γ rays and electron beams can initiate polymerisation. Radicals formed into polymeric materials during sterilisation by such radiation have a long life, especially in the bulk of the material, and can initiate new polymerisation. Such an initiation process has been used widely to modify polymeric surfaces by grafting another polymer.

3.4.2 Reaction with monomer: propagation and termination

After its generation, the primary radical can react with a monomer molecule (M), as shown in Equation 3.10.

$$A \rightarrow 2R^{\bullet} \quad R^{\bullet} + M \rightarrow R-M^{\bullet}, \text{ example: } R^{\bullet} + CH_2{=}CHR' \rightarrow R-CH_2-\overset{\displaystyle H}{\underset{\displaystyle R'}{C^{\bullet}}}$$

$$(3.10)$$

In the propagation phase, monomer molecules react successively and very quickly on the radical centre (Equation 3.11). The rate of each elementary addition is approximately constant.

$$R\text{-}M^\bullet + n\,M \to R\text{-}M\text{-}M^\bullet \to R\text{-}M\text{-}M\text{-}M^\bullet$$
$$\to R\text{-}M\text{-}M\text{-}M\text{-}M^\bullet \text{etc} \dots \to R\text{-}(M)_n\text{-}M^\bullet \qquad (3.11)$$

The average length of the chains can be evaluated before termination:

- If the initial concentration of initiator is constant, then doubling the initial concentration of monomer doubles the average chain length.
- If the initial concentration of monomer is constant, then multiplying the initial concentration of initiator by four halves the average chain length.

The final chain length depends on the mechanism of termination. In the termination phase, free radicals react in pairs and chain growth is stopped. Depending on the monomers and the conditions of the reaction, two termination processes can occur, as shown in Equation 3.12.

$$2R\text{-}(M)_n\text{-}CH_2\text{-}HR'\,C^\bullet \to \text{Either} \quad R\text{-}(M)_n\text{-}CH_2\text{-}CHR'\text{-}CHR'$$
$$-CH_2\text{-}(M)_n\text{-}R$$
$$\text{Or} \quad R\text{-}(M)_n\text{-}CH_2\text{-}CH_2R' +$$
$$R\text{-}(M)_n\text{-}CH{=}CHR' \qquad (3.12)$$

The type of termination is influenced mainly by the steric hindrance of the groups present on the active site.

3.4.3   Transfers

As free radicals are highly reactive, many side reactions can occur. As the radical is transferred from the end of the growing chain to another place or molecule, such reactions are named transfer reactions. The transfer agent T (monomer, solvent, initiator, inhibitor or polymer) reacts with the radical. The initial chain growth is stopped. Depending on the type of the newly formed radical, either a new chain is initiated and starts to grow, or the radical is inactivated, as shown in Equation 3.13.

$$R\text{-}(M)_n\text{-}M^\bullet + T \to R\text{-}(M)_n\text{-}M + T^\bullet \qquad (3.13)$$

Examples of transfers include the following:

- **Transfer to chlorinated solvents (Equation 3.14):** Chlorinated solvents are very efficient radical transfer agents. As one initial radical leads to two chains, the resulting chains are shorter than in the absence of transfer. This kind of transfer reaction can be used to control the molecular weight of polymers, or to introduce reactive groups (in this case, chlorine) at one end of the chain.

$$-\text{CH}_2\text{-CH}^\bullet + \text{CCI}_4 \rightarrow -\text{CH}_2\text{-CH-CI} + {}^\bullet\text{CCI}_3 \qquad (3.14a)$$
$$\qquad\quad | \qquad\qquad\qquad\qquad\qquad | $$
$$\qquad\quad R \qquad\qquad\qquad\qquad\qquad R$$

$${}^\bullet\text{CCI}_3 + \text{CH}_2{=}\text{CH} \rightarrow \text{CI}_3\text{C-CH}_2\text{-CH}^\bullet \qquad (3.14b)$$
$$\qquad\qquad\qquad | \qquad\qquad\qquad\qquad | $$
$$\qquad\qquad\qquad R \qquad\qquad\qquad\qquad R$$

- **Transfer to polymer – example of 'backbiting', leading to low-density polyethylene (LDPE) (Figure 3.3):** At the temperature used for the reaction, the polyethylene chain is very flexible and can fold easily. By 'backbiting', the radical borne by the chain end is transferred on the fourth carbon before the chain end, and the chain grows on this new location. Such a transfer results in the generation of a branched polymer with about one butyl group for every 100 methylene units. As a result, the long-range order is decreased in the material, i.e. crystallinity is decreased, resulting in lower compacity and density (LDPE) compared with completely linear, highly crystalline polyethylene (HDPE), which is produced by another method (see Section 3.6.3).
- **Transfer to inhibitor:** Inhibitors are transfer agents able to react with radicals, generating new radicals, but these new radicals are too stable to initiate polymerisation and thus polymerisation is stopped. Quinones are an important class of inhibitors frequently used for the storage of monomers in order to inhibit 'spontaneous' initiation of polymerisation.

The action of oxygen is rather anomalous, as it can act as an initiator but also as an inhibitor. For this reason, the medium of polymerisation is usually degassed and polymerisation performed under an inert atmosphere, e.g. nitrogen or ideally argon. Oxidants such as $FeCl_3$ and $CuCl_2$ are strong inhibitors.

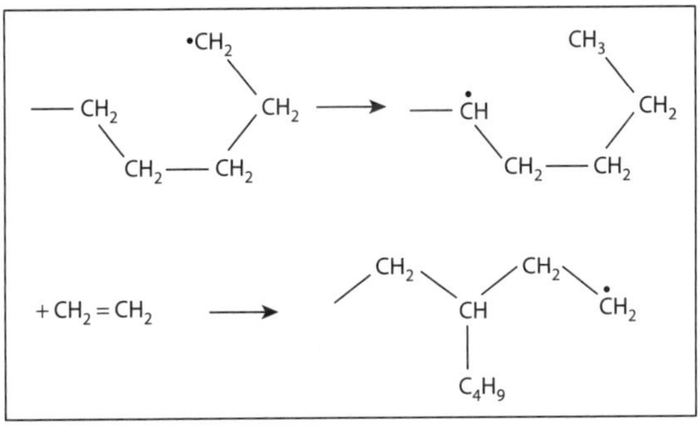

Figure 3.3   Transfer to polymer chain by 'backbiting', leading to low-density polyethylene (LDPE).

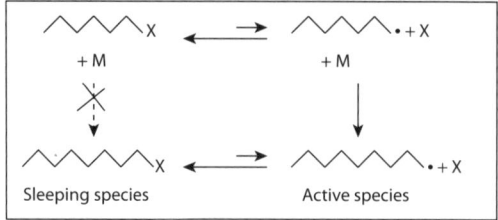

Figure 3.4 Equilibrium between 'sleeping' and active species in controlled radical polymerisation.

3.4.4 Controlled radical chain polymerisation

In a classical free radical chain polymerisation, the slowest step is usually the initiation, for instance in the case of thermal decomposition of a peroxide. In the reaction medium, new radicals are continuously generated, initiating new chains. Growth and termination of chains are very fast, and the active centres are rapidly inactivated, as the termination rate is proportional to the square of radical concentration $(R_t = k_t[\mathrm{M}^\bullet]^2)$. Such a reaction is not controlled, resulting in a large distribution of molecular weight of polymers synthesised by classical free radical chain polymerisation.

New methods have been developed to control the termination phase in radical polymerisation and to yield polymers with a narrower distribution of molecular weight. Some compounds, such as nitroxides (used in nitroxide-mediated stable free radicals, NSFR), thiocarbonylthio derivatives (used in reversible addition fragmentation transfer, RAFT) and organometallic complexes (used in atom transfer radical polymerisation, ATRP), when added to the reaction medium, make equilibrium possible between a very low concentration of active centres and a higher concentration of 'sleeping' species, as shown in Figure 3.4. Termination reactions are limited, allowing control of radical polymerisation and the generation of types of polymer that could not be obtained by classical radical polymerisation. These methods are currently in active phases of industrial development.

3.5 Limitations of polymerisation

Active centres can be generated on many potential monomers, but propagation can be limited by several factors:

3.5.1 Limitation by steric hindrance

Propagation can be limited by steric hindrance. An example is given by styrene and related derivatives, as shown in Figure 3.5. Polymerisation of styrene, i.e. phenylethylene, is easy; polymerisation of α-methylstyrene, i.e. 1,1-methylphenylethylene, is a little more difficult; polymerisation of 1,1-diphenylethylene is impossible. This is due to the fact that the possibility

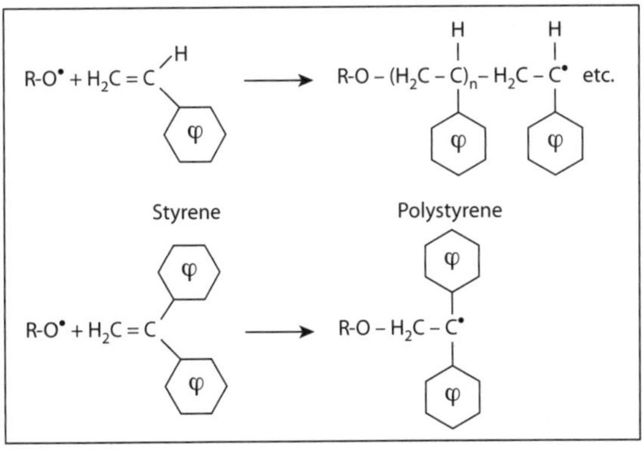

Figure 3.5 Limitation by steric hindrance of polymerisation of some styrene derivatives.

of an efficient collision between the radical and a molecule of monomer is very limited by the presence of two bulky phenyl groups on the same carbon.

3.5.2 Limitation of radical polymerisation by polarity of bonds

The possibility of free radical polymerisation is linked to homolytic opening of bonds to generate radicals. Such an opening can occur only between atoms of similar or very close electronegativity. Although the polarity of a carbon–carbon bond can be modulated by substituents, homolytic opening is often possible in the case of C=C double bonds. This is never possible for C=O double bonds or for C–O single bonds, which are highly polarised and can be opened only according to an ionic mechanism leading to formation of $^+$C–O$^-$. Possibilities of polymerisation of some monomers through free radical or ionic polymerisations are shown in Table 3.1.

Type of monomer	Type of bond	Type of initiation		
		Radical	Anionic	Cationic
Styrene	C=C	+	+	+
Vinyl chloride	C=C	+	–	–
Vinyl ester	C=C	+	–	–
Vinyl ether	C=C	–	–	+
N-vinylpyrrolidone	C=C	+	–	+
Acrylate or methacrylate	C=C	+	+	–
Aldehyde	C=O	–	+	+
Ethylene oxide	C–O in cycle	–	+	+

Table 3.1 Influence of bond polarity on the possible types of initiation

3.5.3 Thermodynamic limitation and possibility of depolymerisation

A release of heat ($\Delta H < 0$) and a decrease of disorder ($\Delta S < 0$) are associated with polymerisation, i.e. transformation from free monomer to repeating unit in polymer, as shown in Equation 3.15.

$$CH_2=CHR \rightarrow \text{-(-}CH_2-CHR\text{-)-} \tag{3.15}$$

The possibility of a transformation is associated with a decrease of free enthalpy ($\Delta G < 0$), and equilibrium between a transformation and the reverse transformation is associated with $\Delta G = 0$.

$G = H - TS$, and so $dG = dH - d(TS) = dH - TdS - SdT$.

If a transformation is performed in conditions in which the temperature and pressure are constant, then $SdT = 0$, and $\Delta G = \Delta H - T\Delta S$.

At the temperature for which $\Delta G = 0$, polymerisation is in equilibrium with depolymerisation. Because this equilibrium generally occurs in conditions above room temperature, this temperature is called the ceiling temperature (T_c). If the temperature of the polymer is below T_c, then the thermodynamically stable species is the polymer. Conversely, if the temperature of the polymer increases above T_c, then the monomer becomes the most stable species, i.e. depolymerisation is possible. However, depolymerisation can occur only in the presence of active species, e.g. radicals.

Examples of styrene and α-methylstyrene

Polymerisation of styrene is associated with $\Delta H = -67.3$ kJ/mol and $\Delta S = -10.5$ J/mol.K. Calculation leads to $T_c = 641$ K, i.e. 368 °C. This means that polystyrene is thermodynamically stable below this temperature and can be heated to be transformed into objects, e.g. by moulding, above its glass transition temperature (T_g), located around 100 °C. However, polystyrene objects are not stable in a fire, resulting in depolymerisation, emission of gases and quick burning.

Polymerisation of α-methylstyrene is associated with $\Delta H = -37.6$ kJ/mol and $\Delta S = -10.9$ J/mol.K. Calculation leads to $T_c = 345$ K, i.e. 72 °C. This means that poly(α-methylstyrene) is thermodynamically unstable above this temperature and cannot be heated safely above its glass transition temperature to be transformed into objects.

Modification of polymers with large substituents, e.g. drugs, can change the ceiling temperature.

3.6 Overview of other synthetic methods

It was shown previously that polarisation of some double bonds prevents polymerisation by a free radical mechanism of molecules containing such bonds. Conversely, double bonds that can be opened by ionic mechanisms make ionic chain polymerisation possible in the presence of adequate initiators. Some polymers, especially most biodegradable polymers, can be obtained only through such mechanisms. Characteristics of ionic chain polymerisations depend on the reactivities of the monomer and initiator and on the solvent that is usually present in the reaction medium. In polar solvents, e.g. water, alcohols, ethers and chlorinated solvents, the reactive species are solvated ion pairs in equilibrium with solvated free ions. Depending on the polarity of the medium, the concentration of solvated free ions can vary widely, but ions are much more reactive than ion pairs. In apolar solvents, e.g. hydrocarbons, reactive species are weakly dissociated solvated ion pairs and thus are weakly reactive. Consequently, rates of polymerisation are faster in polar solvents than in apolar solvents. Some chelating agents capable of increasing the dissociation of ion pairs can be added to increase the polymerisation rate in such solvents.

3.6.1 Anionic chain polymerisation

Polymers prepared by opening of double carbon=carbon bonds

The first anionic polymerisations were performed in the 1930s by Ziegler in Germany, in order to prepare synthetic rubber. The so-called BuNa was prepared by polymerisation of butadiene initiated by metallic sodium. The detailed mechanisms of anionic polymerisation were described in the 1950s by Szwarc. The common feature of anionic chain polymerisations is the fact that at least one anionic group stabilised by a small cation is located at one end of the growing chains. The initiating species are bases according to the definitions of either Brønsted or Lewis, for instance HO^- in water, CH_3O^- in methanol, R_3N, H_2N^-, organometallic compounds such as derivatives of lithium, magnesium, tin and zinc. The mechanism comprises nucleophilic attack and transfer of the electrons at the end of the chain, as shown in Equation 3.16.

$$B^- + CH_2 = \overset{\overset{\displaystyle H}{|}}{\underset{\underset{\displaystyle R}{|}}{C}} \rightarrow B - CH_2 - \overset{\overset{\displaystyle H}{|}}{\underset{\underset{\displaystyle R}{|}}{C^-}} \rightarrow etc \rightarrow B - (-CH_2 - \overset{\overset{\displaystyle H}{|}}{\underset{\underset{\displaystyle R}{|}}{CH}} -)_n - CH_2 - \overset{\overset{\displaystyle H}{|}}{\underset{\underset{\displaystyle R}{|}}{C^-}}$$

$$(3.16a)$$

$$2\,Na + 2\,CH_2 = \overset{\overset{\displaystyle H}{|}}{\underset{\underset{\displaystyle R}{|}}{C}} \rightarrow Na^{+-}\overset{\overset{\displaystyle H}{|}}{\underset{\underset{\displaystyle R}{|}}{C}} - CH_2 - CH_2 - \overset{\overset{\displaystyle H}{|}}{\underset{\underset{\displaystyle R}{|}}{C}}{}^{-+}Na \rightarrow etc$$

$$(3.16b)$$

Reactivity in anionic chain polymerisation of monomers possessing a double carbon=carbon bond is increased by the presence of electro-attractive groups on one of these carbon atoms. Depending on the reactivity of the monomer and on the solvent used, different types of initiator can be used.

The propagation rate depends mainly on dissociation of ion pairs and thus on the polarity of the reaction medium. If the rate of initiation is faster than the rate of propagation, then all the chains are initiated at the same time and grow at a similar rate. In this case, polymeric chains can possess a similar length, i.e. polymolecularity is low ($M_w \cong M_n$).

Depending on the reaction medium, termination can be rather slow, and the active site located at the end of the chain can remain active for a few minutes when all of the monomer has been transformed into polymer; for this reason, 'living polymers' can be described. This phenomenon can be taken advantage of when preparing block copolymers (see Section 4.1) or for terminating the chains with groups that can be activated in a further step (telechelic polymers). Examples of telechelic polymers are given in Equation 3.17.

$$B-(\text{-CH}_2-\text{CH-})_n-\text{CH}_2-\text{CH}^- + (1)\,\text{CO}_2 + (2)\,\text{H}^+,\text{H}_2\text{O}$$

with R substituents

$$\to\ B-(\text{-CH}_2-\text{CH-})_n-\text{CH}_2-\text{CH}-\text{COOH}$$

with R substituents

(3.17a)

$$B-(\text{-CH}_2-\text{CH-})_n-\text{CH}_2-\text{CH}^- + \text{Br}-\text{CH}_2-\text{CH}=\text{CH}_2$$

with R substituents

$$\to\ B-(\text{-CH}_2-\text{CH-})_n-\text{CH}_2-\text{CH}-\text{CH}_2-\text{CH}=\text{CH}_2$$

with R substituents

(3.17b)

Some monomers, such as alkylcyanoacrylates in which the double bond is highly polarised by the presence of two electro-attractive groups on the same carbon, are very reactive and their polymerisation can be initiated at room temperature by HO^- in water, according to Equation 3.18.

$$\text{HO}^- + \text{CH}_2 = C\overset{C\equiv N}{\underset{COOR}{}} \to \text{HO}-\text{CH}_2-C^-\overset{C\equiv N}{\underset{COOR}{}} \to \text{etc}$$

$$\to\ \text{HO}-(\text{-CH}_2-C\text{-})_n-\text{CH}_2-C^- \quad \text{with } C\equiv N \text{ and COOR substituents}$$

(3.18)

Propagation is very fast and termination is due to hydrated protons. The length and number of chains are highly dependent on the pH of the aqueous medium. This fast polymerisation of the shortest esters initiated in the presence of water vapour is used for obtaining quasi-instant gluing (e.g. Loctite®). Increasing the length of the esters decreases the polymerisation rate. Butyl and higher esters are major components of surgical glues and liquid agents for therapeutic embolisation, and they have also been used to prepare nanoparticulate drug carriers (see Section 4.4.6).

Polymers prepared from aldehydes or by ring opening

Several molecules containing a bond between two atoms of different electronegativity – either a double bond or a single bond included in a cycle with a sufficiently high ring strain – can be used as monomers in anionic polymerisation.

Polymerisation of formaldehyde

In aqueous medium, aldehydes are in equilibrium between monomeric and oligomeric forms. This is typically the case for formaldehyde. To obtain high-molecular-weight polymers, formaldehyde can be easily polymerised through ionic polymerisation. Initiation by methanolate ions is shown in Equation 3.19 and poly(methylene oxide) is obtained.

$$CH_3O^- + n\ CH_2{=}O \rightarrow CH_3O{-}CH_2{-}O^- \dots etc$$
$$\rightarrow CH_3O\text{-}(\text{-}CH_2{-}O\text{-})_n\text{-}H \tag{3.19}$$

As the ceiling temperature of the polymer is rather low, depolymerisation is avoided by blocking the chain ends by reaction with carboxylic anhydrides (end-capping). The resulting end-capped poly(methylene oxide), e.g. Delrin®, is highly crystalline (melting temperature $T_m = 175\ °C$) and resistant to wear, shock and chemicals; it has been used for manufacturing tilting disks for valvular heart prostheses.

Polymerisation of ethylene oxide

Ethylene oxide contains a very tight cycle, and polymerisation of this gas is easy, as shown in Equation 3.20. The resulting poly(ethylene oxide) (PEO; see Box 3.2) is soluble in many solvents, including water and acetone.

$$CH_3O^- + n\ CH_2{-}CH_2 \rightarrow CH_3O{-}CH_2{-}CH_2\text{-}O^- \dots etc$$
$$\overset{\diagdown\ \ \diagup}{\underset{O}{}}$$
$$\rightarrow CH_3O\text{-}(\text{-}CH_2{-}CH_2\text{-}O\text{-})_n\text{-}H \tag{3.20}$$

Polymerisation of hydroxyacid cyclic derivatives

An ester bond is present in the main chain of many (bio)degradable polymers. During degradation in vivo, the products generated through hydrolysis are

Box 3.2

The repeating units of poly(ethylene oxide) (PEO) and poly(ethylene glycol) (PEG) are similar. As the methods used to synthesise these polymers are different, however, the chain ends and the range of molecular weight are different. PEO is obtained through anionic polymerisation. Only one end of the chains of PEO is an OH group, and PEO can be obtained within a wide range of molecular weight. PEG is obtained through cationic polymerisation (see Section 3.6.2). Both chain ends of PEG are OH groups, and the molecular weight of PEG is usually lower than the molecular weight of PEO.

then metabolised (see Section 4.2.3). Such polymers have been synthesised for many years and were originally proposed as biodegradable materials for deep sutures. Glycolic and lactic acids, which are α-hydroxyacids, could theoretically be polymerised by step polymerisation through dehydration. However, usually only low-molecular-weight polymers, i.e. oligomers, and cyclic dimeric forms, respectively called glycolide and lactides, are obtained, as shown in Figure 3.6. More recently, preparation of high-molecular-weight poly(α-hydroxyacids) by step polymerisation has been claimed.

The cyclic forms can be opened by nucleophilic attack of various initiators. Polymers often called poly(glycolic acid) and poly(lactic acid)s or, more properly, polyglycolide (PGA) and polylactides (PLA), or their copolymers (PLGA) can be obtained according to the main mechanism, as

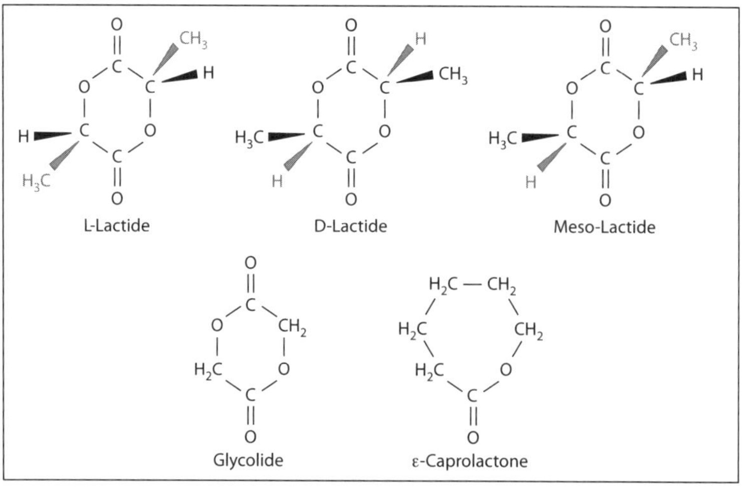

Figure 3.6 Some cyclic monomers leading to biodegradable polymers.

shown in Equation 3.21.

$$\text{Ionic initiator } R^- + \text{lactide} \rightarrow R-(-CO-\overset{*}{C}H-O-CO-\overset{*}{C}H-O-)_n^-$$
$$\underset{CH_3}{|} \qquad \underset{CH_3}{|}$$

$$(3.21)$$

Among the initiators, tin (II) bis-2-ethylhexanoic acid (stannous octano-ate) has been the most used for preparing biomedical and pharmaceutical polymers because of its low toxicity.

Following the development of PLGA, poly(ε-caprolactone) (PCL) has been synthesised by ring-opening polymerisation and also developed as a degradable polymer. Other synthetic polymers based on hydroxyacids such as malic acid and its derivatives have been proposed.

Besides these biodegradable polyesters prepared by chemical synthesis, a new class of biodegradable polyesters produced through biotechnology, the poly(alkanoates), is currently under development (see Section 4.2).

Polyamides obtained by ring-opening polymerisation

Polyamides are now synthesised mainly by ring-opening polymerisation. This is typically the case of polyamide 6, known as Nylon 6, which is prepared by ring opening and polymerisation of ε-caprolactam, the cyclic amide very close to ε-caprolactone.

Silicones

Polysiloxanes, also referred to as silicones, are known for their very high flexibility (as their glass transition is around −127 °C) and their high stability in diverse environments, including the biological environment. Poly (dimethylsiloxane) (PDMS) can be produced by ring-opening polymerisation of the cyclic tetramer octamethylcyclotetrasiloxane, as shown in Figure 3.7.

3.6.2   Cationic chain polymerisation

The active cationic reactive centres are borne by the end of the growing chain and are stabilised by small anions. However, the active cationic centres that

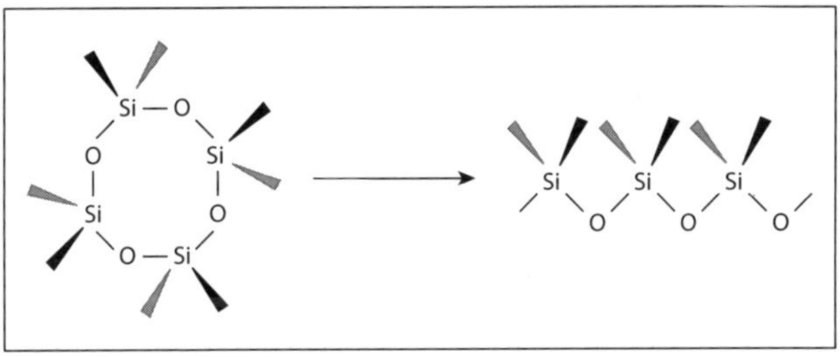

Figure 3.7   Synthesis of poly(dimethylsiloxane) (PDMS) by ring-opening polymerisation.

correspond to a lack of electrons are far less stable than the active anionic centres, and many reactions of transfer and termination can take place. As a consequence, molecular weights of polymers obtained by cationic polymerisation are usually rather low.

Monomers for cationic polymerisation comprise molecules with carbon=carbon double bonds bearing electro-donor substituents, e.g. isobutylene, and also small cycles. Cyclic ethers such as tetrahydrofuran, which is used as a solvent in anionic polymerisation, can act as a monomer in cationic polymerisation. Typically, chlorinated solvents are used in cationic polymerisation as the medium of polymerisation.

The initiating species are acids according to the definitions of either Brønsted or Lewis.

Syntheses of (PEG) and poly(tetramethylene oxide) (PTMO) can be initiated by $TiCl_4$ in the presence of traces of water, as shown in Equation 3.22. PEG and PTMO, which possess one hydroxyl group at each chain end, can be used as prepolymers for synthesis of poly(ether urethane)s.

$$TiCl_4 + H_2O \rightarrow (TiCl_4OH)^-, H^+$$

With ethylene oxide:

$$\begin{array}{lcl} (TiCl_4OH)^-, H^+ + n\begin{array}{c} CH_2 - CH_2 \\ \diagdown \;\; \diagup \\ O \end{array} & \rightarrow & \begin{array}{l} H\text{-}(\text{-}O - CH_2 - CH_2\text{-})_n\text{-}OH \\ (PEG) \end{array} \end{array} \tag{3.22a}$$

With tetrahydrofuran:

$$\begin{array}{lcl} n\begin{array}{ccc} CH_2 & - & CH_2 \\ | & & | \\ CH_2 & & CH_2 \\ & \diagdown \; O \; \diagup & \end{array} & \rightarrow & \begin{array}{l} H\text{-}(\text{-}O - CH_2 - CH_2 - CH_2 - CH_2\text{-})_n\text{-}OH \\ (PTMO) \end{array} \end{array} \tag{3.22b}$$

Ethyleneimine, which possesses the same tight structure as ethylene oxide, polymerises easily through a cationic mechanism. As the detailed mechanism is quite complex, poly(ethyleneimine) (PEI) is usually a branched polymer containing primary, secondary and tertiary amine groups in the approximate ratio 1 : 2 : 1. Synthesis by cationic polymerisation of linear PEI designed to be used for gene delivery has been reported.

3.6.3 Stereo-specific polymerisation

In the previously described methods of polymerisation, monomer addition takes place on an active centre in which spatial configuration is randomised.

As a consequence, configuration of the resulting polymers is also randomised. An example is given by atactic propylene obtained by radical polymerisation, which is highly amorphous.

Conversely, stereo-regular constant or alternate spatial configurations can be obtained if configuration of the active centre is either constant or changed alternately at each addition. To obtain such an effect, Ziegler and Natta, who won Nobel Prizes in 1963, developed a method to generate the initiating species on solid surfaces. In the initial patent, they claimed: 'The catalysts are composed of compounds resulting from reaction of alkoylated derivatives of a metal belonging to groups from 1 to 3 with a compound comprising a transition metal belonging to groups from 4 to 8.' In a typical example, the reagents are $AlEt_3$ and $TiCl_4$ and the mechanisms of polymerisation are likely ionic.

Polypropylene obtained by Ziegler–Natta polymerisation is isotactic and highly crystalline ($T_m \approx 170\ °C$) and thus is endowed with very interesting mechanical properties.

Despite the fact that polyethylene does not possess any tacticity, ethylene can be polymerised in the presence of stereo-specific initiators. Polyethylene obtained by this method is linear and highly crystalline (HDPE), whereas polymerisation of ethylene obtained by radical polymerisation leads to a branched and thus more amorphous polymer (LDPE), as shown in Section 3.4.4.

3.7　Polymerisation reaction processes

The conditions in which polymerisation takes place are very important, concerning for instance the physical form of the polymer that is obtained, the purpose of the form, the 'quality' of the polymeric material, and the costs in economical and environmental terms. Polymers can be prepared:

- in homogeneous systems, i.e. mass or bulk, or in solution
- in heterogeneous systems, i.e. suspension, emulsion or interfacial polymerisation.

3.7.1　Polymerisation in homogenous systems

Bulk polymerisation

The system involved in the bulk polymerisation process is the simplest from the point of view of composition and is used for large-scale radical polymerisation. In this process, the initiator is mixed with the monomer, usually under pressure of an inert gas, and the mixture is heated to induce generation of free radicals by thermal decomposition of the initiator. Depending on whether the monomer is a gas or a liquid, the system can be homogenous or heterogeneous

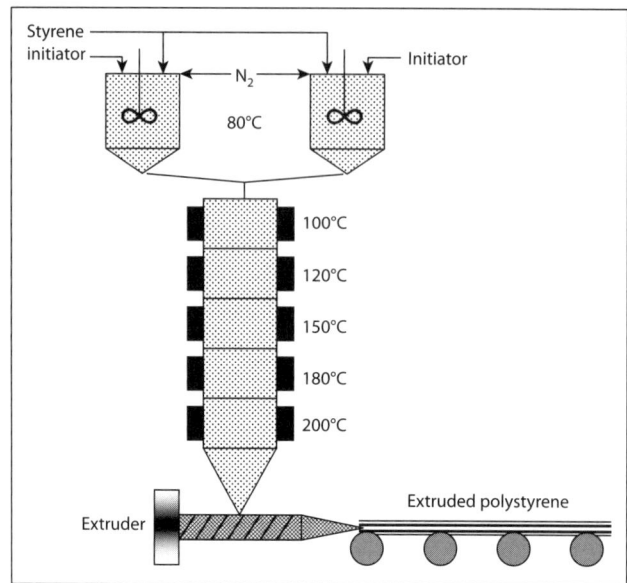

Figure 3.8 Industrial bulk polymerisation of styrene directly followed by extrusion.

at the end of polymerisation. An example of industrial bulk polymerisation is illustrated in Figure 3.8.

From an industrial point of view, this process has many advantages. The monomer is converted into polymer without the need to eliminate by-products. Continuous production of large amounts of polymer is possible. As polymerisation is exothermic, the polymer is usually in a molten state at the end of conversion, and its direct transformation into extruded products is easy.

However, this process is not devoid of drawbacks. As the medium is a bad heat transmitter, the heat generated by polymerisation has to be controlled carefully with efficient mixing in order to avoid heat spots leading to a 'caramelised' polymer. In addition, the viscosity of the polymerisation medium increases with conversion of the monomer into the polymer and is very high at the end of monomer conversion. The increasing temperature of the system contributes to the maintenance of viscosity at a level that makes mixing possible. However, as the concentration of the monomer in the system decreases from the beginning to the end of polymerisation, polymolecularity is rather high. In addition, traces of unconverted monomer can remain in the final product. Such a process is used to produce large amounts of cheap technical-grade polymers useful for instance as materials in civil engineering.

Polymerisation in solution

In the solution polymerisation process, monomer and initiator are dissolved in a solvent and the solution is stirred. Thus, some of the drawbacks cited above, especially those linked to the high viscosity at the end of conversion in the bulk polymerisation process, are solved in the present process. Complete conversion of monomer is easier and polymolecularity is not as wide as in the bulk process. The process in solution is also required in many ionic polymerisations.

However, new drawbacks are generated by the presence of solvent in this process. Side reactions such as transfer to solvent are possible. The solvent has to be eliminated as much as possible and recycled. Solvent residues can remain in the polymer. From an industrial point of view, this process is used only when the presence of solvent cannot be avoided.

3.7.2 Polymerisation in heterogeneous systems

There are different methods of polymerisation in heterogeneous systems. In general, such systems of polymerisation include two phases that either coexist from the beginning of the polymerisation or form during polymerisation because of phase separation of the forming polymer. This is in contrast with polymerisation in solution, which remains homogenous from the beginning to the end of the polymerisation. Compared with polymerisation in bulk or in solution, the main advantages for polymerisation in heterogeneous systems is that these systems provide much better conditions to control the polymerisation reaction and hence the final characteristics of the produced polymer. Low viscosity is maintained in the system, making control of stirring and temperature during the entire polymerisation easier. As a consequence, the polymerisation occurs more homogenously from beginning to end than in the previously described systems, giving polymers of lower polymolecularity and copolymers of higher homogeneity in their composition and structure. At the end of polymerisation, the polymer is generally provided as beads, or sometimes as capsules, with many industrial applications. The size of the beads, which can vary from several nanometres to a few millimetres in diameter, depends greatly on the polymerisation system, which influences the mechanism of particle formation. It is noteworthy that emulsion polymerisations are now the most widely used methods applied in industry to prepare polymers and to obtain latexes.

The principal characteristics of the different modes of polymerisation in heterogeneous systems are summarised in Table 3.2.

Polymers can be produced by applying the various types of polymerisation mechanism described above, i.e. all radical polymerisations including controlled polymerisation and ionic polymerisation. In addition to producing polymers with well-defined characteristics, polymerisation in heterogeneous systems can be used to produce well-defined polymer particles including very well-structured composite nanoparticles. For instance, particles with a magnetic core and nanoparticles showing a core-shell-type nanostructure can be

Table 3.2 Main processes of polymerisation in heterogeneous systems

Process	Main characteristics of initial system	Main characteristics of reaction	Main characteristics of final system
Suspension	Monomer with dissolved initiator roughly dispersed in a continuous phase with a low amount of surfactant	Polymerisation initiated in monomer droplets; droplets converted into polymer particles	Large polymer particles (diameter 10–1000 μm)
Dispersion	Monomer and initiator dissolved in appropriate solvent to prepare homogenous solution	Polymerisation initiated in solution; insoluble polymer precipitates as particles	Polymer particles of several micrometres in diameter
Emulsion	Monomer droplets stabilised by low amount of surfactant, dispersed in continuous phase in which the initiator is dissolved; monomer slightly soluble in continuous phase	Polymerisation initiated in continuous phase; growing chains formed in continuous phase precipitate nucleating polymer particles; chains continue to grow in nucleated particles; polymerisation 24–48 h	Diameter of largest particles is a few micrometres; larger particles can be obtained by seeding and feeding with a further amount of monomer; composite or structured particles can be obtained
Mini-emulsion	Tiny monomer droplets dispersed in continuous phase with surfactant and hydrophobic compound; emulsions produced using high shear rates or ultrasound; initiator dissolved in either monomer droplets or continuous phase	Polymerisation initiated in mini-emulsion droplets; each mini-emulsion droplet behaves like a nano-reactor; high rate of polymerisation	Particles in the size range 5–500 nm, with a narrow size distribution; high molecular weight of resulting polymers; composite or structured particles can be obtained
Micro-emulsion	Swollen monomer micelles dispersed in a continuous phase; fairly large concentrations of surfactants required; initiator dissolved in continuous phase	Polymerisation initiated in the course of nucleation of monomer micelles; process characterised by continuous nucleation during entire reaction; fast rate of polymerisation (< 30 min)	Particles of very small size (diameter < 100 nm) and narrow distribution; polymer with ultra-high molecular weight (> 10^7 g/mol); copolymers with well-defined, homogenous composition

synthesised by these methods. Particles with even more complex nanostructures can be synthesised. Such micro- and nanoparticles, including capsules, have a use in drug-delivery systems with controlled biodistribution and drug-releasing patterns and as tools for diagnosis by imaging methods.

Suspension polymerisation

In the process of suspension polymerisation, the monomer is dispersed by vigorous stirring into a medium in which it is not soluble. As many monomers are hydrophobic, the medium is most often water. An important feature is the presence of initiator in the monomer droplets. A surfactant is used to stabilise the droplets and standardise their size. Mineral salts are added to the water to decrease the solubility of the monomer in water as much as possible.

This process has many advantages, as thermal control is excellent in water and the viscosity of the medium remains low and constant. Each droplet of monomer is converted directly into a polymer bead. Provided that the size of the droplets is well controlled, polymer beads of defined size, e.g. in the range 10–1000 μm, are obtained at the end of conversion. This permits easy storage and feeding of moulding machines for transformation into objects. An example of an industrial process for suspension polymerisation is presented in Figure 3.9.

The dispersing medium has to be eliminated and recycled. When an aqueous medium is used, the beads have to be washed to eliminate salts and surfactants and then dried.

This process is not easy to adapt to continuous production and is energy-consuming, but it allows production of large amounts of good-quality polymers.

Inverse suspension polymerisation is a convenient way to obtain microspheres of hydrophilic polymers. More details about the use of microspheres for therapeutic embolisation are found in Section 4.3.8.

Emulsion, mini-emulsion and micro-emulsion polymerisations

Emulsion polymerisation was initially developed for producing synthetic rubber from butadiene and styrene during the Second World War. The system

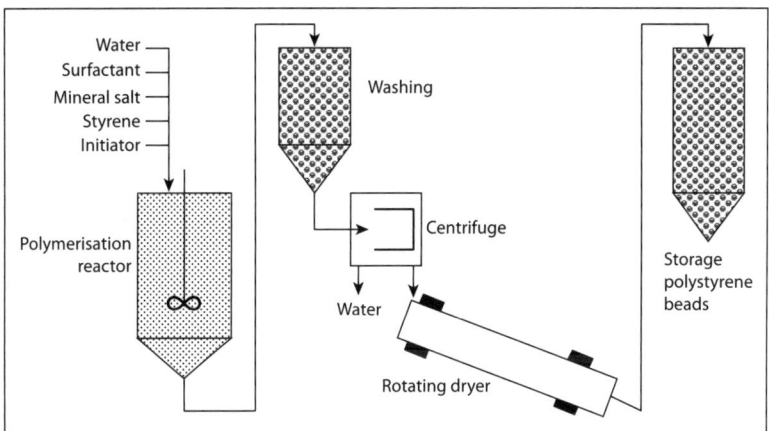

Figure 3.9   Industrial suspension polymerisation of styrene.

used in emulsion polymerisation is very close to the previously described system in the sense that the monomer is dispersed in a medium, usually water, in which its solubility is low or very low, a surfactant is present and the medium is stirred. Unlike in the suspension polymerisation process, however, nothing is done to avoid the presence of soluble monomer in water, as the initiator is water-soluble. Thus, polymerisation is initiated in water and the polymeric chains stabilised by surfactants grow in the aqueous phase. The monomer is present in equilibrium between rather large droplets acting as reservoirs, micelles of monomer, monomer in low concentration in water, and micelles of growing polymer. Depending on the concentration of surfactant in the medium, the polymeric micelles can more or less combine together, leading to formation of a colloidal suspension of submicronic particles, i.e. latex or nanoparticles, usually in the size range 50–1000 nm. A model of emulsion polymerisation is presented in Figure 3.10.

To obtain larger particles, it is possible to use a seed process and to induce polymerisation of a further amount of monomer on the seed particles. Note that this process can be used to obtain composite or structured particles.

Mini-emulsion is a variant of emulsion polymerisation. Tiny stabilised monomer droplets are dispersed in a continuous phase. Emulsions are produced by using either high shear rates (high pressure homogeniser) or ultrasound. Such high rates of agitation are required to reach a steady state given by the balance between droplet fission and fusion. The high stability of these emulsions can be explained by the inhibition of inter-droplet mass transfer phenomenon, i.e. Oswald ripening. The choice of surfactant and the addition

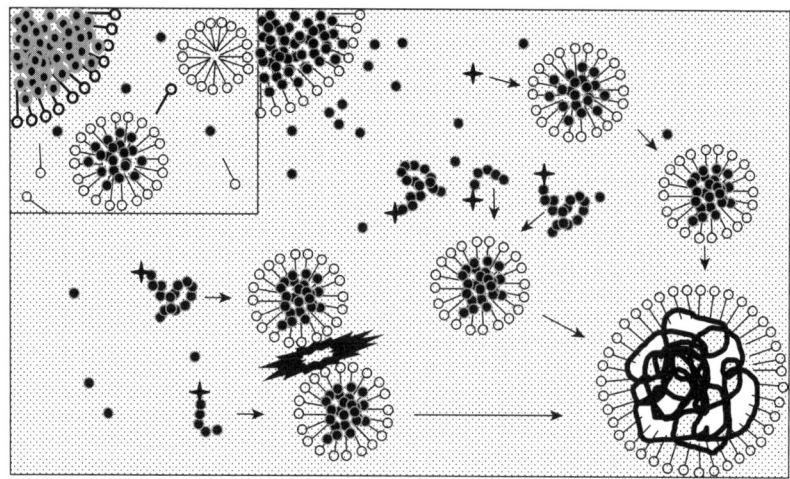

Figure 3.10 Preparation of latex (nanoparticles) through emulsion polymerisation. Insert: in the absence of initiator, equilibrium between monomer droplets, monomer in solution, and micelles of surfactant with or without monomer. Main figure: after initiation by the active species (star), distribution of monomer between the different forms, either solution, or micelles or particles.

of a hydrophobic compound are critical in the formulation of such polymerisation systems. The hydrophobic compound can be chosen from among transfer agents or initiators of polymerisation therefore being active in the polymerisation process, but its principal role is to counterbalance the Laplace pressure of the droplets, responsible for fusion of droplets. This process can also be used to obtain composite or structured particles.

Micro-emulsion is another variant of emulsion polymerisation. Such emulsions are thermodynamically stable systems including swollen monomer micelles dispersed in a continuous phase. In general, they require fairly large concentrations of surfactants to be produced compared with the other dispersed polymerisation systems. Hence, the interfacial tension of the oil/water is generally close to zero. Polymers with ultra-high molecular weight, i.e. above 10^7 g/mol, can be obtained, as can copolymers with a very well-defined, homogenous composition. Whereas polymerisation can take 24–48 h in the normal emulsion process, it proceeds at a fast rate in micro-emulsion, as total conversion can be obtained in less than 30 min. Polymer particles of very small size (diameter < 100 nm) and narrow distribution can be obtained by this process.

Recovery of solid polymer can be obtained by coagulation of the latex. As the size of the particles is submicronic, recovery by filtration without precipitation is not possible. Separation without precipitation cannot be obtained by usual centrifugation but requires ultracentrifugation. The emulsion polymerisation process is very well adapted for production of large amounts of polymeric colloids used in the paint industry by polymerisation of acrylic and methacrylic monomers, i.e. acrylic paints. Similarly, poly(alkylcyanoacrylate) nanoparticles can be obtained by such a process.

It is noteworthy that each particle is covered at the end of synthesis both by the hydrophilic fragment resulting from decomposition of the initiator, e.g. sulphate groups, and by the surfactant. Both entities participate in the stability of the colloidal suspension. Emulsion polymerisation of a hydrophobic monomer in aqueous medium is sometimes referred as oil-in-water (o/w), whereas emulsion polymerisation of a hydrophilic monomer, e.g. an acrylamide, in a non-polar organic solvent is referred to as inverse emulsion polymerisation or water-in-oil (w/o). More details about the use of nanospheres for drug delivery can be found in Section 4.4.6.

Interfacial polymerisation

Similarly to suspension and emulsion polymerisation, the system used in interfacial polymerisation is heterogeneous, but polymerisation takes place at the interface between both phases. Such a system can be easily illustrated in a practical laboratory course by reaction of a diamine soluble in an aqueous alkaline medium present in the upper part of a beaker, with a diacid chloride soluble in a non-miscible organic solvent such as chloroform present in the lower part of the beaker. A tiny film of polyamide is formed at the interface and can be recovered. Other polymers can be prepared by such a process, but the large amount of solvents that must be used and recovered limits its commercial utility for preparing large amounts of polymers.

However, this is not the case when considering the encapsulation of drugs, proteins, nucleotides and even cells for biotechnology. More details about the use of nanocapsules for drug delivery can be found in Section 4.4.6.

3.8 Copolymerisation

Despite the fact that many polymers obtained by step polymerisation are real alternate copolymers, most copolymers are prepared by chain polymerisation. Chain copolymerisation is very important from a technological point of view, as it increases the possibility of preparing polymers endowed with properties that cannot be obtained with homopolymers. In addition, as the probability of obtaining significant cohesive properties by mixing polymers to prepare blends or alloys is very low, copolymerisation can provide covalent binding between separated phases. Random or alternating copolymers can usually be obtained by a classical radical chain polymerisation in a single step, while preparation of block and graft copolymers usually needs at least two steps.

3.8.1 Random and alternate radical copolymerisation

When two monomers A and B are mixed and radical polymerisation is initiated, four propagation reactions are possible:

$$—A^{\bullet} + A \rightarrow —AA^{\bullet} \text{ rate constant } k_{AA}$$
$$—A^{\bullet} + B \rightarrow —AB^{\bullet} \text{ rate constant } k_{AB}$$
$$—B^{\bullet} + A \rightarrow —BA^{\bullet} \text{ rate constant } k_{BA}$$
$$—B^{\bullet} + B \rightarrow —BB^{\bullet} \text{ rate constant } k_{BB}$$

Thus, composition of the copolymers depends on the reactivity of monomers A and B with the reactive centres and on the composition of the monomer mixture, which can vary with conversion.

Reactivity ratios can be defined as follows: $r_A = k_{AA}/k_{AB}$ and $r_B = k_{BB}/k_{BA}$.

Simple cases: $r_A = r_B$

When $r_A = r_B$, the composition of both the mixture of monomers and the copolymer does not depend on conversion.

When $r_A = r_B = 1$, this means that A or B has a similar reactivity towards $—A^{\bullet}$ and $—B^{\bullet}$. As a result, instant composition of the copolymer is ideally random.

When $r_A = r_B < 0.01$, this means that the reactivity of A on $—B^{\bullet}$ is far higher than on $—A^{\bullet}$, and the reactivity of B on $—A^{\bullet}$ is far higher than on $—B^{\bullet}$. The resulting copolymer is strongly alternate.

When $r_A = r_B > > 1$, the copolymer tends to contain blocks, and the limit is simultaneous homopolymerisation of both monomers, but this case is very uncommon.

General case: r_A and r_B are different from each other

Let us consider that monomer A is bound faster than B to active centres. The result is that the concentration of A in the monomer mixture decreases when conversion increases. Consequently, the composition of copolymers formed at the beginning and at the end of conversion is very different when nothing is done to compensate for the preferential consumption. From an industrial point of view, such heterogeneity in the composition of a batch of copolymer can be a real drawback.

Copolymerisation is not limited to mixtures of two monomers, and the simultaneous polymerisation of three monomers, or terpolymerisation, is commercially used to further improve properties of copolymers. Quantitative treatment of nine propagation reactions is quite complex and beyond the scope of this book.

3.8.2   Synthesis of block and graft copolymers

Synthesis of block copolymers with well-defined structure has received considerable attention, as their properties are potentially of great interest (see Section 4.1). Until recently, the possibilities were limited to the use of either sequential addition of monomers in 'living' anionic polymerisation systems, or coupling of polymers possessing reactive ends, e.g. telechelic polymers. Advances in radical controlled polymerisation have opened new perspectives.

Graft copolymers contain a long sequence composed of one polymer, i.e. the backbone, with branches or grafted sequences composed of another polymer. Different methods, such as radical chain transfer, irradiation, redox initiation and ionic initiations, have been used to induce grafting on to different backbones such as cellulose in order to modify their properties.

3.9   Modifications of polymers

A large number of polymers cannot be obtained by polymerisation of monomers but are obtained by chemical modification of polymers from either natural or synthetic origin. The first objects manufactured from polymers were obtained from chemically modified natural polymers. The chemical modifications are usually performed through classical reactions of organic chemistry, such as esterification, hydrolysis or etherification. However, the reactivity of chemical groups linked to polymers is not similar to the reactivity of the same groups present in small molecules, as the distance between polymer-linked

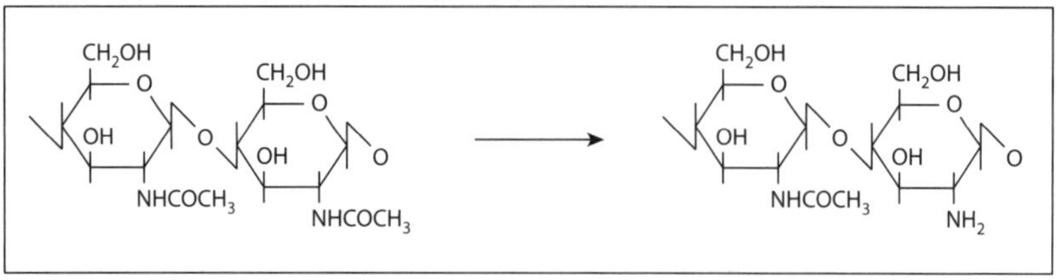

Figure 3.11 Repeating units in chitin and chitosan (partly de-acetylated chitin).

groups cannot be changed, resulting in 'neighbouring' effects. Moreover, physical characteristics of polymers, such as crystallinity and hydrophobicity, have a strong influence on the reactivity of polymer-linked groups.

Polysaccharides are natural polymers that are highly diverse and used widely as they are or after modification in the biomedical and pharmaceutical fields. Among the polysaccharides, cellulose is the most abundant, as it represents about one-third of all plant matter. Cellulose fibres have been used for centuries without major modification, but for many uses cellulose has been chemically modified to be easily manufactured. Chitin, the major constituent of crab shells, is probably the second most abundant polysaccharide. Before being used, chitin has to be de-acetylated, resulting in chitosan, as shown in Figure 3.11. Chitin de-acetylated over 70% is water-soluble.

3.9.1 Modifications of cellulose and other polysaccharides

Cellulose and dextran, shown in Figure 3.12, are natural polymers of glucose. Their molecular weights can be very high, up to $1–2 \times 10^6$ g/mol. Dextran, in which the glucose units are linked by $(1{\rightarrow}6)$ linkages, is water-soluble. Despite the high hydrophilicity of cellulose, which can retain 70% of its weight in water, cellulose is not water-soluble. The structure of cellulose is very regular and the β-$(1{\rightarrow}4)$ linkages are rigid. Thus, formation of a large number of strong hydrogen bonds between chains is possible. This results in a high crystallinity, insolubility and strong cohesive properties; in addition,

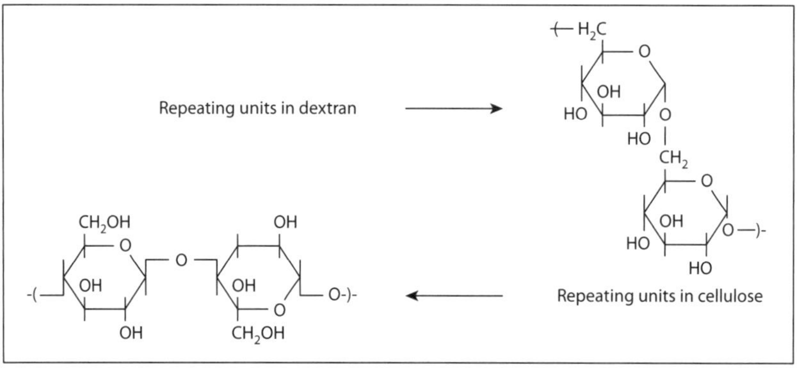

Figure 3.12 Repeating units in some natural polymers of glucose, i.e. dextran and cellulose.

when heated, cellulose decomposes without flowing or melting. The OH groups of cellulose are poorly accessible and not very reactive.

These properties impair the use of native cellulose in the manufacture of useful products, except those made of threads. Modifications of cellulose usually require the cellulose to be solubilised. In the viscose process, cellulose is treated with 18–20% aqueous sodium hydroxide. The mass is aged to allow oxidative degradation of the chains in order to reduce molecular weight. Then the alkali cellulose is treated with carbon disulfide, leading to the soluble sodium xanthate derivative of cellulose, as shown in Equation 3.23.

$$\text{Cell-OH} + \text{NaOH} \rightarrow \text{Cell-ONa (partly)}$$
$$\text{Cell-ONa} + \text{CS}_2 \rightarrow \text{Cell-OCS}_2\text{Na (xanthate)}$$

$$(3.23)$$

Coagulation of xanthate is performed in 10% aqueous sulphuric acid. The xanthic acid derivative that is formed is not stable and is decomposed, and cellulose is regenerated. Viscose rayon fibres and cellophane films have been produced by this method.

Regenerated cellulose films and hollow fibres used in haemodialysers have been prepared by a method known as the cuprammonium process. Cellulose is dissolved in a solution of ammonia and cupric oxide. The complex cupric salts are water-soluble and cellulose is regenerated by treatment with acid. Cuprophan® is prepared by this process.

Many cellulose esters have been developed. They include acetates, acetopropionates, acetobutyrates and nitrates. As the crystallinity of cellulose is suppressed by such substitutions, the esters are thermoplastic and can be manufactured by usual methods, e.g. extrusion or moulding. Properties of these compounds depend on the type of substituent and on the degree of substitution. Cellulose nitrates were the first modified polymers. Depending on the degree of substitution, different applications have been developed: Highly nitrated cellulose is a well-known explosive, whereas a little less substituted cellulose is used as solid fuel for rockets and the least substituted cellulose is a thermoplastic called celluloid. Celluloid was used to make films for early movies and moulded objects, e.g. dolls and table tennis balls. However, as celluloid is highly flammable, other esters have almost completely replaced cellulose nitrates for manufacturing everyday objects.

Cellulose acetates are now the most important derivatives and are obtained by reaction of acetic anhydride on cellulose. As this reaction occurs in a heterogeneous system, some chains are completely substituted, even at the beginning of the reaction, whereas others are not substituted at all. Thus, the triacetate is first prepared and less acetylated derivatives are prepared by controlled hydrolysis of the triacetate. Cellulose acetates are used widely in everyday life. In the biomedical field, partially acetylated cellulose is used as a constituent of haemodialysis membranes (see Section 4.3.6). In pharmaceutical technology, the mixed esters are used as excipients for the oral route (see Section 4.4).

Cellulose ethers, e.g. the methyl, carboxymethyl and diethylaminoethyl (DEAE) ethers, are prepared by successive reactions with concentrated aqueous sodium hydroxide and then with the halide derivative, as shown in Equation 3.24.

$$\text{Cell-OH} + \text{NaOH} \rightarrow \text{Cell-ONa (partly)} \qquad (3.24a)$$

$$\text{Cell-ONa} + \text{ClCH}_2\text{COONa} \rightarrow \text{Cell-O-CH}_2\text{COONa} \qquad (3.24b)$$

$$\text{Cell-ONa} + \text{ClCH}_2\text{CH}_2\text{N}(\text{C}_2\text{H}_5)_2 \rightarrow \text{Cell-O-CH}_2\text{CH}_2\text{N}(\text{C}_2\text{H}_5)_2 \qquad (3.24c)$$

Cellulose ethers have found many applications in industry, including the pharmaceutical industry. Cellulose membranes partially substituted with DEAE groups, Hemophan®, have been used in haemodialysis devices.

Many graft copolymers can be obtained by creating active radical centres capable of initiating polymerisation of vinylic or acrylic monomers on the cellulose backbone. The properties of cellulose are completely modified by the presence of these grafted chains.

All of these modifications can be applied to other polysaccharides and to hydroxyl-bearing polymers.

3.9.2 Modifications of poly(vinyl acetate)

As the monomer vinyl alcohol does not exist, because it is not stable, poly-(vinyl alcohol) can be prepared from poly(vinyl acetate), for instance by transesterification in methanol, as shown in Equation 3.25.

$$\text{-(-CH}_2 - \text{CH-)-} \; + \text{CH}_3\text{OH} \quad \rightarrow \quad \text{-(-CH}_2 - \text{CH-)-} \; + \text{CH}_3\text{OCOCH}_3$$
$$\mkern30mu | \mkern180mu |$$
$$\text{O} - \text{COCH}_3 \mkern110mu \text{OH}$$

$$(3.25)$$

Poly(vinyl formal) and poly(vinyl butyral) are prepared by reaction of poly-(vinyl alcohol) with the corresponding aldehydes, as shown in Equation 3.26.

$$\text{-(-CH}_2 - \overset{\displaystyle \text{CH}_2}{\overset{\displaystyle /\;\;\;\backslash}{\text{CH} - \text{CH-)-}}} + \text{H}_2\text{C}=\text{O} \quad \rightarrow \quad \text{-(-CH}_2 - \overset{\displaystyle \text{CH}_2}{\overset{\displaystyle /\;\;\;\backslash}{\text{CH} - \text{CH-)-}}} + \text{H}_2\text{O}$$

$$(3.26)$$

Bibliography

General

Allen G, Bevington JC, eds (1989). *Comprehensive Polymer Science*. London: Pergamon Press.
Brandrup J, Immergut JH, Grulke EA, eds (1999). *Polymer Handbook*, 4th edn. New York: John Wiley & Sons.

Synthesis, methods and processes

Braun D, Cherdron H, Rehahn M, Ritter H, Voit B (2005). *Polymer Synthesis: Theory and Practice, Fundamentals, Methods, Experiments*, 4th edn. Berlin, New York: Springer.
Candau F, Pabon M, Anquetil JY (1999). Polymerizable microemulsions: some criteria to achieve an optimal formulation. *Colloids Surf A Physicochem Eng Asp* 153: 47–59.
Landfester K (2001). Polyreactions in miniemulsions. *Macromol Rapid Commun* 22: 896–936.
Mecking S (2007). Polymer dispersions from catalytic polymerisation in aqueous systems. *Colloid Polym Sci* 285: 605–619.
Odian G (2004). *Principles of Polymerization*, 4th edn. Hoboken, NJ: Wiley-Interscience.
Pichot C, Daniel JC, eds (2006). *Latex Synthétiques: Elaboration-Propriétés-Applications*. Paris: Lavoisier.

4

Special properties of polymers, case studies and detailed examples of applications

4.1   Properties of block copolymers: phase separation in solution and at solid state

Homopolymers are usually not miscible; hence, blending homopolymers generally leads to phase-separated large domains. As there are only weak interactions between phases, such systems are weakly cohesive. In block copolymers, blocks are also phase-separated but they are linked together by covalent bonds. Thus, solutions and solids composed of such systems possess special properties owing to the presence of the linkages between blocks. The organisation of the micro-domains formed by block copolymers and properties in solutions and in the solid state depend on the composition, structure, molecular weight and properties of the blocks. A few examples of their properties are presented below.

4.1.1   Solution properties

Block copolymers composed of two or three hydrophilic and hydrophobic blocks possess amphiphilic properties and are used widely as non-ionic surfactants. Poloxamers are triblock copolymers polyoxyethylene–polyoxypropylene–polyoxyethylene (PEO–PPO–PEO), commercially known

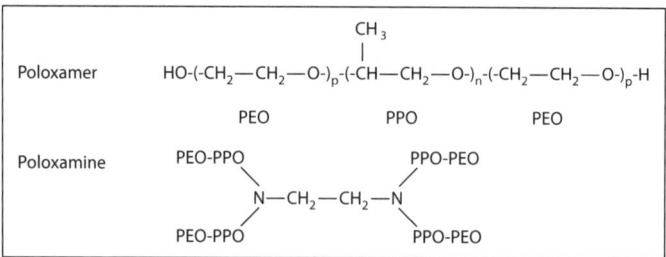

Figure 4.1 Repeating units in poloxamers and poloxamines.

as Pluronics®. Poloxamines, commercially known as Tetronic®, are composed of a central unit of ethylenediamine, denoted Y, on which four arms of PPO–PEO are linked [Y(PPO$_n$–PEO$_p$)$_4$], as shown in Figure 4.1.

Synthesis of poloxamers begins with creation of the hydrophobic block by addition of propylene oxide to propylene glycol. Then the hydrophilic blocks are added by polymerisation of ethylene oxide, as shown in Equation 4.1.

$$HO-CH-CH_2-OH + nCH-CH_2$$

with CH_3 on the first and second CH, and $\diagdown O \diagup$

$$\rightarrow HO\text{-}(\text{-}CH-CH_2-O\text{-})_{n+1}\text{-}H$$

with CH_3

$$+\ 2p\ CH_2-CH_2$$

with $\diagdown O \diagup$

$$\rightarrow HO\text{-}(\text{-}CH_2-CH_2-O\text{-})_p\text{-}(CH-CH_2-O\text{-})_{n+1}\text{-}(CH_2-CH_2-O\text{-})_p\text{-}H$$

with CH_3

$$(4.1)$$

The total molecular weight of poloxamers can vary from 1000 g/mol to 16 000 g/mol, and the hydrophilic segment can comprise between 15% and 90% of the molecule. Box 4.1 describes the code names of poloxamers.

When poloxamers are introduced into water at a low concentration, the soluble species are only isolated hydrated molecules. When the concentration of a copolymer is increased at constant temperature above the critical micelle concentration (CMC), micelles composed of several molecules are formed. In aqueous medium, such micelles are endowed with a core-shell structure composed of a hydrophobic core and a hydrophilic shell. The equilibrium is illustrated in Figure 4.2.

CMC depends on the copolymer, the solvent and the temperature. Unexpectedly, solubility is greater in cold than in warm water. Hydrogen bonds are formed between the oxygen atoms of the macromolecule and

> **Box 4.1**
>
> Composition of the poloxamer molecule is indicated by the code name. The approximate molecular weight of the hydrophobic segment is given by the first two digits of the poloxamer number, multiplied by 100. The approximate percentage of polyoxyethylene (PEO) of the final molecular weight is given by the last digit, multiplied by 10. Some confusion can arise from the fact that the code names of poloxamers and Pluronics® are different. In Pluronics, the physical state is indicated by the associated capital letter.
>
> As an example, poloxamer 407 (Pluronic F127) is a solid derived from a 4000 PPO, comprising around 70% of PEO in the final molecular weight, which is around 12 000; poloxamer 407 is water-soluble.

surrounding water. When the temperature increases, some of these bonds are broken, decreasing the solubility. This effect, together with micelle formation, can result in reversible gelation. For instance, aqueous poloxamer 407 solutions are liquid below 25 °C and can jellify at higher temperatures at a concentration of at least 20%. This phenomenon is even more marked when the polymolecularity of the poloxamer is reduced.

At a constant temperature in aqueous medium, CMC decreases when the length of the hydrophobic chain increases and can become very low. For this reason, nanoparticles are formed readily in aqueous medium from block copolymers possessing fairly long hydrophobic chains. Such large block copolymers can be considered as polymeric surfactants.

Toxicological studies have shown that low-molecular-weight poloxamers are only slightly toxic, whereas those with a high molecular weight can be considered non-toxic. These results allow the use of poloxamers in contact with living tissues. They have been used as additives in contact lenses, artificial tears and ophthalmic drug solutions. For instance, poloxamer 407 has been proposed to increase the efficacy of drugs by increasing the duration of contact with the cornea. A poloxamer 407 of low polymolecularity has been developed

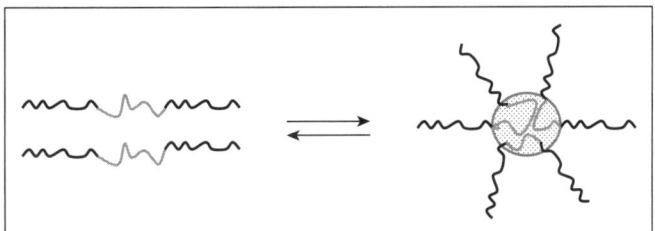

Figure 4.2 Equilibrium between free molecules and micelles above the critical micelle concentration (CMC).

that permits temporary embolisation of a blood vessel without clamping. A cold solution of this poloxamer is injected in the liquid state into the vessel. At body temperature, the vessel is embolised by instant gelation of poloxamer solution. After surgery, gelation is reversed by local cooling, resulting in reopening of the vessel and solubilisation of the poloxamer into the blood.

4.1.2 Block copolymers in phase-separated materials

Because of their unique properties, block copolymers are increasingly used commercially, either as materials themselves or as additives in polymeric alloys. The most developed systems have been copolymers composed of two or three monomer units with two or three blocks. In the solid state, block copolymers are phase-separated, and hence they can be considered as solid emulsions. The different types of structure of the materials and the resulting properties depend on both the structure and the composition of copolymer, as exemplified in the case of biblock (SB) and triblock (SBS) copolymers of styrene and butadiene, illustrated in Figure 4.3.

When the percentage of polystyrene is below 15% of the total volume, spherical nodules of polystyrene are dispersed in the matrix of polybutadiene. The larger the molecular weights, the larger the nodules. When the percentage of polystyrene is between 15% and 33%, cylinders of polystyrene are dispersed in the matrix of polybutadiene. The structure of the material is lamellar when the percentage of polystyrene is between 33% and 66%. When the percentage of polystyrene is increased further, the dispersed phase is composed of polybutadiene in a matrix of polystyrene.

The mechanical properties of the materials composed of the biblock and triblock copolymers are different, as shown schematically in Figure 4.4.

Indeed, in the case of a biblock containing a high percentage of polybutadiene, the nodules of polystyrene are completely independent. The stress/strain response of the material made of such a copolymer is similar to the response of polybutadiene, i.e. a non-vulcanised elastomer, which does not recover its initial length after elongation. In the case of a triblock SBS of

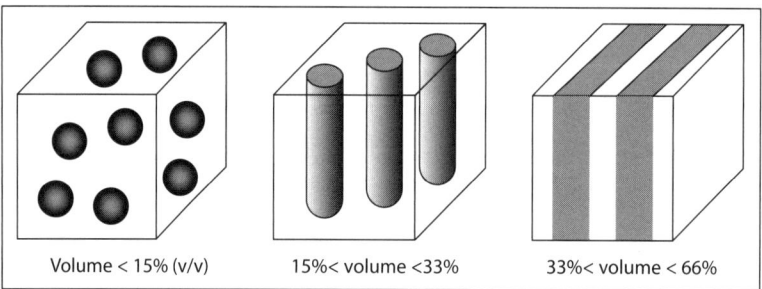

Figure 4.3 Structural organisation of solid block copolymers poly(styrene)-poly(butadiene) as a function of composition.

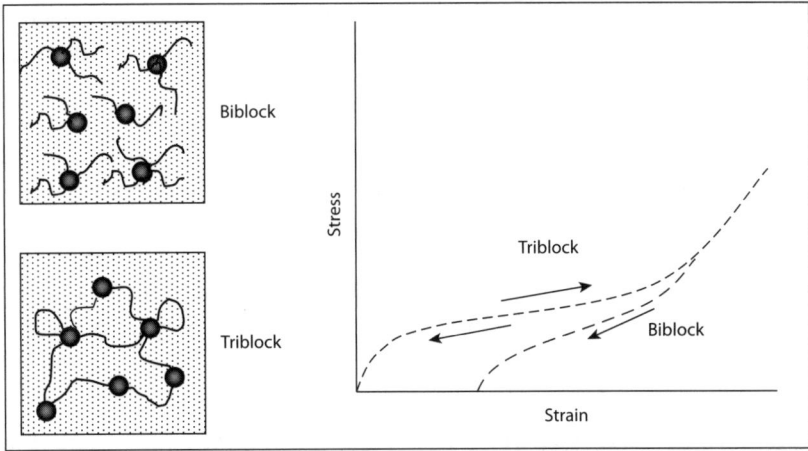

Figure 4.4   Structural organisation and stress/strain behaviour of biblock and triblock copolymers of styrene and butadiene of similar composition.

similar composition, however, polybutadiene chains can act as links between nodules composed of polystyrene, generating physical cross-linking. The stress/strain response is the response of a vulcanised rubber, which recovers its initial length after elongation.

The main advantage of such triblock copolymers is that they can be moulded and recycled simply by heating the material above the glass transition temperature of polystyrene, unlike classical vulcanised rubbers, which cannot be reused without degradation as they are chemically cross-linked. Such SBS-based materials are called thermoplastic elastomers. However, for various reasons, including cost, the commercial use of such polymers is rather limited compared with the use of natural and classical synthetic rubbers.

This is not the case for copolymers containing a majority of styrene units (high-impact polystyrene) and for terpolymers composed of acrylonitrile, butadiene and styrene (ABS), which are used widely as shock absorbers. The latter is a cohesive polymeric alloy stabilised by distribution of the different chains between phases.

This example shows that block copolymers can act as polymeric surfactants to stabilise polymeric mixtures of homopolymers, providing that the constituents of the blocks are similar to those constituting the homopolymers.

4.2   Biodegradable and bioerodible polymers

Biodegradable polymers were developed originally for biomedical and pharmaceutical uses. The aim was to obtain materials for temporary or repeated use and that degraded in vivo with a controlled rate into non-toxic products that could be eliminated through natural ways. For such uses, only small amounts of high-grade polymers were required, and the initial high cost of such polymers was a small issue when compared with the expected properties. Then biodegradable polymers were developed in order to solve environmental concerns, e.g. to avoid non-degradable polymer-based wastes polluting the landscape. In this case, the aim was to obtain materials for general uses, such as packaging and agriculture, and that degraded outside. Unlike for biomedical uses, large amounts of technical-grade polymers and low cost were required.

This chapter focuses on biodegradable polymers used in the health domain. Some examples of biodegradable and bioerodible polymers are presented in Table 4.1, and some of their thermomechanical properties are given in Table 4.2.

Table 4.1 Some biodegradable and bioerodible polymers

Name	Abbreviation	Repeating unit	Polymerisation
Poly(glycolide) or poly(glycolic acid)	PGA	-(-O-CH$_2$-CO-)-	Synthetic
Poly(lactides) or poly(lactic acids)	PLA	-(-O-*CH-CO-)- $\mid$ CH$_3$	Synthetic
Poly(3-hydroxybutyrate)	P3HB	-(-O-*CH-CH$_2$-CO-)- $\mid$ CH$_3$	Biosynthetic
Poly(3-hydroxyvalerate)	P3HV	-(-O-*CH-CH$_2$-CO-)- $\mid$ C$_2$H$_5$	Biosynthetic
Poly(4-hydroxybutyrate)	P4HB	-(-O-CH$_2$-CH$_2$-CH$_2$-CO-)-	Biosynthetic
Poly(malic acids)	PMA	-(-O-*CH-CH$_2$-CO-)- $\mid$ COOH	Synthetic
Poly(ε-caprolactone)	PCL	-[-O-(CH$_2$-)$_5$-CO-]-	Synthetic
Poly(sebacic acid)	PSA	-[-O-CO-(CH$_2$)$_8$-CO-]-	Synthetic
Poly[1,3-bis(p-carboxy-phenoxy) propane]	PCPP	-[-O-CO-φ-O-(CH$_2$)$_3$-O-φ-CO-]-	Synthetic
Poly(butylcyanoacrylate)	PBCA	C$\equiv$N $\mid$ -(-CH$_2$—C-)$_n$- $\mid$ COOC$_4$H$_9$	Synthetic

Table 4.2 Thermomechanical properties of some biodegradable polymers

Polymer	T_g (°C)	T_m (°C)	Modulus (GPa)
PGA	35	225	6.5
PGA (fibres)	–	233	13.4
PLA50	55	a*	2–3.6
PLLA	60	180	2.1
PLLA (fibres)	60	187	8.5–10.4
PCL	−60	55	0.3
P3HB	1	171	2.5
PHB-co-PHV	−5/−1	137–160	0.6–1.4

a* = amorphous.

Designing a true biodegradable polymer is theoretically simple. This can be obtained by introducing into the main chain of the polymer a type of bond that can be cleaved in vivo. Depending on the requirements concerning the site of degradation, such bonds can be sensitive to non-specific hydrolysis, e.g. esters or anhydrides, or to a specific enzymatic cleavage, e.g. peptide bonds. A controlled decrease of molecular weight with time and production of small molecules that are easy to eliminate are expected.

Polyglycolide or poly(glycolic acid) (PGA) wires were proposed under the trade names Dexon® and Ercedex® in the 1960s to replace 'catgut' used for deep sutures. Then polylactides (PLA), also known as poly(lactic acid)s, and copolymers of lactides and glycolide (PLGA) were developed for different fibre-based devices under the trade names Vicryl® and Glactine910®.

As shown in Section 3.6.1, synthesis of these polymers starts from lactides and glycolide, which are dilactones resulting from cyclisation of the hydroxy-acids by dehydration. As an asymmetric carbon is present in lactic acid, two asymmetric carbons are present in lactides. Thus, when starting from the natural L-lactic acid, only one L,L-lactide is expected, whereas three different lactides, L,L-, D,D- and D,L-, are obtained from the synthetic lactic acid (see Figure 3.6). Ring-opening polymerisation of L,L-lactide in non-racemising conditions, for instance by using tin octanoate as the initiator, leads to poly-(L,L-lactide) (PLLA), whereas poly(D,L-lactide) (PLA50 or racemic PLA) is obtained from the racemic mixture of lactides.

Catgut has now been completely replaced by PLA and PLGA wires and meshes, which are degraded at a controlled and reproducible rate. Copolymers of different compositions have found their use in different domains, such as sutures, bone surgery, tissue reconstruction and drug-delivery systems, depending on their thermomechanical properties and

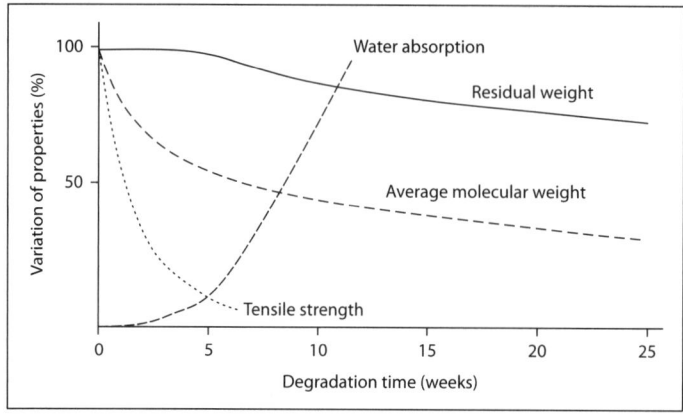

Figure 4.5 Degradation of poly(L,L-lactide) (PLLA) in aqueous medium: variation of several parameters with time.

degradation rate. Another important property that makes such polymers attractive is the fact that they are expected to form final endogenous degradation products that can be metabolised, resulting in water and carbon dioxide. Finally, possible immune responses that may occur when using materials from natural origin are not encountered with PLGA owing to its synthetic nature.

PLA and PLGA have been studied extensively as materials for sutures and later as a basis for polymeric drug carrier systems as micro- and nanoparticles (see Section 4.4.6). To evidence the rate of degradation of PLA, measurements of different parameters have been proposed. It can be seen in the example presented in Figure 4.5 that the weight loss of the material is not very sensitive to degradation. Conversely, degradation is rapidly evidenced by a decrease in the average molecular weight of the polymer and a drop in the mechanical properties of the material.

Crystallinity and water uptake have been shown to be key factors in determining the rate of degradation. As PLLA is the most crystalline and hydrophobic among polylactides, its rate of degradation is the slowest. PLA50 prepared from racemic lactide is also hydrophobic, but it is more amorphous than PLLA and is degraded at a faster rate. However, degradation proceeds faster in amorphous than in crystalline domains of the material. Consequently, the crystallinity of PLA50 increases with degradation, modulating the rate. Finally, degradation of PLGA cannot be extrapolated from degradations of pure PGA and PLAs, as glycolic units are more hydrophilic than lactic units, but more crystalline. Degradation rate of PLGA is maximal for a 50/50 composition of lactic and glycolic units.

The degradation rate also depends on the conditions of preparation of the material, such as quenching and annealing, as such processes can change the crystallinity. Concerning other parameters that are extrinsic to the polymer itself, it has been demonstrated clearly that degradation of PLGA does not depend normally on enzymatic activity. However, degradation is faster in the presence of bacteria in infected tissues. Many other factors can influence the degradation rate, including sterilisation processing, storage conditions, external physicochemical parameters in the environment of the material, e.g. pH, ionic strength, applied stress, and adsorption and absorption of different compounds (e.g. solvents, proteins, lipids).

When polylactides were proposed for use in larger devices such as bio-degradable screws and plates for the temporary internal fixation of bone fractures, attention was drawn to some unexpected features concerning the degradation mechanism. It was shown that the size of the object made from polylactides was an important parameter in the degradation, as explained below. Degradation occurs through hydrolysis, and the final product is lactic acid. However, two initial different mechanisms are possible, according to Equation 4.2 concerning PGA.

$$HO\text{-}CH_2\text{-}CO\text{-}(\text{-}O\text{-}CH_2\text{-}CO\text{-})_n\text{-}O\text{-}CH_2\text{-}COOH + H_2O \quad \rightarrow$$

- either $\quad HO\text{-}CH_2\text{-}CO\text{-}(\text{-}O\text{-}CH_2\text{-}CO\text{-})_{n-1}\text{-}O\text{-}CH_2\text{-}COOH$

$+ HO\text{-}CH_2\text{-}COOH$

$$(4.2)$$

- or $\quad HO\text{-}CH_2\text{-}CO\text{-}(\text{-}O\text{-}CH_2\text{-}CO\text{-})_p\text{-}O\text{-}CH_2\text{-}COOH$

$+ HO\text{-}CH_2\text{-}CO\text{-}(\text{-}O\text{-}CH_2\text{-}CO\text{-})_m\text{-}O\text{-}CH_2\text{-}COOH$

(with $m + p = n$).

In other words, scission is susceptible to occur at the end of the chain, resulting in the production of one molecule of glycolic acid and one chain of polymer just short of one repeating unit. Scission can also occur randomly in the chain, resulting in the production of two shorter polymeric chains. By measuring the average molecular weight of the degradation products, it was shown that the real mechanism is the random one.

Concerning the degradation of objects made of PLA, it was expected that the degradation rate would be faster at the surface and independent of the size of the object. However, it was demonstrated that degradation depended on the size of the object and proceeded faster in the bulk than at the surface. This unexpected phenomenon resulted from a fast accumulation of degraded poly-meric and oligomeric chains inside the object. Degradation started from the surface in the aqueous medium surrounding the object, but water absorption into the bulk of the material was fairly fast (see Figure 4.5). Thus, degradation took place also in the bulk. At each step of hydrolysis, one carboxylic group was generated and such groups were able to act as catalysts of hydrolysis. The shorter polymeric chains and the oligomers that were generated at the surface of the material were eliminated in the surrounding aqueous medium. Such species generated in the bulk of the material could not diffuse easily in the

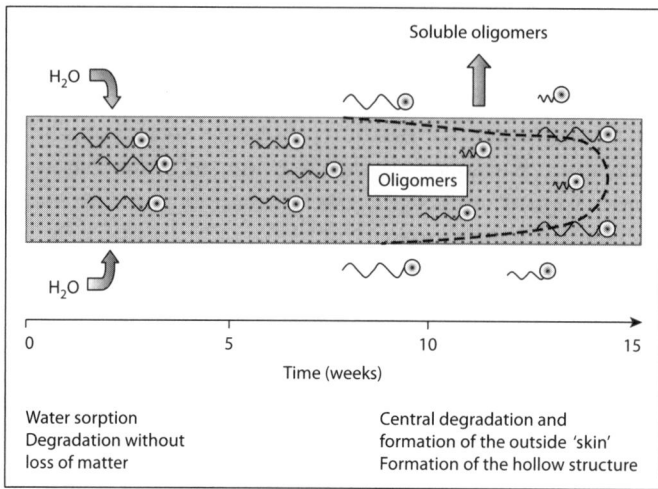

Figure 4.6 Degradation of a large object made of poly(L-L-lactide) (PLLA) by formation of oligomers terminated by a carboxylic group.

polymeric network and remained inside. Owing to the increasing production of carboxylic groups, which were able to catalyse hydrolysis, the rate of degradation was faster in the bulk than at the surface. A hollow structure with an outside 'skin' filled with a honey-like matter was progressively formed, as illustrated in Figure 4.6.

Rupture of the skin resulted in liberation of large amounts of degradation products. As the in vivo elimination rate was surpassed, degradation products were concentrated in the surrounding tissues, resulting in an inopportune inflammatory reaction.

For many reasons, new biodegradable polymers were needed and developed following the PLGA family. Poly(ε-caprolactone) (PCL), which is also obtained by ring-opening polymerisation, has the advantage of being softer than PLGA, as its glass transition is well below room temperature; its degradation rate is also slower. Thermomechanical and degradation properties can be modulated by copolymerisation, increasing the possibility of uses of such synthetic biodegradable polyesters.

Polyhydroxyalkanoates (PHA), shown in Table 4.1, are naturally occurring polyesters produced by microorganisms. Poly(β-hydroxyacids) such as poly(3-hydroxybutyrate) (P3HB) and its copolymers with 3-hydroxyvalerate [poly(3HB-co-3HV)] were isolated a long time ago. They were developed in the 1980s by ICI under the trade name Biopol® for replacing non-biodegradable plastics. Several PHAs are now commercially available and were investigated for biomedical and drug delivery applications. Their degradation rate is generally slower and more gradual than degradation of PLGA. The degradation rate depends on the structure of the polymers and on the sterilisation process. Because of their bacterial origin, their in vivo use in humans has been questioned, but development of purification processes and careful sterilisation has made their use possible.

From a chemical point of view, all of the polyesters presented above have a maximum of two reactive groups per chain, i.e. one at each chain end, which can be modified. Poly(malic acid) and its substituted derivatives were proposed to circumvent this lack of reactive groups. As each repeating unit bears one carboxylic group, it can be modified through many types of reaction. When carboxylic groups are not protected, degradation of the unprotected polymer is expected to be very fast, as carboxylic groups act as catalysts of hydrolysis. A large amount of work is currently being carried out with this family of biodegradable polymers.

Other types of biodegradable polymer such as poly(ortho esters), poly(organo phosphazenes) and polyanhydrides have been described. However, they have been less developed than polyesters.

Bioerodible polymers represent another possibility of obtaining polymers that can be eliminated through natural ways. Such polymers can be obtained by introducing into the lateral chains of a water-insoluble polymer a bond that can be cleaved in vivo, turning the hydrophobic polymer into a water-soluble polymer. Mainly ester bonds have been used. The main characteristic of bioerodible polymers is that the molecular weight remains almost constant during degradation, but solubility is dramatically changed. To avoid accumulation of the degradation products, it is expected that the production rate of the water-soluble polymer could be slower than its elimination rate.

The main family of bioerodible polymers is represented by poly(alkylcyanoacrylate)s (PACA). These polymers have a long history since 1947 as adhesives, especially in areas where a fast cure rate is needed. Polymerisation of alkylcyanoacrylates (ACA) can be initiated in the presence of bases as weak as the hydroxyl ions of water. The propagation rate decreases when the size of the lateral alkyl chain increases. As polymerisation can be very fast, ACAs have been used as surgical glue, as tissue adhesive and for embolisation purposes. As shown in Section 4.4.6, ACAs have also been used extensively for preparing nanospheres and nanocapsules for drug delivery.

Degradation of PACA has been much discussed with regard to possible in vivo toxicity. The main chain is not biodegradable, but hydrolytic degradation leading to production of formaldehyde and alkylcyanoacetate is possible, according to the inverse Knoevenagel reaction. This mechanism depends on the pH, temperature and type of PACA; however, the reaction is very slow in physiological conditions when compared with the hydrolysis of the lateral ester, which occurs faster in vivo. At physiological pH, the hydrolysis rate depends on the length of the alkyl chain and leads to production of water-soluble poly(cyanoacrylic acid) or its salts and to the corresponding alkyl alcohol, as shown in Equation 4.3 in the case of poly(butylcyanoacrylate).

$$
\begin{array}{ccc}
C \equiv N & & C \equiv N \\
| & & | \\
\text{-(-CH}_2\text{-C-)}_n\text{- + H}_2\text{O} \rightarrow & & \text{-(-CH}_2\text{-C-)}_n\text{- + HOC}_4\text{H}_9 \\
| & & | \\
COOC_4H_9 & & COOH
\end{array}
\tag{4.3}
$$

Hydrophobic polymer $\rightarrow$ water soluble polymer + alcohol

This degradation catalysed in vivo by various esterases proceeds at the surface, limiting the rate of production of degradation products. Toxicity could result from a rate of production exceeding the rate of elimination. As the shortest alkyl chain degrades the fastest, the alkyl chain of the monomers used in vivo is at least equal to or longer than a butyl.

4.3   Applications of polymers in biomedical uses

Polymers have been extensively used both as biomaterials, which are constituents of medical devices, and as constituents of drug-delivery systems. Many regulatory requirements must be met in order to use materials in the domain of human health. For instance, sterility is mandatory concerning materials in direct contact with living tissues in the absence of a barrier such as the intact skin. In addition, both polymers and devices have to be biocompatible, and their biocompatibility has to be evaluated by in vitro and in vivo tests.

However, the regulations differ depending on whether the polymer is a constituent of a medical device or part of a medication. If a drug is included in a medical device for an auxiliary action, then the regulations for medical devices are applicable. If the main action is linked to the presence of the drug, then regulations for medications are applicable.

The aim of this chapter is not to discuss regulatory affairs but to give a rationale for helping one choose the appropriate polymers for a given application. The choice of polymer or another material for making a device or drug-delivery system is directed by the function and the requirements. For instance, the requirement of either elimination or stability of the polymer in vivo is a prominent issue. Implanted devices that are supposed to remain functional as long as possible are made from biostable polymers. Injected drug-delivery systems that are administered several times are made from polymers that can be eliminated. In the following sections, some practical examples of existing applications are presented.

4.3.1   Processing and fabrication

In order to be transformed into items such as tubing, catheters and other medical devices, polymers have to be processed by different techniques, such

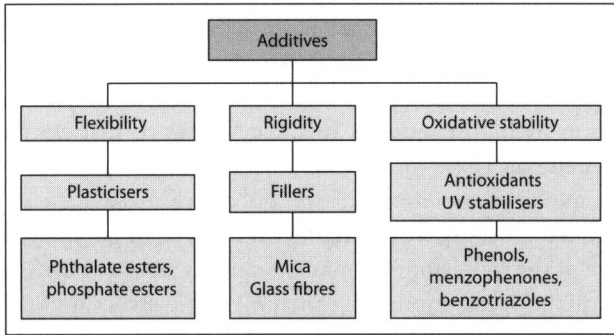

Figure 4.7 Schematic view of different additives used to modify the properties of polymers during processing.

as extrusion, moulding, spinning and dip-coating. To facilitate the processing and improve the properties, several additives are used, for instance to increase the stability of polymers during thermomechanical treatments and to modify their properties. A schematic view of additives used during processing is shown in Figure 4.7.

The addition of such products is important in the manufacture of useful items. However, most of these products are small molecules compared with the size of the polymers and therefore some are susceptible to migrating and inducing unwanted reactions in the surrounding living tissues, as explained later.

4.3.2 Sterilisation of polymers

Before contact with the living tissues of animals or humans, polymers and devices have to be sterilised. Even if fabrication is performed in a 'clean room', the materials and processing machinery are not sterile. In addition, it has been shown that some bacteria that are normally benign and easily eliminated by the body's defence systems become pathogenic and drug-resistant when present on the surface of devices.

Current sterilisation processes are generally not well adapted to polymers, except in the cases of water-soluble polymers and colloids, which can be sterilised by filtration in solution. The simplest process is autoclaving with steam at 120 °C for 20 min. This process can be detrimental to devices that include polymers with thermomechanical properties not compatible with the temperature used in the sterilisation process.

Sterilisation by ethylene oxide is very efficient, whatever the shape of the device, as this molecule is very small and reactive. Some drawbacks are linked to these qualities, however. Ethylene oxide can easily penetrate into polymeric networks, and it may react with chemical groups present in some polymers. In the first case, a sufficient degassing time in sterile conditions is necessary before the device is used in contact with living tissues. In the second case, modifications of the polymer, and especially of its surface, can occur and change the reactions of living tissues in contact with the device.

Sterilisation by high-energy beams, e.g. γ rays or fast electrons beams, is very efficient, as these beams are usually not stopped by materials. However, some covalent bonds of the polymeric network can be broken easily by such a high energy. Depending on the type of polymer and the dose and dose rate of the radiation, permanent chain scission or cross-linking can result from this process, modifying the polymeric structure and properties of the material.

Evaluating the mechanical and surface properties, toxicity and biocompatibility of polymers and devices before and after sterilisation is relevant in order to select for a given polymer or device a sterilisation process that is efficient against bacteria but is as benign as possible for the polymer, the device and the patient.

The drawbacks described above have emphasised the need for new sterilisation processes that are more compatible with polymers. However, these processes are still being evaluated for routine use.

4.3.3 Definition and concepts of biocompatibility

Biocompatibility was a vague concept until it was defined during a consensus conference organised in 1986 under the auspices of the European Society for Biomaterials at Chester as follows: 'The ability of a material to perform with an appropriate host response in a specific application.' This means that there is no 'intrinsically biocompatible' material. This precise definition excludes the common use of vague sentences such as 'The device is made from biocompatible materials', which sounds more like advertising copy than a scientific demonstration. The precise definition means that the animal model in which biocompatibility tests have been performed should be specified, as each animal species, including humans, has its own specificities. The application should be specified, as reactions of living tissues surrounding the material depend on many biological parameters and the type of material. A description of the local and systemic reactions should be provided as a function of time, as tissue responses also vary with this parameter.

Biocompatibility and toxicity

Biocompatibility is not equivalent to non-toxicity. Toxicity, either local or systemic, is related to cell death generally induced by soluble products, whereas biocompatibility is related more to the reactions of living tissues in contact with a solid material. Soluble products can be released by a material. Corrosion of metals and metallic alloys can produce multivalent ions, which are generally toxic. Multivalent ions used for in vivo imaging, e.g. in magnetic resonance imaging (MRI), are carefully chelated in order to avoid toxicity.

It can be deduced from their density that polymeric materials are not as compact as metallic materials. A polymeric material can be thought of as a sponge or a mass of cooked spaghetti, especially when the polymer is amorphous. For this reason, polymeric matrices can load and then release small molecules and can be used as drug-releasing systems. Polymeric materials may also release unwanted soluble products, such as degradation products, residues of monomers, solvents, additives, and ethylene oxide used for sterilisation purposes (see Section 4.3.2). Toxicity of the soluble products can result from lysis of the outer cell membrane, or diffusion into cell organites. Polycationic polymers, e.g. polylysine, either water-soluble or solid, can be considered as potentially toxic, because they are able to react readily with the negatively charged membrane of cells.

Evaluation of toxicity and biocompatibility is performed in graded test systems starting from general ones, i.e. in vitro. Toxicity is usually tested with cell lines growing in the presence of a sufficient amount of the material, and compared with negative and positive controls. Toxicity should be expressed by reference to the weight and surface area of the material. Toxicity of aqueous or lipidic extracts can also be evaluated. When possible, tests of toxicity should be performed with the sterilised material or device, as sterilisation processes can result in the generation of toxic products (see above). Tests of mutagenicity using relevant cells isolated or in living tissue explants in contact with the material can be performed.

When a permanent blood contact is involved in the application, in vitro tests such as measurements of haemolysis of erythrocytes or thrombogenicity induced by contact with the material are usually performed. Such tests are not necessary when permanent blood contact is not involved.

If the results of the in vitro tests are satisfactory, then in vivo tests in small animal models such as mice, rats, guinea pigs or rabbits are performed at different durations with a statistically significant number of animals, including controls. If these results are satisfactory, then the device is tested in large animal models relevant to the application, such as pigs or sheep. Finally, the device is tested in clinical trials. Different procedures for all these tests have been described and normalised.

A toxic material cannot be biocompatible, but contact of a non-toxic solid material with living tissues results inevitably in non-specific and sometimes specific tissue reactions. A schematic presentation of the reactions involved and of some proteins and cells cooperating in these reactions is shown in Figure 4.8.

In order to facilitate the understanding of reactions, two cases have been considered: either (i) there is no permanent contact with blood, expressed as 'tissue compatibility'; or (ii) the contact with blood is permanent, expressed as 'blood compatibility'.

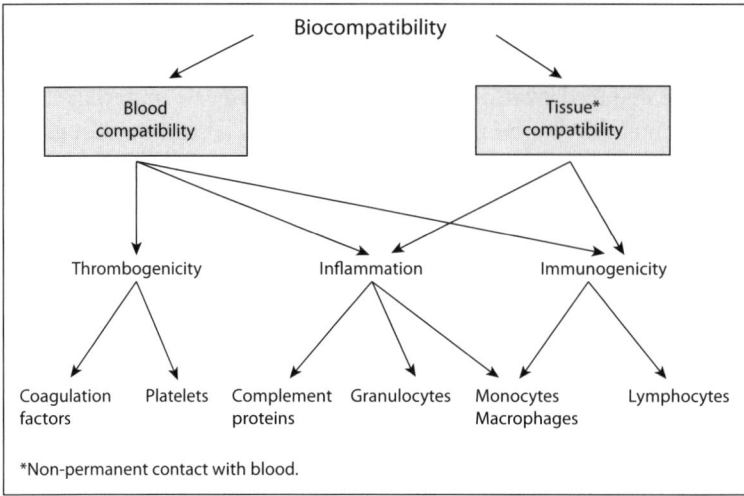

Figure 4.8 Schematic representation of possible reactions to contact between materials and some proteins and cells involved in the reactions. For the sake of simplicity, water and ions are not included.

Tissue compatibility

In this case, the reactions linked to the permanent presence of blood are excluded, even if a transient contact occurs during surgery. Two types of reaction can occur: inevitably inflammation and sometimes immunogenicity.

The unavoidable inflammatory response

Following the surgical trauma at the insertion of implanted materials, a non-specific tissue reaction inevitably occurs around the inserted material. The aim of the inflammatory reaction is to allow elimination of dead cell debris and further tissue repair. From the point of view of the inflammatory response, a material of optimal biocompatibility should neither add to the basic response in intensity and duration, nor prevent the tissue repair. All of these non-specific reactions occurring on the material's surface involve efficient cooperative processes between ions, proteins and cells.

Histologists have classified the inflammatory and healing processes as a function of the types of cell present around the implant. The **acute inflammatory phase**, normally lasting for a few days, is characterised by the presence of polymorphonuclear neutrophils (PMN). This phase is followed within 2 weeks by the **chronic inflammatory phase**, characterised by the presence of macrophages and lymphocytes. If the material is well tolerated, then this is followed by the **healing process**, characterised by the presence of fibroblasts and the growth of new capillaries, resulting in a thin capsule of fibrosis. If the material is not well tolerated, then inflammation is prolonged, with giant macrophagic cells and development of a thick capsule of fibrosis. Hence, it results that tissue compatibility of materials has to be evaluated at the different phases, for instance after 2–3 days, after 10–15 days and after 2–3 months of implantation.

The possible specific response

A specific immune response, i.e. a specific biological reaction to a substance regarded as non-self, is not usually involved during contact with synthetic materials. However, the use of materials from natural origin, such as proteins, polysaccharides, and natural rubber and its derivatives, may induce reactions with pre-existing antibodies or formation of antibodies of different classes against some typical epitopes displayed on the surface of the material.

Two examples of such reactions are given. The first is concerned with natural rubber. Natural rubber latex from *Hevea brasiliensis* has been used for a very long time and the rubber itself should not pose any danger to health. However, natural rubber particles are surrounded by a protective film composed mainly of lipids and proteins. The lipids are similar to the common lipids in the body, but the proteins are quite different and hence are recognised as foreign by the immune system. Frequent exposure to these foreign proteins may cause sensitisation in the user, leading to an allergic response. The rise in the prevalence of latex hypersensitivity in the 1980s was probably due to the increased production of gloves by inexperienced manufacturers, induced by an increased demand coupled to protection against viral problems.

The second example is concerned with regenerated cellulose haemodialysis membranes and is presented in Section 4.3.6.

As shown in the examples above, the presence of antigenic sites can be direct, resulting from the material itself, or from contaminations present on the surface. It can also be indirect, resulting from changes of conformation of proteins adsorbed on the material and becoming antigenic. Thus, immunogenicity of polymeric materials has to be considered as possible, even if the probability is low as far as synthetic polymers are concerned.

Blood compatibility

Reactions involved in blood compatibility include inflammation and immunogenicity, but the fastest reaction is often thrombogenicity. As blood is a liquid medium, the rate of all reactions is increased as diffusion is much faster in blood than in other tissues, which can be considered as 'jellified' media. In addition, blood is usually not static in vivo and some rheological parameters such as type of flow, i.e. laminar or vortex, and shear rate on the surface, strongly modulate reactions of blood. The influence of flow was noted as early as the mid nineteenth century by Virchow in the case of the interactions of blood with blood vessels. In his pioneering work, Virchow showed that interactions between blood and the inside surface of blood vessels depended on the blood itself (normal or pathologic), the flow (continuous or not) and the surface of the vessel (damaged or undamaged). From these early observations,

Table 4.3 Examples of polymers used in blood-contacting devices

Device	Purpose	Conditions	Polymer used
Blood bags	Storage of blood	Static blood; absence of divalent ions chelated by citrate ions	Any endowed with suitable thermomechanical properties; not expensive (disposable)
Haemodialysers	Replacement of deficient kidneys for blood purification	Flowing blood; anticoagulated with heparin	Flexible polymers for tubing; porous polymeric membranes: modified cellulose, PAN copolymers, polysulfone
Large arterial prostheses	Replacement of deficient large arteries, e.g. aorta or femoral artery	Flowing blood; high shear rate; low ratio of contacted surface/blood volume	Woven or knitted PET for Ø > 6 mm; expanded PTFE for Ø > 4 mm
Small arterial prostheses	Replacement of deficient coronary arteries	Flowing blood; high shear rate; high ratio of contacted surface/blood volume	Currently none

PAN, polyacrylonitrile; PET, poly(ethylene terephthalate); PTFE, poly(tetrafluoroethylene).

it can be deduced that compatibility of blood with the surface of a material is not intrinsic, as it depends on parameters that are independent of the material.

The use of different polymers in contact with blood is shown in Table 4.3. It is clear that some polymers could be considered as 'blood-compatible' when used in some conditions of flow but not in others. This is typically exemplified in the case of knitted or woven poly(ethylene terephthalate), e.g. Dacron®, which can be used as a constituent of vascular prostheses in humans for replacing arteries larger than 6 mm in diameter but cannot be used for replacing smaller arteries and induces blood coagulation in static blood.

As illustrated in Figure 4.9, the interactions between blood and a material surface depend on the blood and on many parameters determined by the structure and composition of the material. The interactions are modulated both by rheological parameters and by the ratio between the contacted surface area and the volume of the contacting blood.

Concerning blood, reactions depend strongly on the presence of divalent ions (calcium and magnesium), on the presence of many proteins (e.g. factor VIII) and on the presence of platelets mainly in the case of flowing blood. This explains why reactions of blood in vivo, i.e. in blood circulating in contact with a material, are difficult to predict from static in vitro experiments. Indeed, such experiments are performed in conditions in which coagulation is blocked, for instance in blood plasma depleted in divalent ions or anticoagulated with heparin, or in serum that is devoid of at least fibrinogen.

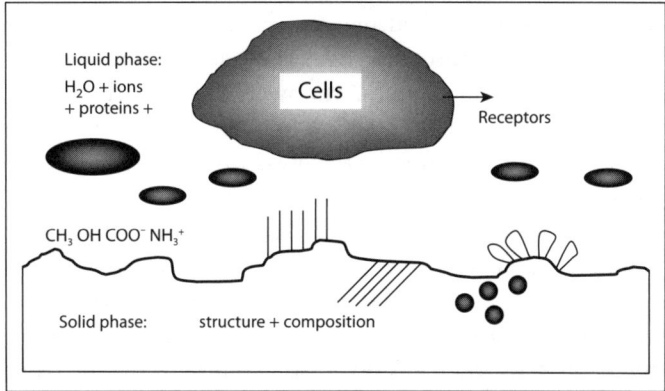

Figure 4.9   Model of a blood/material interface. The liquid phase, i.e. static or flowing blood, contains water, ions, proteins and cells. The solid phase is characterised by structural parameters, i.e. size, surface area, rigidity, crystallinity and conformation, and by composition dependent parameters, i.e. types of chemical group, hydrophilicity/hydrophobicity, charge and homogeneity of distribution.

Concerning the surface contacted by the blood, it has been shown for many years that the only blood-compatible surface is the healthy endothelium, which is composed of a monolayer of very active endothelial cells. Concerning all materials, structural parameters (e.g. size, surface area, roughness, rigidity, crystallinity and conformation of molecules on the surface) and also physicochemical parameters (e.g. type of chemical group determining hydrophilic/hydrophobic balance, type of electrical charge, degree of ionisation, ions binding and the existence of micro-domains) have an influence on the interactions between the blood and the surface. Thus, no suitable vascular prosthesis for coronary artery has been found to solve major health problems such as myocardial infarction.

The influence of the size of the material in contact with the blood in vivo is a good illustration of the non-specific reactions that permit natural protection against foreign bodies. When submicronic particles, e.g. nanoparticles for drug delivery, are injected in the bloodstream, they are rapidly opsonised, i.e. coated with proteins, and phagocytised. Conversely, if the material is too large to be phagocytised, e.g. microparticles for embolisation, then formation of a thrombus results from contact with the blood. These reactions are generally independent of the material, with a few important exceptions shown in Section 4.4.6. However, the ultimate fate of a material in vivo depends strongly on the physicochemical features of its surface.

4.3.4   Polymers for hip and knee prostheses

The hips and knees support the weight of the body and make walking possible. The force applied to these parts can be markedly increased during walking, compared with the weight of the immobile person, especially when the speed of walking is increased or when playing sport. The bone constituting the original femoral neck supports the changes of applied force with flexibility, as the healthy bone is a living material endowed with the structure of a natural composite material. Walking is possible when the joints can move freely. Free movements of joints are favoured by the presence in the joint of continuously lubricated cartilage.

With progression of osteoporosis, the femoral neck becomes brittle and breaks. Cartilage degraded in some pathologies can become unable to play its role in the joint. In both cases, replacement by a total hip prosthesis is needed. Concerning the femoral neck, materials supporting such applied forces should resist compression and bending. Polymeric composites reinforced by carbon fibres were proposed as materials for such prostheses, as they are light and flexible. However, release of carbon fibres by the prosthesis in the surrounding tissues led to the withdrawal of such materials. Thus, the stems and necks of hip prostheses are presently made of metals, increasingly titanium alloys.

Polymers can be used in the sliding parts of joints. Poly(tetrafluoroethylene) (PTFE) was proposed, thanks to its excellent sliding properties. However, PTFE does not resist friction under compression and is rapidly crushed, leading to loosening of the prosthesis. Ultra-high-density polyethylene is used in the hip when the head of the femoral part is made of stainless steel, and in the joint of the tibia in the knee prosthesis.

Poly(methylmethacrylate) is used to seal prostheses into the bones in vivo. As shown in Section 3.4.1, radical polymerisation of methylmethacrylate (MMA) can be initiated at body temperature by decomposition of benzoyl peroxide (BPO) catalysed by dimethyltoluidine (DMT). In a typical example, two vials have been prepared ready for use at the temperature of the operating theatre. The first vial contains MMA and DMT. The second vial contains BPO, micro-beads of PMMA and a radio-opaque agent, e.g. ZrO_2, to evidence the presence of polymer. Depending on the room temperature, the surgeon has instructions concerning the times for mixing, filling the syringe, injecting the mixture, and maintaining immobilisation of the bone and prosthesis. For instance, at 21 °C, the indicated times are 40 s for mixing, 5 min for filling the syringe and 9–12 min for injection and immobilisation. Thus, sealing such prostheses is a fast process, but the main issue is to avoid too high an increase in temperature in the surrounding living tissues. Indeed, polymerisation is an exothermic process, and the amount of monomer should be limited in order to reduce the emission of heat. To have a sufficient amount of polymer for sealing, the mixture is supplemented with PMMA.

4.3.5   Polymers for breast prostheses

This example has been chosen as typical of the misuse or lack of knowledge of materials used for implantation. As silicones (more precisely, poly(dimethylsiloxane) rubber) are very soft, compliant and rather inert, bags made of silicone rubber and filled with a liquid or a gel have been used extensively for making breast prostheses. Many serious health problems have occurred, and the use of implanted 'silicones' has led to controversy and lawsuits. The occurrence of anti-silicone antibodies was even claimed in a paper, but fortunately this was not true.

Silicone rubber is very soft and compliant, but this material is rather fragile because its structure is loose, and it can be torn easily if it is too thin. Silicone rubber is also highly hydrophobic. When filled with aqueous liquids, there are no leaks through the wall, whereas oily liquids such as silicone oils can diffuse readily through the wall. In addition, powdery materials such as talc, which may be present on surgical gloves, stick easily to the surface of silicone rubber, inducing strong inflammatory reactions in the tissues surrounding the prosthesis.

When implanted, silicone rubber is slowly calcified and thus rigidified through a mechanism that has not been elucidated. Despite this drawback, there is presently no alternative to the use of silicone rubber, but it should be used only under appropriate conditions, i.e. the bags should be thick enough and filled with aqueous solution, and there should be no talc on the surgical gloves.

4.3.6   Polymers for haemodialysers

Haemodialysers are external assistance devices designed to replace the filtering function of deficient kidneys. A schematic illustration of haemodialysis is shown in Figure 4.10.

The first haemodialyser was designed by Kolff during the Second World War in the Netherlands. The original idea was to circulate the patient's heparinised blood in a long enough dialysis bag in order to permit:

- exchange of small molecules with a dialysis bath
- elimination of excess water and salt, and of metabolic wastes
- retention of proteins in the blood circuit.

The only type of semi-permeable tubing suitable and available at that time was the cellophane 'skin' used for sausages. Kolff evaluated that a surface area of about 1 m^2 was suitable for an efficient and fast enough dialysis. This same surface area is still the reference for haemodialysis membranes. A mandatory requirement is that albumin should not cross the membrane.

Following Kolff's pioneering work, the design of the circuit was improved and the original cellophane tubing was replaced by flat Cuprophan® membranes and then hollow fibres. Despite having good filtering qualities and being of low cost, Cuprophan has been used less and less. Indeed, during haemodialysis sessions with such membranes, it has been shown that problems such as fever and nausea have occurred. In a few cases, life-threatening respiratory distress occurred, even if this was the first dialysis for the patient,

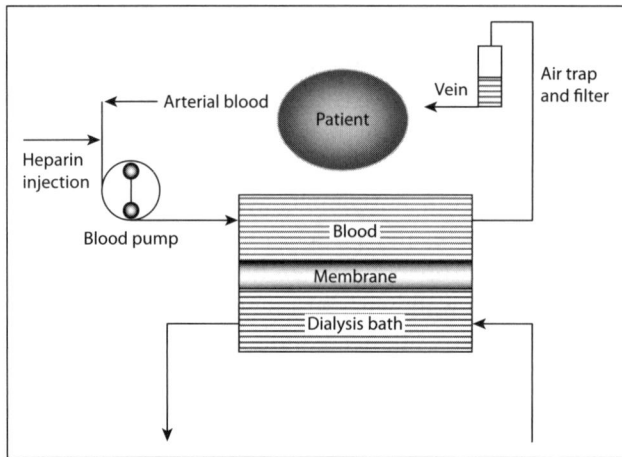

Figure 4.10 Schematic representation of extracorporeal haemodialysis. Arterial blood is taken from a fistula created in the arm of the patient. After anticoagulation by heparin, blood is pushed into the haemodialyser by a non-haemolytic pump. Blood comes into contact with a semi-permeable membrane (surface area approx. 1 m^2). Water, salts in excess and metabolic wastes are eliminated into the dialysis bath circulating against the bloodstream on the other side of the membrane. The dialysis bath contains ions that can diffuse through the membrane into blood to re-equilibrate the ionic content. After elimination of bubbles and possible clots by filtering, cleaned blood is re-injected into the patient.

the so-called 'first-use syndrome'. A fast decrease of the circulating neutrophils was observed, resulting from leukocyte activation and sequestration of the aggregates in lungs of the patients. Strong activation of the alternative pathway of complement, resulting in release of inflammatory mediators such as interleukin 1, was associated with the physiological reactions. This occurred in spite of the presence of soluble heparin in the circuit to avoid blood coagulation.

In a model system, it was shown that complement was also activated by contact with cross-linked dextran, i.e. Sephadex®. The extent of activation depended on the individual patient, with a factor varying between one and ten in healthy people but being higher in patients undergoing haemodialysis using Cuprophan membranes. For a given individual, the amplification factor in the presence of regenerated cellulose is proportional to the factor evidenced in the presence of Sephadex. Thus, it is thought that a natural antibody able to cross-react with both polysaccharides and to amplify complement activation was present at various levels in certain individuals, inducing strong physiological reactions. The origin of such antibodies is still hypothetical.

To decrease the reactions and the duration of haemodialysis sessions, new types of membrane have been proposed. It has been shown that modifications of the cellulose membrane by substitution of some hydroxyl groups by acetate, or by diethylaminoethyl (DEAE) groups in Hemophan®, resulted in

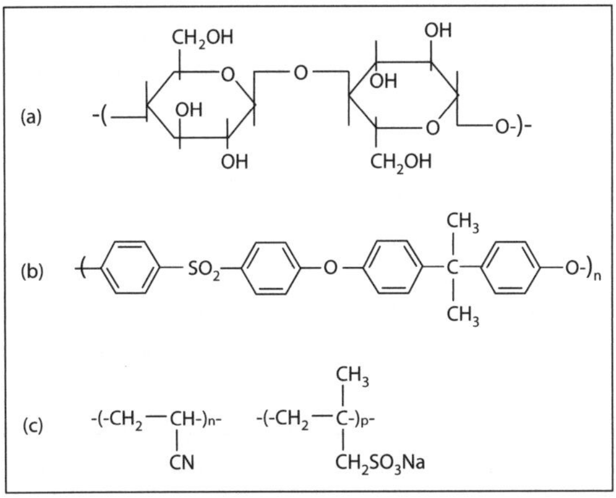

Figure 4.11 Polymeric materials used in haemodialysis membranes: (a) regenerated cellulose (cellophane, Cuprophan®) and modified cellulose derivatives in which some OH groups are modified by binding acetyl or diethylaminoethyl (DEAE) groups (in Hemophan®); (b) polysulfone; (c) poly (acrylonitrile-co-methallylsulphonate) copolymers (AN69S®).

reduction of complement activation and its physiological consequences. Different synthetic polymeric and more porous membranes, e.g. copolymers of acrylonitrile and methallylsulphonate (AN69S®) and polysulfone, have been proposed for haemodialysis and are increasingly used. The polymers used to prepare haemodialysis membranes are presented in Figure 4.11.

4.3.7 Polymers for ophthalmology

The main requirement for polymeric materials used in contact with the eye (contact lenses) or inside the eye (e.g. intraocular lenses) and located on the optical path is isotropic transparency to visible light. Such a requirement has been met by PMMA, which is amorphous. In 1950, Ridley published a study performed in pilots of the British Royal Air Force who had received aeroplane windshield fragments in the eyes. The fragments of PMMA, e.g. Perspex®, were generally well tolerated. Thus, for years PMMA has been the polymeric material of choice for meeting both requirements of isotropic transparency and tolerance.

Contact lenses made from PMMA have been manufactured and worn by a large number of people. However, PMMA lenses were not comfortable, patients could use them for only a few hours a day, and the eyes became red at the end of the day. This indicated that the cornea cells suffered because of a lack of oxygen, resulting in the development of small blood vessels in the eye in order to supply oxygen.

These drawbacks were due both to the rigidity of PMMA and to its impermeability to oxygen. As PMMA is very rigid, the radius of curvature of the lens has to be perfectly adapted to that of the eye. In addition, cornea cells that normally receive oxygen through tears cannot receive oxygen through PMMA. To remedy these drawbacks, manufacturers developed lenses based on acrylic and silicon polymers, which are less rigid and have an increased permeability to oxygen. However, tear proteins and lipids are still adsorbed on these hydrophobic materials.

The real breakthrough was the invention at the beginning of the 1960s of hydrophilic soft lenses, by Wichterle in Prague. Made from poly(2-hydroxyethyl methacrylate) (PHEMA), these lenses contained about a third of their weight in water (see Section 2.2.2). They were soft, compliant and permeable to oxygen, making them more comfortable to wear. As they were rather hydrophilic, adsorption of proteins and lipids on their surface was decreased. However, they required careful disinfection, as bacteria could develop in such hydrogels. As the lenses were very fragile and the process of disinfection and rinsing was tedious, long-wear and single-use lenses have now been developed.

Other materials have been proposed, such as silicones, with the advantages of being highly flexible and less fragile than the PHEMA-based lenses, and permeable to oxygen, but with the inconvenience of being highly hydrophobic. Surface treatments have been designed to increase their surface hydrophilicity. Contact lenses are now worn daily by many people, but the instructions for use must be followed carefully in order to avoid severe problems such as abscess of the cornea. No artificial cornea is currently available.

With an ageing population, the occurrence of cataract has increased. This disease results in opacification of the natural crystalline lens. The only way to treat this kind of blindness is to extract the opacified lens and to replace it either externally by very thick glasses, or internally by intraocular lenses (IOLs). PMMA that has been modified by the addition of an ultraviolet-filtering additive to protect the retina has been used to manufacture the optic part of the device.

Some difficulties occurred with maintaining the optic part at the correct place in the eye. Three positions are possible: behind the iris as the natural lens (i.e. posterior chamber), or on the iris or in front of the iris (i.e. anterior chamber). It was shown that the iris was irritated when the IOL was placed on it. Concerning the other positions, the supporting part has to be flexible enough to adapt itself to the size of the patient's eye. As PMMA is a rigid material, the supporting part has been made of a more flexible polymer, e.g. polypropylene, but inflammation occurred at the junction between the polymers. The problems were solved by manufacturing IOLs in one piece of PMMA with long, thin branches in order to obtain sufficient flexibility.

Nowadays, IOLs are mainly composed of PMMA, but some foldable IOLs are in development to facilitate the work of the surgeon and minimise bleeding at the incision, which could contribute to possible inflammation. The only unsolved problem is re-opacification due to cells growing on the surface of the IOL, which needs laser treatment. The reason for this phenomenon is unknown. Some IOLs are shown in Figure 4.12.

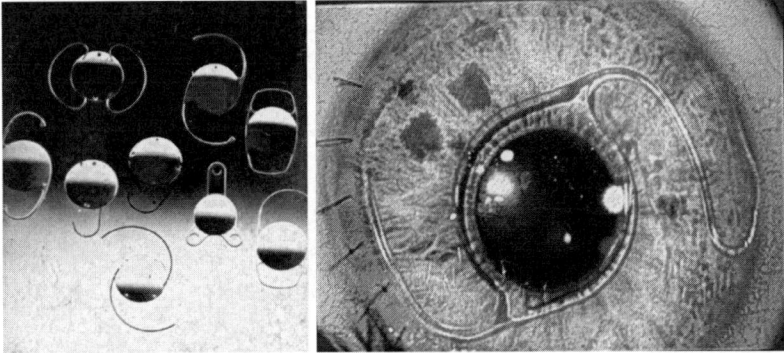

Figure 4.12 Intraocular lenses alone (a) and in the eye (b).

4.3.8 Catheters and microparticles for therapeutic embolisation and chemoembolisation

Dedicated to Pr. A. Jayakrishnan and Dr. A. Laurent.

Therapeutic embolisation has been a pioneering method within the methods known as interventional radiology and mini-invasive techniques. Such techniques using radiology and catheterisation as tools have the great advantage of avoiding surgery in many cases; for instance, they are currently used to reopen stenosed coronary arteries. The aim of therapeutic embolisation, however, is to obliterate blood vessels supplying blood to a pathological territory, e.g. arteriovenous malformation (AVM), uterine fibroids or other vascularised benign tumours. Embolisation can be used temporarily to occlude a vessel before surgery, or for long-term treatment when surgery cannot be used safely, e.g. in the brain or spinal cord, as shown in Figure 4.13.

Chemo-embolisation has been developed for the treatment of vascularised malignant tumours. Its aim is to combine a local delivery of drug at and around the site of embolisation with a shortage of blood supply. It is currently used mainly in the treatment of hepatic carcinoma.

Different devices have been used as tools for embolisation purposes. The vascular system is accessed typically through the femoral system under local anaesthetic. Under systemic heparinisation, a catheter system is advanced with direct visualisation by radiography. Then the vascular system is imaged by injection of an angiographic dye. The images are stored in a computer to serve as reference. Depending on the precise use and on the diameter of the vessels to be occluded, various types of balloon, coil, particle, glue (e.g. PACA) and solutions of jellifying polymers are used. A micro-catheter can be selectively advanced into the vessels and the occlusive material delivered.

Microparticles, i.e. particles with a size usually in the range 50–1000 μm, have been used widely for embolisation of small vessels, and many types of material have been tried. As polymers can be adapted to the many requirements concerning embolisation, polymeric microparticles are mainly used for this purpose. The microparticles should preferably be spherical in order to

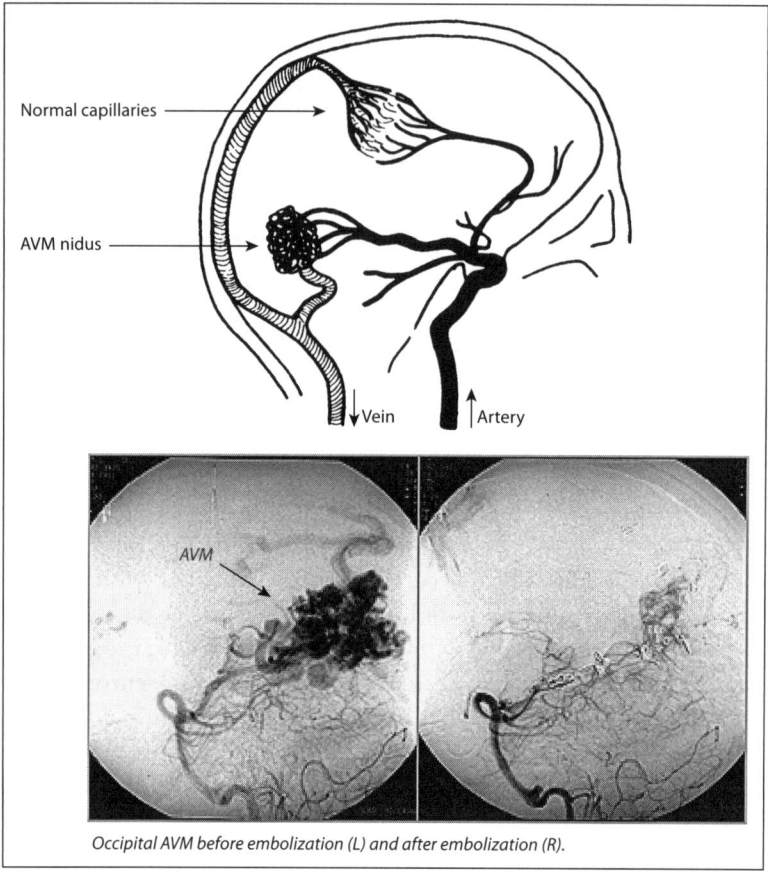

Normal capillaries

AVM nidus

↓Vein   ↑Artery

Occipital AVM before embolization (L) and after embolization (R).

Figure 4.13 Intracranial arteriovenous malformation (AVM) and a radiological view before and after embolisation, visualised by the presence or absence of a contrast agent.

provide optimal occlusion. The size of the spheres should have a narrow distribution in order to control the size of the vessel to be occluded. As the arterial wall is elastic, the sphere diameter should be approximately 1.5 times the diameter of the artery to be occluded. To avoid fractionation of the particles capable of inducing hazardous distal occlusions, the material has to be mechanically stable. The material must be soft, as it is delivered through micro-catheters that are smaller in diameter than the particle; in addition, the material must be elastic enough to recover its initial diameter as soon as possible at the exit of the catheter. To avoid sticking and aggregates forming in the catheters, the surface of the spheres must be smooth and hydrophilic. Finally, the microspheres should not induce a strong inflammatory reaction in the surrounding tissues. An example of such microparticles is presented in Figure 4.14. The efficacy of embolisation is controlled by injection of a contrast agent and comparison with reference images. To make possible in vivo follow-up of the particles, it would be preferable to detect them directly by X-rays or MRI.

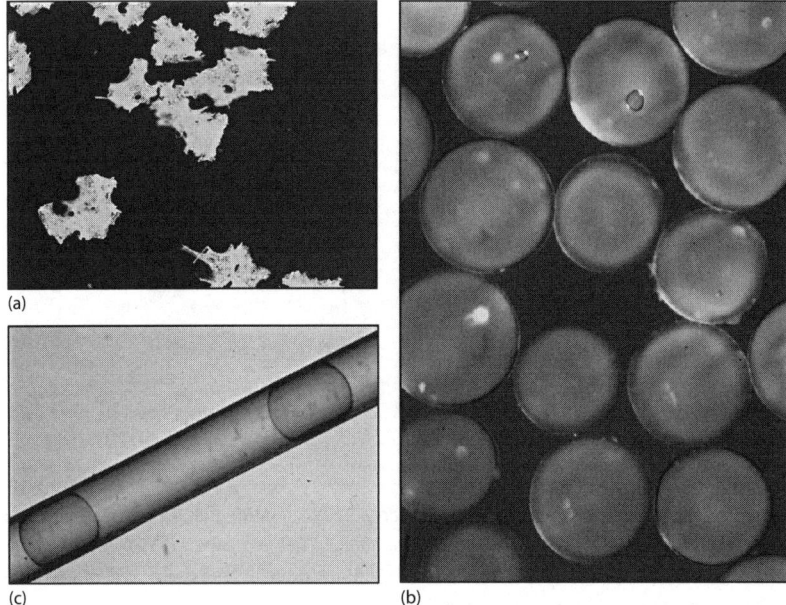

Figure 4.14   Microparticles for embolisation; clockwise: (a) early PVA particles, (b) soft hydrated microspheres in suspension and (c) soft hydrated microspheres in a catheter.

The most developed particles in the 1980s were based on cross-linked poly(vinyl alcohol) (PVA), e.g. Ivalon®. As the particles were not spherical, the main drawbacks resulted either from blockage of catheters, or from too proximal and insufficient embolisation. Spherical particles were developed in order to avoid such drawbacks. They have been made from PVA or from other polymers in different countries: poly(2-hydroxyethyl methacrylate), partially hydrolysed poly(methylmethacrylate) and substituted poly(acrylamides) (Trisacryl®). All of these particles are spherical and are made from hydrophilic, non-degradable materials; some are microporous, but others are macroporous. The latter structure was proposed both to add more flexibility to the microspheres and to permit loading with additives such as drugs, gelatin and radio-opaque agents. However, radio-opacity was achieved at the expense of other more useful properties, and such radio-opaque microspheres have not been developed commercially. Microspheres with the required properties and containing a super paramagnetic compound that can be detected by MRI have been developed; an example is given in Figure 4.15.

A high selectivity of the site of embolisation has been achieved by using microspheres with a very narrow size distribution. Such a property has made possible selective embolisation of uterine fibroids without side embolisation of the uterus itself, which would impair pregnancy.

Microparticles made from biodegradable polymers have been proposed for temporary embolisation and for drug-delivery purposes, e.g. chemo-embolisation. The main problem with PLGA-based microparticles is the

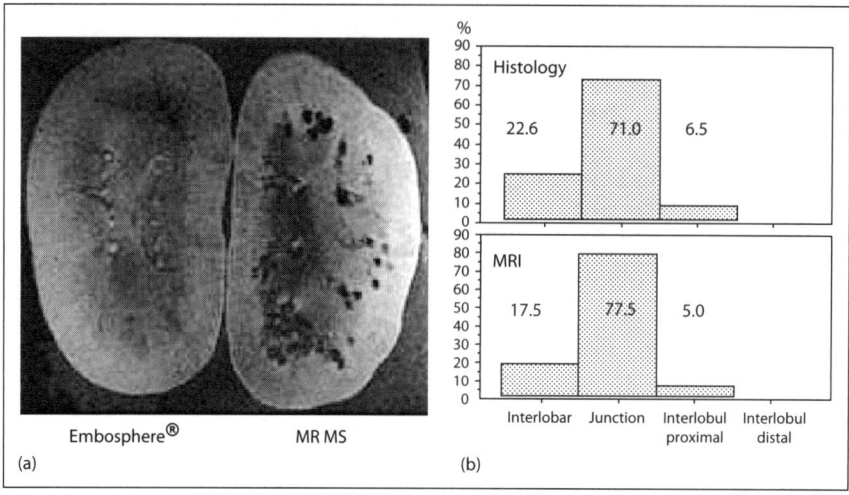

Figure 4.15 (a) Comparison of magnetic resonance imaging (MRI) of kidneys embolised either with normal Embospheres® (left kidney) or microspheres of similar diameter (500–700 μm) labelled with colloidal superparamagnetic iron oxide (MR MS) (right kidney). (b) Arterial level of occlusion of right kidney evaluated either by histology or by MRI.

inflammatory response that results from the large amount of degradation products, which are released faster than they can be eliminated. An important piece of work has been performed on microspheres based on natural polymers. These pose less toxicity and many are susceptible to biodegradation. However, the presence of antigenic determinants in such polymers is possible. Microspheres made from albumin, casein, gelatin, chitosan, starch, alginate and dextran have been proposed, and review papers are available.

Despite the fact that the presence of microspheres made from non-degradable polymers in pathological arteries induces a generally acceptable inflammatory response, embolisation is not definitive. In fact, revascularisation invariably occurs, excluding this foreign body from the lumen of the vessel at a rate that depends on the material, the animal and the embolised tissue. The molecular mechanisms occurring in this process are unknown.

4.4 Applications of polymers in pharmaceutical uses

4.4.1 Excipients for formulation of conventional dosage forms

Among the various ingredients that are commonly used as excipients in the formulation of dosage forms, polymers are widely used in pharmacy. These polymers are of semi-synthetic or synthetic origin. They are used because of their ability to confer various original functionalities, which can be finely tuned and cannot be achieved using other excipients. It should be noted that, except for parenteral delivery, degradability is not a major concern for most of these applications. Because of the breadth of the subject, only some examples of applications are given here.

Excipients for tabletting

Formulation of tablets requires the use of various excipients in order to confer a series of functionalities to these conventional dosage forms. A few polymers are currently used as excipients for tablets in various purposes. Cellulose and starch, which can be considered as natural excipients, can be used as diluents when the drug content is low. When tablets have to be prepared by the wet-granulation technique, the addition of a binder is used to agglutinate the powder particles and form grains that are more easily compressed and form strong enough tablets. Common binders include starch used in the form of starch paste, and cellulosic ethers such as carboxymethylcellulose (CMC) and hydroxypropylcellulose (HPC). Alternatively, poly(vinylpyrrolidone) (PVP) (Figure 4.16) in the proportion of a few per cent of the final preparation can be used as a binder.

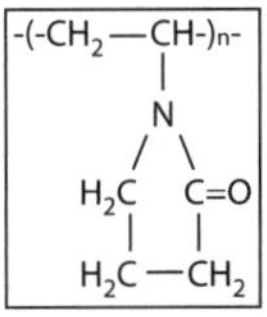

Figure 4.16 Repeating unit of poly(N-vinyl-2 pyrrolidone).

A series of linear homopolymers of vinylpyrrolidone synthetically produced by free radical polymerisation are commercially available. These products have a mean molecular weight ranging from 4000 g/mol to about 1 300 000 g/mol. As this is the case for many commercial brands, these values are only averages and their polydispersity may be rather large. PVP is freely soluble in water and in many solvents, including ethanol, making it an interesting excipient not only as a binder but also in various applications, including as a film-forming material, a thickener and an adhesive agent.

Because conventional tablets need to be rapidly disintegrated in water or gastric fluids in order to allow drug dissolution and absorption, it is generally necessary to add a disintegrating agent in the formulation. Pre-gelatinised starch or chemically modified starch, such as sodium starch glycolate (Figure 4.17) can be used for this purpose. The latter semi-synthetic polymer is called a 'super-disintegrant' owing to its capacity to induce fast tablet disintegration when used at levels as low as 2%. Sodium starch glycolate is the sodium salt of a carboxymethyl ether of starch; the molecular weight of commercial brands typically ranges from 500 000 g/mol to 11 000 000 g/mol. It is insoluble in water and most solvents.

Alternatively, purely synthetic polymers such as cross-linked homopolymers of N-vinyl-2 pyrrolidone are commercialised under the trade name

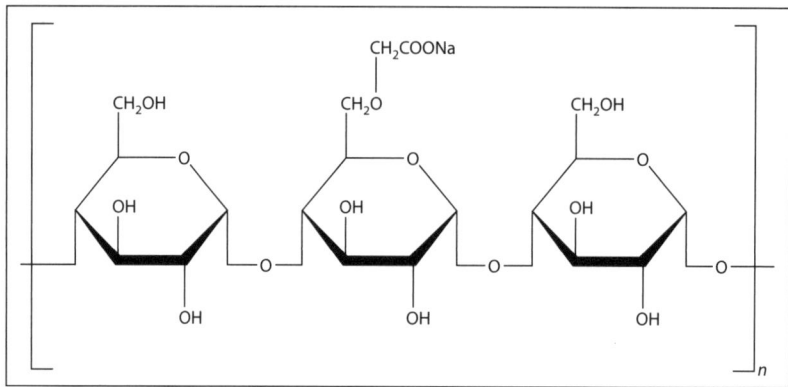

Figure 4.17   General structure of sodium starch glycolate.

Polyplasdone®. These polymers are completely insoluble in water, acids, alkalis and all organic solvents. As they are highly hygroscopic and able to swell rapidly in water without forming gels, they are also very efficient disintegrating agents.

Finally, instead of conventional lubricants, low-molecular-weight (typically a few thousand g/mol) polyethylene glycol (PEG) grades can be used as lubricants in very specific circumstances when water solubility of the whole of the ingredients is required, e.g. in effervescent tablets.

Excipients for semi-solid preparations

Many semi-solid preparations, such as ointments, creams, gels and toothpastes, lotions, oral suspensions and transdermal gel reservoirs require the use of thickeners or suspending agents. Polymeric excipients have very interesting functionalities for such applications. Hydrophilic polymers are used widely for thickening water solutions or forming gels; semi-synthetic cellulose ethers and synthetic polymers such as carbomers (poly(acrylic acid) derivatives) belong to this category. Carbomers are a good example of a widely used family of such hydrophilic polymers.

Carbomers were first prepared and patented in 1957. Commonly known under their trade name Carbopol®, these polymers are composed of homopolymers of acrylic acid loosely cross-linked with polyalkenyl ethers or divinyl glycol. Poly(acrylic acid) homopolymers corresponding to the general structure shown in Figure 4.18 are loosely cross-linked together by various molecules bearing hydroxyl groups, such as sugars or glycol derivates.

The carboxyl groups provided by the acrylic acid backbone of the polymer are responsible for many of the product's benefits. The molecular weight of

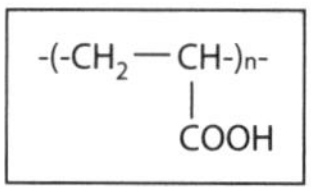

$$-(-CH_2-CH-)_n-$$
$$\overset{|}{C}OOH$$

Figure 4.18   Repeating unit of poly(acrylic acid).

the repeating unit of Carbopol polymers, defined as the moiety containing a single carboxylic group, is considered to be 76 g/mol on average. The calculation of the amount of base requested for neutralising these polymers can be based on this average value.

Commercial grades are available as fluffy white powders consisting of primary polymer particles of about 0.2–6.0 μm average diameter. Due to cross-linking, and once swollen and flocculated, the agglomerates cannot be broken into smaller particles; instead, each particle can be viewed as a network of homopolymeric chains interconnected via cross-linking or entangled together. In the presence of water, the numerous carboxylic groups are hydrated by water molecules, allowing swelling of the polymeric chains (Figure 4.19). Other H-bond-forming substances such as glycerol or diamines can be used for increasing swelling. Alternatively, due to the presence of acidic functions, these polymers can be neutralised by mineral or organic bases.

Because the apparent pKa of carboxylic groups in these polymers ranges from 6.0 to 6.5, the carboxylate groups on the polymer backbone are ionised at physiological pH, resulting in repulsion between charges and increasing swelling of the polymer. Therefore, Carbopol polymers exhibit very good water sorption properties and, depending on the grade, they can swell in water up to 1000 times their original volume at neutral pH. Being water-insoluble polymers, individual powder particles form microgels after hydration, which are biologically fairly inert. Macroscopically, agglutination of these microgels leads to viscous and firm gels in water.

Depending on the nature of the cross-linker, the degree of cross-linking and the manufacturing conditions, various grades of Carbopol are available.

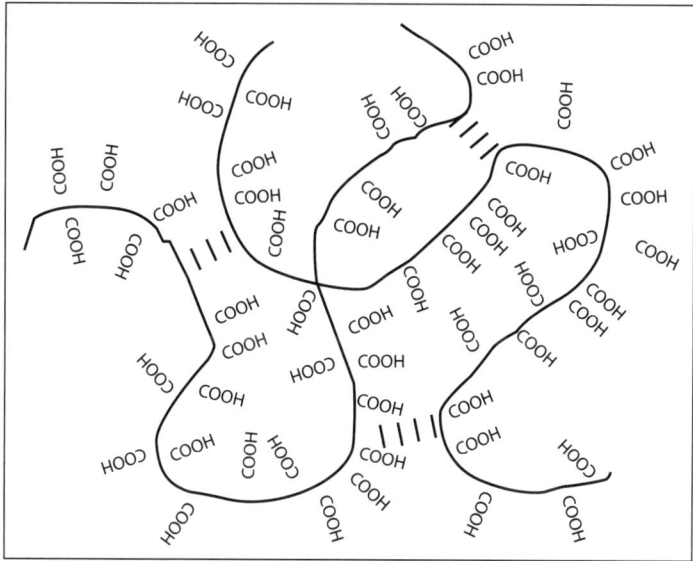

Figure 4.19   Cross-linked polyacrylic acid polymers (Carbopol®).

The molecular weight of these cross-linked polymers cannot be precisely determined. However, the molecular weights between adjacent cross-links are approximately inversely proportional to the density of the cross-linker. These molecular weights may be calculated from the functionality of the cross-linking monomer, the relative ratio of acrylic acid to cross-linking monomer, and the efficiency of the cross-linking reaction. Therefore, for practical purposes, commercial grades are characterised mainly by the rheological characteristics of the macroscopic dispersions in water. Rheological properties are dependent on the particle size, the molecular weight between cross-links and its distributions, etc., making available an interesting range of commercially available products.

Historically, Carbopol 934 P grade consisted of poly(acrylic acid) homopolymeric chains loosely cross-linked with allyl sucrose and polymerised in benzene. Similarly, Polycarbophil® was cross-linked with divinyl glycol and polymerised in benzene. In order to switch to less toxic solvents, other grades were prepared. New grades, such as Carbopol 71G, 971 P and 974 P, are cross-linked with allyl penta-erythritol and polymerised in ethyl acetate. Differences in the process of polymerisation are reflected in the application properties, such as the degree of swelling and the rheological properties of hydrogels, which can vary from one grade to the other.

Being supported by extensive toxicological studies, water-swellable Carbopol polymers have been used in a wide range of pharmaceutical applications. These polymers are well tolerated, and low toxicities and irritation have been demonstrated. Due to their extremely high molecular weight, they cannot diffuse through epithelia or skin. Specifically, they are used widely as thickeners at very low concentrations in order to produce a wide range of viscosities and flow properties, with high yield values in topical lotions, creams and gels, oral suspensions and transdermal gel reservoirs or suspensions of insoluble drugs in oral suspensions.

Apart from poly(acrylic acid) polymers, other polymers are used widely in the formulation of semi-solid pharmaceutical dosage forms, including natural gums and cellulosic ethers (see Section 4.4.2), PVP and PEG. Different grades of PEG (Macrogol®) can be used as thickeners or gelling agents. Interestingly, grades with different molecular weights can be mixed together to adjust exactly the rheological properties of the mixture.

4.4.2 Polymers as excipients for controlled release by the oral route

The emergence of the concept of controlled-release delivery systems as an effective way to enhance patient compliance and extend the lifecycle of a drug has led to the need for novel ways of controlling drug-release profiles. Polymers offer the opportunity to develop functional excipients able to efficiently control the release of drugs in a specific location and according to a preset time profile. The use of polymers in pharmaceutical preparations was developed during the 1970s and 1980s, corresponding to a rising need for the minimisation of toxic side-effects and for the lifecycle management of drugs. The basic idea of controlled drug-delivery systems consists of delivering a drug encapsulated in a dosage form accordingly to a preprogrammed amount versus the time profile, conceived in such a way that plasmatic drug levels or organ drug levels can be maintained in a therapeutic window defined by the minimal effective concentration and the maximal tolerated concentration. This strategy has led to a reduction of plasmatic drug peaks and valleys typically associated with immediate-release dosage forms, which is not only beneficial for the patient but also interesting in reducing health costs.

Controlled-release delivery systems can be categorised into matrix or reservoir delivery systems. Such delivery systems are based on natural or synthetic polymers. Matrix systems consist of microscopic or macroscopic polymeric materials in which a drug is dispersed either in a molecular state or as crystalline particles. Delivery of the therapeutic agent can occur via diffusion or erosion of the bulk material. In reservoir systems the drug is placed in the so-called reservoir, which can be semi-solid or solid and is surrounded by an external membrane that controls outside diffusion of the drug and therefore the release profile. The general organisation of controlled-release delivery systems and the type of polymer to be used is influenced strongly by the route of administration.

Delivery systems for oral delivery are typically based on natural polymers or their derivatives, e.g. cellulose and cellulose ethers, as well as on hydrophilic synthetic non-degradable polymers, e.g. poly(vinyl pyrrolidone) and poly(alkylmethacrylates). Development of new applications in this area has mostly been based on the finding of optimal formulations by selecting or mixing adequate commercial grade polymers, and on the development of original fabrication processes of solid dosage form, rather than on the design of novel polymers. However, the use of polymers for parenteral applications, including injection or implants, is relatively new and is an active research field in the search for innovative polymers.

The aim of this section is to give a broad overview of the polymers that have been commonly used in controlled delivery by the oral route but not to develop the rationale underlying the formulation of these types of systems. The development of matrix or reservoir systems is based on the properties of the materials themselves, e.g. their swelling, diffusion and barrier properties, and suitable polymers must be chosen for the specific properties of the materials they form, e.g. tablets, microgranules and films, in the presence of physiological fluids. Commonly used polymers in this area are presented according to this classification.

Hydrophilic polymers for matrices formulation

Matrix systems provide controlled release of the drug via diffusion or erosion mechanisms. Insoluble polymers such as polyethylene or poly(alkylmethacrylates) can be used. In such cases, matrices are formed by tabletting or hot melt extrusion processes, in which the drug to be released is generally dispersed as a powder. Because of the inertness of these matrices in contact with gastrointestinal fluids, drug release is governed mainly by diffusion, while the matrices remain almost intact during intestinal transit. However, much more commonly, controlled release is achieved by using water-soluble polymers that encapsulate the active ingredient in specific patterns (e.g. layers, cores, three-dimensional structures). The release of the active ingredient over time can be controlled mainly by diffusion. Typically, the matrix is swollen by water, which then dissolves the solid-state drug contained in the matrix, resulting in a further progressive diffusion through the swollen network. Alternatively, polymer can be dissolved in the gastrointestinal tract, leading to progressive erosion of the matrix and progressive release of the active ingredient. The rate of release can be adjusted by mixing or layering hydrophilic polymers with varying swelling/dissolution kinetics and by the use of innovative fabrication designs.

For common applications, polymers for controlling oral delivery are non-absorbable due to their high molecular weight and their hydrophilicity, making useless the use of degradable polymers from a toxicological standpoint. Thus, cellulose derivatives or hydrophilic gums are commonly used, especially methylcellulose (MC) (Figure 4.20) and hydroxypropylmethylcellulose (HPMC) (Figure 4.21).

Cellulose ethers have the polymeric backbone of cellulose, a natural carbohydrate that contains a basic repeating structure of anhydroglucose units. During the manufacture of cellulose ethers, cellulose fibres are treated with caustic solution, which in turn is treated with methyl chloride or propylene oxide. The chemical reaction yields a fibrous product, which is purified and ground to a fine powder. Commercial grades vary chemically and physically for matching the desired applicative properties.

The major chemical differences are in the degree of methyl substitution, hydroxypropyl substitution and polymerisation of the cellulosic backbone.

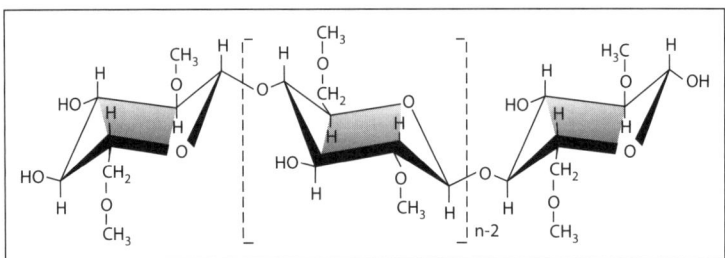

Figure 4.20 General structure of methylcellulose.

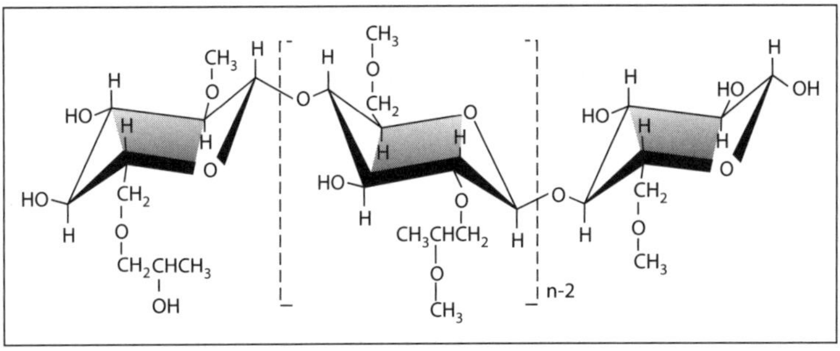

Figure 4.21   General structure of hydroxypropyl methylcellulose.

Although the molecular weights and polydispersity of these products can be determined, e.g. by intrinsic viscosity determinations, these data are generally unknown and commercial grades are characterised indirectly by the viscosities of 2% solutions of the polymer in water. These products possess varying ratios of hydroxypropyl and methyl substitution, a factor that influences properties such as organic solubility and the thermal gelation temperature of aqueous solutions. As an example, the percentages of methyl groups and hydroxypropyl groups in the K HPMC grades commonly used for matrices formulation are 19–24% and 7–12%, respectively. For more detailed information, the reader is referred to the technical bulletins of the commercial producers.

Apart from these widely used products, other cellulosic ethers such as HPC, hydroxyethylcellulose and CMC are often used in the formulation of controlled pharmaceutical delivery systems.

Controlled release in specific regions of the gastrointestinal tract

Specific polymers have been designed to release drugs into specific regions of the gastrointestinal tract. For this purpose, methacrylic polymers with pH-dependent solubility have been used widely. As described above, commercial-grade polymers characterised by their solubility at different pH can be used to adjust the level of delivery in the intestine. Further, azopolymers have been developed to target the colon, which is of great interest for the local treatment of inflammatory diseases and colitis. An example of azopolymer is presented in Figure 4.22.

The diazoic bond is stable in the gastrointestinal fluids, except in the colonic environment because of the presence of colonic bacterial flora, which produce enzymes able to cleave such bonds. Such polymers can be used to form matrices or coatings that are progressively eroded, allowing localised release of the drug.

Bioadhesive polymers for mucosal delivery

Following administration, bioadhesive dosage forms are intended to adhere at the surface of a mucosa, either to prolong the duration of activity of a drug locally or to enhance the permeation of the drug and thus enhance its systemic

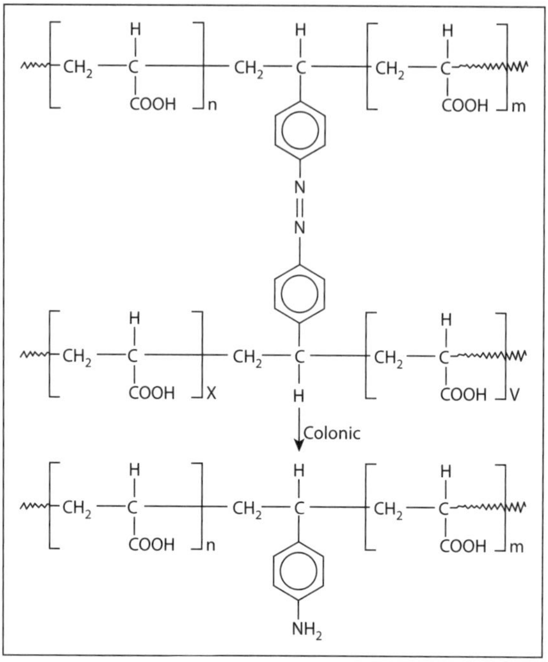

Figure 4.22 Example of azopolymer (after Kakoulides EP et al., *J Control Rel*, 52: 291–300, 1998). (with permission).

availability. Moreover, efficient protective effects against degrading conditions prevailing in physiological fluids, e.g. pH and enzymatic activity, can be obtained by incorporating the drug into such dosage forms. Many routes of administration can benefit from bioadhesive dosage forms, including the oral, buccal, vaginal, ocular, nasal and pulmonary routes. Bioadhesive or mucoadhesive properties can be conferred to various dosage forms, using specific polymers able to interact efficiently with mucosal surfaces. Because of the hydrophilic nature of this substrate and the ubiquitous presence of fluids on these surfaces, commonly used polymers should be able to form hydrogels in contact with mucosal surfaces. Usually, dosage forms such as tablets and microspheres are intended to be administered in a dry state. When placed in contact with a mucosal surface, a hydrogel is rapidly formed. Then, polymeric chains encounter the mucosal surface, which is lined with a mucous layer formed by a very large network of glycoproteins that creates a kind of 'natural' hydrogel. In the first stage of contact, the jellifying dosage form should wet this surface. Further, diffusion of the polymeric chains into the glycoprotein network is expected, increasing the possibility of interactions at the molecular state. Simultaneously, the polymeric chains should be able to develop molecular interactions with specific chemical groups belonging to the mucosal substrate. Various interactions can be developed at the interface, including electronic interactions and H-bonding, as shown in Figure 4.23.

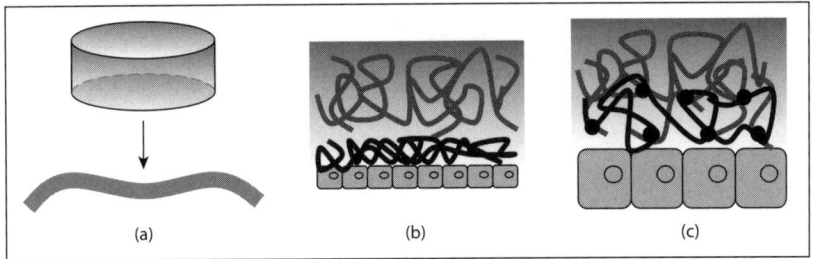

(a)   (b)   (c)

Figure 4.23 Schematic events following bioadhesion of a matrix tablet at a mucosal surface: (a) initial contact of the dry polymeric matrix with the mucosal surface; (b) polymeric chains are progressively hydrated at the matrix surface and in contact with the mucous layer lining the mucosa; (c) progressive chain interdiffusion between bioadhesive polymer chains and mucous glycoproteins encourages intimate contact and favours development of adhesive interactions, schematically depicted as black spots at the molecular level.

The strength of the interaction depends simultaneously on the interfacial behaviour of the polymeric chains and the rheological properties of the hydrogel, making the molecular properties of the polymers key parameters for optimised bioadhesion. Not surprisingly, hydrophilic polymers represent good candidates for such applications. Polymers containing carboxylic groups, such as poly(acrylic acid) and poly(methyl vinyl ether-co-maleic anhydride) (PVM/MA; Gantrez® AN), shown in Figure 4.24, exhibit excellent mucoadhesive properties, but other neutral polymers, including PVP, PVA and cellulosic ethers such as MC, HPMC, sodium CMC, HPC and other cellulose derivatives, can also be used as efficient ingredients for the formulation of bioadhesive dosage forms.

Alternatively, cationic polymers such as chitosan and chemically modified chitosan can be used because of their capacity to interact strongly with anionic electric charges borne by glycoproteins in the mucous layer.

Important factors of adhesion are the chain linearity, chain flexibility and molecular weight of the polymer, which should be high enough (up to millions) for facilitating chain interdiffusion at the interface and also formation of highly viscous hydrogels. The presence, density and spatial availability of chemical groups able to interact by forming with substrate and under the physiological conditions are equally important parameters.

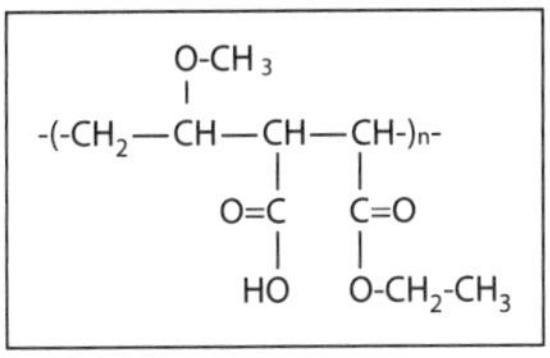

$$-(-CH_2-CH-CH-CH-)_n-$$

with $O-CH_3$ on the first CH, and $O=C$/HO and $C=O$/$O-CH_2-CH_3$ below the central CH groups.

Figure 4.24 Chemical structure of poly(methyl vinyl ether-co-maleic anhydride) (PVM/MA, or Gantrez® AN).

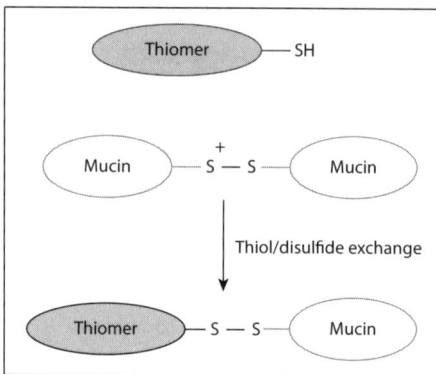

Figure 4.25 Schematic representation of mucoadhesive interactions of thiomers with mucin glycoproteins.

Further, the rheological properties of the bulk hydrogel are important, as the strength of mucoadhesion depends partly on these properties. From this point of view, formulation is of importance in order to obtain rheological synergies favourable to adhesion, which can be obtained by polymer blending, e.g. two cellulosic ethers or two grades of a single cellulosic.

Based on this, advanced polymers have been designed more specifically to improve mucoadhesive applications. For example, thiomers are thiolated polymers constructed by grafting thiol groups on a hydrophilic polymer. The presence of thiomers makes possible formation of disulfide bridges between the natural mucins, which are rich in thiolated amino acids and the thiomers, thus reinforcing adhesion, as shown in Figure 4.25. Additionally, such polymers have been shown to exhibit antiproteasic activities, which are expected to be useful for enhancing peptide delivery.

Alternatively, acid-based polyanhydrides such as poly(fumaric anhydrides) and poly(maleic anhydrides) have raised interest because of the capacity of anhydrides to progressively hydrolyse in the presence of physiological fluids, leading to the production of high amounts of carboxylic groups on the surface of the dosage form, which have been shown to enhance bioadhesiveness of the matrix, thus increasing its residence time at the mucosal surfaces.

Finally, it should be mentioned that many attempts have been proposed to enhance adhesion by grafting adequate ligands at the surface of the polymeric matrices, either made of inert or degradable polymers. Indeed, when matrices are in the form of micro- or nanoparticles, specific ligands able to recognise specific receptors at the mucosal surface can be presented at the surface of the delivery device. The rationale for such an approach is to simultaneously increase the intensity and the duration of adhesion and to localise the adhesion on mucosal areas bearing specific receptors.

4.4.3   Polymers for coating applications

In pharmacy, polymeric film coating is currently applied to various dosage forms, including tablets, pellets and microgranules, for decorative, protective and functional purposes. These coatings can be used to protect the active ingredient against exposure to environmental factors. Very often, for safety and marketing reasons, it is necessary to improve the appearance and enhance the mechanical strength of the dosage form, in particular for many tablets. Tablets may be coated in order to give a glossy, coloured finish, which may also be printed with the trade name for safety reasons. Finally, polymer coating is one among many technologies employed to modify the release of oral solid dosage forms. One such method is the use of insoluble or semipermeable polymer films to surround the dosage form and alter drug release.

Whatever the application, polymers for coating can be used either as solutions in organic solvents such as ethanol or hydroethanolic mixtures, or as water dispersions. For technological simplicity and to minimise the amount of residual solvents in the final products, the latter technique is of interest and is far more developed. Thus, polymers for coating are generally commercially available as preformulated water dispersions, sometimes including plasticisers, colorants and opacifiers. However, powders are also available, which have to be further treated before being used for coating. Film coating is achieved by a spray atomisation technique using coating pans or turbines, in which polymer-containing solutions or dispersions are atomised with air and delivered to the substrate surface as fine droplets. These droplets spread on the surface; solvent evaporation causes the droplets to pack closely and to coalesce to form the film. Finally, polymer chains may entangle to some extent. Thus, the final properties of polymer films depend not only on the physicochemical characteristics of the polymers but also on the coating formulation employed, the substrate variables and the processing conditions.

Important properties of coatings include solubility/insolubility in physiological fluids, drug diffusibility through water-insoluble films, water vapour and oxygen permeability, and thermal, mechanical and adhesive characteristics. These characteristics can be evaluated either directly on isolated films or indirectly after deposition on the considered dosage forms.

Polymer and film solubility/insolubility in physiological fluids

Depending on the application, a variety of polymers with varying solubility in physiological fluids are available. Some currently used polymers and their solubility and ordinary uses in formulation are presented in Table 4.4. When coatings are requested, for example to improve the external aspect or to enable easy swallowing of tablets, fast-dissolving films are needed. Commonly, low-molecular-weight grades of cellulosic ethers such as HPMC are used for this purpose. These polymers are water-soluble and

Table 4.4 Polymers used for coating applications

Polymer	Solubility	Common use	Usual presentation
Ethyl cellulose	Insoluble in water, regardless of pH; soluble in some organic solvents	Controlled-release coatings	Aqueous dispersions (20–30% solids)
Cellulose acetate phthalate	pH-dependent solubility in water; soluble in alcohols, hydrocarbons and some ketones	Enteric coating	Used either as aqueous dispersion (30% solids) or in solvent-based coatings
Hydroxypropylmethylcellulose phthalate	pH-dependent solubility in water	Enteric coating	
Poly(methyl methacrylate) copolymers, e.g. Eudragits®	Insoluble or pH-dependent solubility; soluble in solvents	Controlled release and enteric coating	Powders or aqueous dispersions
Hydroxypropylmethylcellulose (HPMC)	Soluble in water	Masking taste; moisture barrier for immediate-release dosage forms	Mostly sold as preprepared formulations, including plasticisers and colourants
Methylcellulose	Soluble in water; very low viscosity	Tablet and pellet coating	Powder or as preprepared formulations, including plasticisers and colourants
Hydroxypropylcellulose (HPC), e.g. Klucel®	Soluble in water	Tablet or pellet coating combined with other cellulosic ethers	Powder
Hydroxypropylethylcellulose (HPEC)	Soluble in water	Tablet or pellet coating	Powder

non-ionised, making their films easily dissolved following administration of the dosage form and contact with gastric or intestinal fluids.

Enteric coatings, i.e. coatings that are insoluble at the acidic pH encountered in the stomach but are readily soluble at intestinal pH, can be achieved using polymers bearing carboxylic groups. Because of their pH-dependent solubility, some cellulosic derivatives, e.g. cellulose acetate phthalate (Figure 4.26), can be used for such applications.

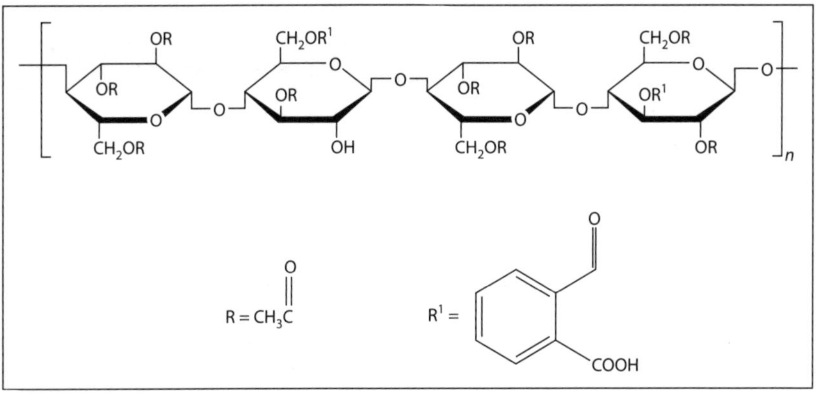

Figure 4.26 General structure of cellulose acetate phthalate.

Alternatively poly(alkylmethacrylates) have been tailored for this purpose. Eudragit® L and S are anionic copolymers of methacrylic acid and methyl-methacrylate that are water-soluble only above gastric pH, making it possible to mask and protect the dosage form during gastric transit and to unmask the dosage form at intestinal pH. By varying the ratio of monomers, it is possible to accurately tune the pH of dissolution of these copolymers in such a way that drug delivery can be triggered at a specific level along the gastrointestinal tract, depending on the physiological pH prevailing at the considered level. Some types of Eudragit are shown in Figure 4.27 and discussed in Tables 4.5 and 4.6.

Finally, insoluble polymers can be used for controlled-release applications, regardless of the pH. Ethyl cellulose or different Eudragit grades corresponding to copolymers of acrylate and methacrylate bearing no ionisable groups can be used for forming insoluble films at the surface of microgranules, or other dosage forms, and with varying permeability to the drug contained into the dosage form.

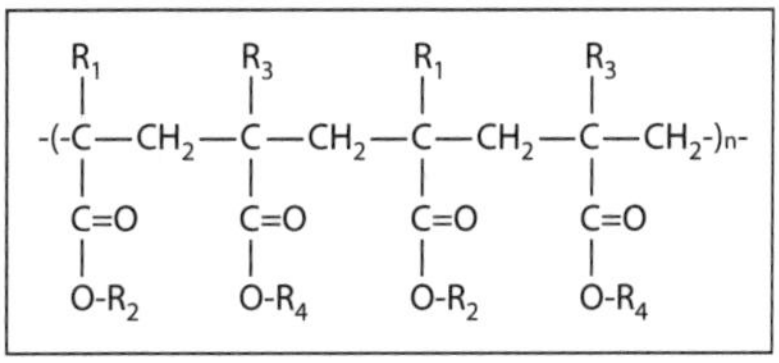

Figure 4.27 General structures of Eudragit®. Variations are given in Table 4.6.

Water vapour permeability

Water vapour permeability can be measured to determine the effectiveness of a film coating to act as a barrier to water. Several variables have been shown to influence water vapour permeability, and considerable variations can be observed when modifying the film composition, film thickness and film preparation technique. By using different experimental setups, it is possible to measure the water vapour transmission rate (WVTR, generally expressed in $g/m^2/day$) of

Table 4.5 Eudragit®: a series of methacrylate-based coating materials with a variety of functional properties

Polymer characteristics	Commercial grades, pH of dissolution and applications
Anionic copolymers of methacrylic acid and alkyl methacrylates with available –COOH groups	Eudragit L 100-55 (powder), soluble above pH 5.5
	Eudragit L 30 D-55 (aqueous dispersion), soluble above pH 5.5 (delivery in upper intestine)
	Eudragit L 100 (powder) soluble above pH 6.0 (delivery in jejunum)
	Eudragit S 100 (powder), soluble above pH 7.0 (delivery in ileum)
	Eudragit FS 30D (aqueous dispersion), soluble above pH 7.0 (delivery in ileum), requires no plasticiser
Cationic copolymer bearing dimethylaminoethyl ammonium groups	Eudragit E 100 (powder or granules), soluble in water up to pH 5.0, swellable and permeable above pH 5.0
Cationic copolymers of acrylate and methacrylates bearing quarternary ammonium groups	Eudragit RL 30D (aqueous dispersion), insoluble and pH-independent polymer for sustained-release formulations, high-permeability films
	Eudragit RL PO (powder), insoluble and pH-independent polymer for sustained-release formulations, high-permeability films
	Eudragit RL 100 (granules), insoluble and pH-independent polymer for sustained-release formulations, high-permeability films
	Eudragit RS 30D (aqueous dispersion), insoluble and pH-independent polymer for sustained-release formulations, low-permeability films
	Eudragit RS PO (powder), insoluble and pH-independent polymer for sustained-release formulations, high-permeability films
	Eudragit RS 100 (granules), insoluble and pH-independent polymer for sustained-release formulations, high-permeability films

isolated or coated films. This latter method is especially useful for investigating the influence of excipients in the tablet core on water vapour permeability.

Oxygen permeability

Oxygen permeability is a measure of the effectiveness of the coating material to act as a barrier to oxygen and is especially important when working with active pharmaceutical ingredients that can be degraded by oxidative

Table 4.6 Composition of main Eudragit® grades, accordingly to the formula presented in Figure 4.27

Eudragit grade	Composition
Type E	R1, R3 = methyl
	R2 = dimethylaminoethyl
	R4 = methyl, butyl
Type L	R1, R3 = methyl
	R2 = H (50% methacrylic acid)
	R4 = methyl
Type S	R1, R3 = methyl
	R2 = H (30% methacrylic acid)
	R4 = methyl
Type RL	R1, R3 = methyl
	R2 = methyl, ethyl
	R4 = trimethylammoniumethacrylate (10%)
Type RS	R1, R3 = methyl
	R2 = methyl, ethyl
	R4 = trimethylammoniumethacrylate (5%)
Type E 30D	R1, R3 = H, methyl
	R2, R4 = methyl, ethyl
Type L 30D	R1, R3 = H, methyl
	R2 = H (50% methacrylic acid)
	R4 = methyl, ethyl

processes. Film composition and film thickness have been shown to significantly influence oxygen transmission. This parameter is determined more easily on isolated films using similar techniques as for water vapour permeability, although it is possible with coated dosage forms. Deposition of a light HPMC-based coating used to produce a high gloss and pearlescent appearance in tablets is enough to slow down the rate of oxygen permeation through an applied film compared with uncoated tablets.

Various methodologies for determining the permeability of materials or polymeric films to water vapour or oxygen have been described. The reader is referred to the references given at the end of the chapter.

Thermal properties

The glass transition temperature (T_g) is an important polymer property that is closely related to the mechanical properties of the polymer films. The T_g is the temperature at which the mechanical properties of a polymer change from a brittle to a rubbery state (see Section 2.3.3). Film coatings need to be simultaneously strong enough and highly flexible in order to remain intact on rough surfaces or when dosage forms such as tablets present angular profiles. There have been numerous studies on T_g to evaluate polymer properties, polymer miscibility and long-term interactions with excipients. The introduction of plasticisers mixed with the polymer is a common strategy to decrease T_g and make the film less brittle. Dynamic mechanical analysis (DMA) is another type of test that can be used to study the relationship between T_g and the mechanical properties of the film.

Another interesting parameter is the minimum film-forming temperature (MFFT), which is the minimum temperature at which a polymeric material is able to coalesce to form a film. At temperatures below MFFT, a white opaque or powdery material is formed, whereas a clear, transparent film is formed at temperatures equal to or greater than MFFT. The MFFT has implications in coating processes. The temperature in the mass during coating must be above the MFFT in order to ensure film formation.

Mechanical testing

Polymer films must be mechanically strong enough such that they do not break or fracture during processing, packaging, shipping or storage. Prediction of these properties is not an easy task, since commonly used experimental techniques such as tensile testing, which are used to assess the mechanical strength of polymer coatings, are performed more easily on isolated films than on deposited films. Alternatively, compression or puncture testing can be carried out directly on the films borne by their substrate.

Adhesion between the polymeric film and substrate is a major concern. Poor adhesion could result in flaking or peeling of the coating from the substrate core. Moisture could accumulate at the film–substrate interface and compromise the mechanical protection provided by the coating. Polymer adhesion is related to both film–substrate interfacial interactions and internal stresses within the film. Polymer adhesion can be evaluated by peel tests or butt joint tests. Apart from the specific properties of the polymers, excipients used in tablet formulations can influence film–tablet adhesion. Since adhesion between a polymer and the tablet surface is due primarily to hydrogen bond formation, hydrophobic agents may decrease adhesion by presenting a surface consisting of mainly apolar hydrocarbon groups, which depends on the nature and concentration of the excipient.

Polymer coatings and drug interactions

For many pharmaceutical applications, polymeric coatings and most dosage forms are water-soluble. During application of the coating layers on the substrate, dissolution of the outermost surfaces of the substrate can occur quite easily, resulting in mixing and migration of the drug or excipient into the coating film. This phenomenon can affect the mechanical, adhesive and drug-release properties of the polymer film. Similar migrations can occur during the shelf life of the products, even in the presence of very low amounts of water and regardless of the water solubility of the polymeric coating. This negative effect can often be limited by depositing a preventive HPMC sub-coating as a sandwich layer between the drug-containing dosage form and the functional polymeric coating.

4.4.4 Adhesive polymers for skin delivery

The domain of medical adhesives is broad and can be divided into different categories, including structural adhesives for assembly of medical devices, tissue adhesives (e.g. surgical glues) and pressure-sensitive adhesives (PSAs), mostly designed to adhere at the surface of the skin. Typical applications for PSAs in the healthcare industry include wound coverings and closures, surgical drapes, ostomy (i.e. a surgically created opening in the body for the discharge of body wastes) mounts and pouches, electrocardiograph electrode mounts, electrosurgical grounding pads, and transdermal drug delivery systems.

Adhesion to skin

Skin is a very demanding and variable substrate for adhesive bonding. Various applications are based on the use of PSAs. The minimal requirements for PSAs are (i) to adhere easily to varying skin types for a prolonged period of time, (ii) to be removable without leaving adhesive residue or causing skin damage and pain and (iii) to be not irritating to the skin.

Skin is a rough surface, requiring PSAs to have the capacity to spread and to flow easily. For this reason, PSAs should have a T_g or softening temperatures ranging from $-20\,^{\circ}\mathrm{C}$ to $-60\,^{\circ}\mathrm{C}$, meaning that these materials are soft materials at skin temperature. Once the PSA has spread at the surface of the skin, optimal adhesion is dictated by two main properties: the surface energy of the PSA–skin, and the bulk rheological properties of the adhesive polymer. Formulation of PSAs for skin applications is rather difficult since it requires good, prolonged adhesion at the skin surface and simultaneously easy removal with minimal trauma, regardless of the duration of application.

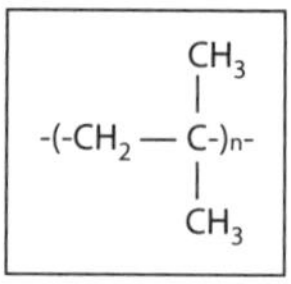

$$-(-CH_2 - \underset{\underset{CH_3}{|}}{\overset{\overset{CH_3}{|}}{C}}-)_{n}-$$

Figure 4.28   Repeating unit of poly(isobutylene).

The surface energy of the adhesive has to be lower than that of skin. The surface energy of the skin is dependent on temperature, relative humidity due to transepithelial water loss (TEWL), sudation and sebum secretion. It is in the range 40–60 mJ/m^2; that of the non-polar components under normal conditions is higher than that of the polar components. For the sake of comparison, acrylic medical-grade PSAs may have surface energies in the range 25–30 mJ/m^2.

Adhesion results from the combination of an adequate surface energy couple between the PSA and skin and rheological properties. Adhesion is commonly measured by a peeling test, which involves the measurement of the force required to peel an adhesive, spread on to a flexible backing, from a substrate whose surface properties are well characterised.

Polymers used in the formulation of medical grade PSAs

Natural rubber and poly(isobutylene) (Figure 4.28) were the earliest polymers used for formulating medical PSAs due to their high peel strength, elongation and ease of acceptance by skin tissue.

Poly(isobutylene) has a low T_g, producing naturally flexible materials that are naturally tacky masses. Poly(isobutylene) (molecular weight 80 000– 100 000) such as Vistanex™ are used for the preparation of medical tape. This polymer needs to be tackified, which can be achieved by mixing with polybutyl rubber or other low-molecular-weight poly(isobutylene) or mineral oils. However, for more demanding applications, these are now largely replaced with modern, synthetic polymers, which are used in the formulation of medical-grade PSAs, depending on the applications, as described in Table 4.7.

Acrylic polymers are used widely due to their wide tailoring possibilities and their low allergenicity. Poly(acrylates) come from the polymerisation of acrylic acid esters. The group borne by acrylate can be an alkyl group or be varied in functionality, with a varying hydrophilic/hydrophobic nature, in order to confer original properties to the adhesive. The length of the chain is used as a variable to adjust the adhesive properties. Moreover, the presence of a methyl group in poly(methacrylates) is known to produce a higher T_g (see Section 2.3.3).

Acrylic copolymers are normally synthesised by free radical polymerisation to produce random copolymers of molecular weight typically in the range 200 000–1 000 000 g/mol. They are typically composed of mixtures of different monomers, the proportions being adjusted for a specific T_g value. Some acrylic monomers (commonly called 'hard monomers') are known to produce

Table 4.7 Polymers used in the formulation of medical-grade pressure-sensitive adhesives (PSAs)

Polymer	Application	Requested functionality
Silicone (PDMS)	Transdermal drug-delivery systems	Chemically inert, biocompatible, high drug permeability
Poly(vinyl ether)	Skin patches, surgical dressings	Moisture permeability
Poly(vinyl pyrrolidone)	Ostomy	Moisture absorption
Polyacrylates	Transdermal drug-delivery systems	Chemically inert, ability to control drug release
	First-aid dressings	Quick adhesion, adherence during normal daily activity
	Electromedical devices	Long-term adhesion
	Surgical dressings	Moisture permeability
	Incise drapes	Sterilisable, wet stick
	Surgical tapes	Sterilisable
Hydrophilic gels	Electromedical applications	Moisture absorption, quick adhesion
Natural rubber and poly (isobutylene)	First-aid dressings	Adherence during normal daily activity, quick adhesion

hard homopolymers characterised by high T_g, and others ('soft monomers') are known to produce homopolymers with low T_g. Table 4.8 summarises the T_g of acrylic homopolymers prepared from typical monomers used in medical PSAs.

Various functionalities can be imparted to these adhesives, including high moisture vapour transmission rate (MVTR), which is of importance for

Table 4.8 Glass transition temperatures (T_g) of acrylic homopolymers derived from typical monomers used in medical pressure-sensitive adhesives (PSAs)

Monomer	T_g of homopolymer	Rigidity of segment
n-Butyl acrylate	−54 °C	Soft segment
2-Ethylhexyl acrylate	−70 °C	Soft segment
Acrylic acid	106 °C	Hard segment
Vinyl acetate	30 °C	Hard segment
n-Butyl methacrylate	20 °C	Hard segment

prolonged duration of adhesion, for wet stick or for when adhesion on the wet skin is requested. Enduction processes are generally used for preparing adhesive devices, often requiring the use of solvent-based acrylic adhesives. Attempts have been made to develop alternative strategies, including the preparation of acrylic dispersions by emulsion polymerisation and the development of hot-melt adhesives.

Silicones form the third category of PSAs. They have been used since the 1960s for bandages and medical tapes. Silicone adhesives are typically prepared from poly(dimethylsiloxane) and silicone resins, which are cross-linked to impart sufficient mechanical resistance to the adhesive. As silicone adhesives contain no plasticisers, no tackifiers and no stabilisers, they have excellent skin compatibility and make non-irritating, non-sensitising materials. Silicone adhesives are found in transdermal delivery systems because of their high permeability to drugs, allowing control of the delivery of various ingredients to the skin and subsequently yielding pharmacokinetic profiles extending over a few days.

4.4.5   Ion-exchange resins

Immobilisation of drugs on ion-exchange resins has been proposed in pharmaceutical formulations for different applications such as taste-masking, improving drug stability, enhancing dissolution, and providing a sustained-release effect for orally active drugs. Ion-exchange resins are water-insoluble cross-linked polymers containing salt-forming groups in repeating position on the polymer chain. These insoluble polymeric porous particles or hydrogels contain basic or acidic groups, which can form ionic complexes with the oppositely charged drugs. Thus, the drug is bound to ion-exchange resin particles via electrostatic interactions. Once administered, and because they are insoluble in physiological fluids, ion-exchange resins are not absorbed from the gastrointestinal tract and do not have significant associated side-effects.

Taste-masking represents an interesting application of ion-exchange resins, since drugs do not display their original taste characteristics in a bound state. Most of the bitter drugs have an amine as a functional group, which is the cause of their taste. If the amino functional groups are blocked by complex formation with cationic resins, then the bitterness of these drugs can be drastically reduced. Once the drug is administered, and as the pH and ionic strength of the physiological fluids in the gastrointestinal tract change with time and location, the drug can be desorbed from the resin, possibly providing a sustained-release effect.

Strong acid anionic resins such as sulphonated styrene-divinyl benzene copolymers can be used to mask the taste of basic drugs with a bitter taste. They can be used almost throughout the entire physiological pH range above

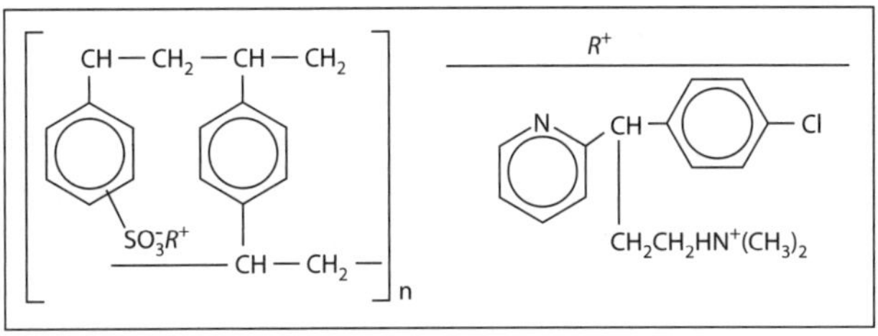

Figure 4.29 Sulphonated styrene-divinylbenzene copolymer complex with chlorphen amine.

pH6. Similarly, strong base cationic exchange resins are efficient throughout the entire pH range, while the weak base cationic exchange resins are functional below pH7. The apparent pK_a values of resins based on sulphonic, phosphoric and carboxylic acids as exchanger groups are in the range 1–2, 3 and 4–6, respectively. The apparent pK_a values of resins bearing quaternary, tertiary or secondary ammonium groups are in the ranges > 13, 7–9 and 5–9, respectively. The rate at which the drug can be released from its complex with the resin in the physiological fluids is significantly influenced by the apparent pK_a value of the resin.

Insoluble adsorbates or resinates are formed through weak ionic bonding of the resin with oppositely charged drugs, as shown in Figure 4.29. They are prepared either by soaking the purified resins in a solution of ionised drug or by passing a concentrated solution of drug through an ion-exchange-packed column until the effluent concentration is the same as in the eluent concentration. Drug complexation depends on the particle size, porosity and swelling, depending on the cross-linking degree, acid/base strength and available capacity of the resin. At the end of the preparation process, resinates are produced in the form of powders, which can be formulated to form solid dosage forms, such as tablets or capsules. In some cases, and because release can be very rapid in the presence of ions in saliva, a preventive coating with a semi-permeable membrane such as ethyl cellulose can be requested.

4.4.6 Polymers for controlled delivery following parenteral administration

Polymeric implants

Parenteral delivery of drugs can be foreseen for various reasons, for example circumventing impaired oral absorption and achieving controlled release for a long duration. For this latter application, implants have been conceived for delivering drugs during an extended period of time, from months to years. Such applications are very demanding, since the polymers used for preparing implants must not only control the delivery of the drug but also be biocompatible and non-toxic. The preparation should be easily delivered, meaning that soft or liquid preparations are of interest from this point of view. In order to avoid surgical removal, implant applications require the polymer to be biodegradable and to yield low-toxicity degradation products, which should not create any inflammation and should be cleared rapidly from the body. Moreover, the polymer must be able to encapsulate and efficiently control drug release during an extended period. Finally, specific mechanical properties (rigidity versus flexibility) may be requested. Because no single polymer is able to fulfil all of these criteria, a family of polymers has been progressively created by industry and academia, and nowadays a broad choice of polymers series is available to the formulator. Research in this area is focused increasingly on the development of polymers conceived specifically for exactly matching the requested criteria for specific delivery cases.

Poly(α-hydroxyacid)s are the leading biodegradable polymers that have been developed. The poly(α-hydroxyacid)s series of polymers includes PLA and PLGA as well as other polymers such as polycaprolactone and poly (butyric acid) (see Section 4.2). These well-known polymers have been studied extensively for implant applications, and many drug-delivery systems based on these polymers are now commercialised.

Apart from these polymers, some polyanhydrides have undergone active clinical development. Polyanhydrides involving sebacic acid (hydrophilic component) and carboxyphenoxypropane (hydrophobic component) have been used to develop a matrix for Gliadel®, a commercial product for the sustained release of carmustine, an anti-cancer drug used in the treatment of brain tumours. Other anhydrides have also been investigated, such as poly-(erucic acid dimer : sebacic acid 50 : 50) copolymers for the development of implants for the antibiotic treatment of osteomyelitis.

Specifically designed polyphosphoesters (Figure 4.30) have been developed for applications in drug delivery and tissue engineering. Their composition can be modified to obtain polymers with a wide range of properties and useful versatile mechanical properties, making it possible to formulate injectable gels, elastomeric films and amorphous solids. The phosphate groups make the polymer more soluble in common organic solvents and improve the polymer flexibility. Finally, the phosphate groups impart hydrophilicity to the polymer, which reduces protein adsorption on the device surface.

Polyphosphazenes (Figure 4.31) contain alternating phosphorus-nitrogen double and single bonds and side-chain functionalities that can be varied to

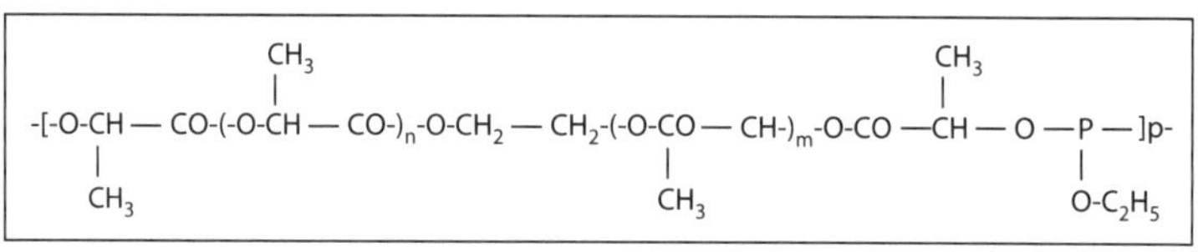

Figure 4.30 Example of polyphosphoester.

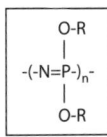

Figure 4.31   General structure of polyphosphazenes.

obtain various series of polymers with a wide range of properties, including water solubility and degradability. Polyphosphazenes have been synthesised by reaction of poly(dichlorophosphazene) with organic nucleophiles such as alkoxides, aryl-oxides or amines. Water-soluble polyphosphazenes have attracted special attention due to the possibility of formulating sensitive drugs such as proteins and vaccines via a completely aqueous process.

Other series of polymers have also been investigated extensively, including hydrolytically labile poly(orthoester)s, poly(aminoacids) and pseudopoly-(amino acid)s.

Polymer–drug conjugates and targeting by water-soluble polymeric conjugates

Polymer–drug conjugates were born in the mid 1970s thanks to the development of monoclonal antibodies by Milstein and Köhler and to the Ringsdorf vision of what a polymeric drug carrier should be. The driving forces were searches for new drug-delivery platforms to improve the therapeutic index of drugs active against severe diseases but presenting major limitations. Typically, some drug candidates exhibit a short half-life in the bloodstream due to either a rapid degradation or rapid clearance rate. The smallest molecules distribute evenly in the body, diffusing in both diseased and healthy tissues. In consequence, only a small amount of the administered drug reaches the target tissue, and hence the therapy is associated with severe side-effects.

Several advantages were foreseen by using polymer–drug conjugates to improve the therapeutic efficacy of those drugs:

- Better control of the biodistribution of the drug by associating a targeting moiety; this led to the earlier strategy development of antibody–drug conjugates
- Improvement of the targeting efficacy based on multivalent interactions with target cells
- Protection against degradation
- Reduction of the immunogenicity of proteinic or peptidic drugs
- Prolonged retention of the drug in the blood compartment thanks to the reduction of renal clearance for the smallest drug molecules.

Then it appeared that conjugation of drugs with a polymer or macromolecule enhanced its passive distribution in favour to tumour tissue. This enhanced permeation and retention (EPR) effect was explained by differences

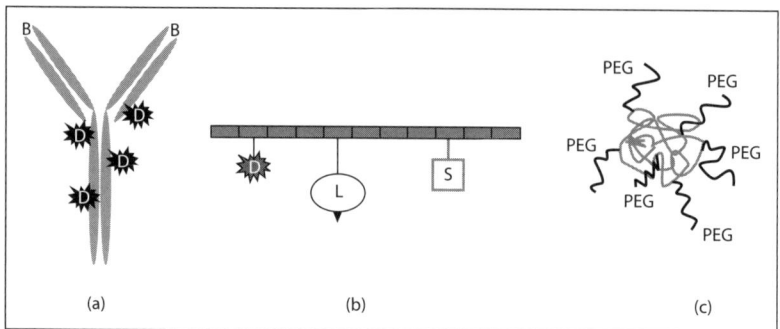

Figure 4.32 Schematic representation of the three kinds of polymer–drug conjugates.
(a) Antibody–drug conjugates with a mean of four drug molecules (D) per antibody. Each antibody has two binding sites (B) for high specificity of recognition for the corresponding antigen.
(b) Polymer–drug conjugate built according to the original model of Ringsdorf. Many drug molecules (D), ligands for specific targeting (L) and chemical groups to adjust the solubilising properties of the conjugate (S) can be grafted on the polymer backbone (grey oblongs), which serves as a carrier.
(c) PEGylated peptides or proteins are therapeutic peptides or proteins on which chains of poly(ethyleneglycol) (PEG) have been grafted.

in the biochemical and physiological characteristics between healthy and malignant tissues that allowed entry and accumulation of macromolecules only in solid tumours and not in healthy tissues. Another interesting benefit is the enhancement of the solubility of new cytotoxic drugs designed by the pharmaceutical industry. Many of these molecules displayed extremely high potential as anticancer agents in cell culture but their clinical development was hampered because their solubility characteristics made them extremely difficult to administer in vivo. In addition, their toxicological profile combined with their lack of specificity required them to be associated with a targeting strategy in order to improve their biodistribution towards diseased tissues.

Three types of polymer–drug conjugate have been described, as presented in Figure 4.32: antibody–drug conjugates, synthetic polymer–drug conjugates and PEGylated-peptides and proteins. All of these are built from the covalent coupling of drug molecules to a macromolecule. Therefore, from an industrial standpoint, polymer–drug conjugates can be considered more like new chemical entities. This implies that their development needs to follow the development route requested for a new drug. Indeed, the drug molecule is modified by the covalent attachment to the macromolecule. Thus, the resulting drug-delivery system cannot be considered as a conventional formulation in which the drug molecule remains chemically intact and is simply entrapped in the formulation. It is noteworthy that, despite this constraint, several marketed compounds are currently used in clinics and the Food and Drug Administration (FDA) has approved more macromolecular drugs than small molecules for a couple of years. In fact, the development of the first marketed compounds from these macromolecular drug conjugates has overcome many

challenging milestones, including the difficulty of obtaining a perfectly reproducible batch-to-batch synthesis of a polymer–drug conjugate with precise
physicochemical characteristics. It has also been demonstrated that it is
possible to validate all steps of the production by developing appropriate
methods of analysis.

Antibody–drug conjugates

The rationale behind the development of antibody–drug conjugates was to
increase the specificity of the biodistribution of the drug (Figure 4.32a). Such
conjugates result from the covalent attachment of drug molecules to antibodies. In such a construct, the two partners have to show perfect complementary actions. The antibody, which is mostly not cytotoxic, brings the high
specificity of targeting, while the drug, generally a cytotoxic agent with a very
poor selectivity for tumours, brings the cell-killing ability. Although most
classical coupling reactions can be used, precautions must be taken to preserve
both the antibody recognition specificity and the drug activity.

In practice, humanised monoclonal antibodies are used to avoid induction
of an immune response. Other advantages of using these antibodies are their
long half-life in the blood circulation (up to several days) and their non-
toxicity during circulation. Some of them show a low cytotoxic effect when
they interact with the corresponding antigens found on the target cell surface.
However, as they are highly specific for a single antigen found only on the
surface of the target tumour cells, their role is supposed to carry very specifically the cytotoxic agent. Antibodies showing an affinity towards its antigen
of 1 nM expressed as the dissociation constant are considered as suitable to be
used as a targeting tool. The linkage of the drug to the antibody is often
achieved through a spacer. Based on the experience acquired by authors
who have developed drug–antibody conjugates over the past 30 years, the
linker between the drug and the antibody needs to be stable during circulation
in blood but should be cleaved to release the original drug molecule after
arrival at the destination.

Several types of linker have been investigated, including acidic sensitive
bonds, covalent bonds cleavable by esterases or proteases, and disulfide
bonds. Spacers including a disulfide bond present many advantages and have
been used to synthesise antibody–drug conjugates of the last generation. They
can be stable during the period of storage of the drug conjugate and remain
intact in the blood. As required, they can be cleaved to release the drug in the
intracellular medium of cancer cells because the amount of glutathione
responsible for the scission of disulfide bounds is important in the intracellular
medium (millimolar range versus micromolar range in the extracellular
medium). In general, an average of four drug molecules can be grafted per
antibody. The grafting occurs on the most accessible lysine residues among
the 80 available on the antibody. Although this method of targeting presents

high potential for cytotoxic drugs to develop very efficient treatments with drugs presenting an adverse toxicological profile, the low number of drug molecules grafted per antibody may represent a limitation for the efficacy of the treatment.

In a very similar approach, it was suggested to use transferrin as a carrier and targeting tool for anticancer drugs. The rationale behind this idea was to use transferrin as the targeting moiety to recognise cells overexpressing the receptor for transferrin on their surface and allowing the drug to penetrate into cells via the internalisation route specific to the transferrin receptor.

Synthetic polymer–drug conjugates

Conjugates obtained from synthetic polymers were developed as alternative carriers for drug targeting. These polymers are tailor-made according to the original model suggested by Ringsdorf (Figure 4.32b) as a function of the drug-targeting goal. They were extensively developed as tools for intralysosomal delivery of cytotoxic agents presenting major limitations for clinical applications. In general, the polymer backbone can host many drug molecules, which are linked to the polymer backbone through a spacer containing a bond, which can be cleaved when the conjugate has reached the target. Targeting moieties including small ligands, antibodies or antibody fragments are grafted on the same polymer chains, as are groups ensuring that the polymer remains fully soluble in biological media. High-molecular-weight species have been designed. This is required to promote passive targeting of the carrier to tumour tissue from the general circulation thanks to the EPR effect. However, the molecular weight should not exceed 100 000 g/mol in order to ensure endocytic internalisation by cells. In addition, the molecular weight of non-biodegradable polymers should be below 40 000 g/mol in order to allow final elimination by renal filtration. Nevertheless, higher-molecular-weight polymers can be designed by including cleavable bonds, which reduce the molecular weight, to allow internalisation by cells or final elimination. Once in the tumour, the targeting moieties grafted on the polymer ensure a high specificity of recognition of the target cells. In general, the affinity is also very high thanks to multivalent interactions between the carrier and the target cell because several targeting moieties can be carried on a single polymer–drug conjugate.

Besides the molecular weight requirements, other features are required to design an effective polymer–drug conjugate. The polymer used as the carrier must be non-toxic and non-immunogenic. The spacer between the drug molecule and the polymer should include a cleavable bond in order to allow release of the intact drug molecule only at arrival at the target site. Finally, the addition of solubilising groups may be required in case the original polymer becomes insoluble in biological fluids after grafting of the drug and the targeting moiety.

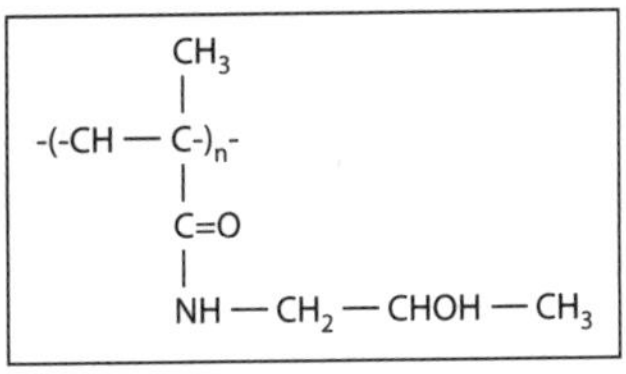

$$-(-CH-\underset{\underset{\underset{NH-CH_2-CHOH-CH_3}{|}}{\underset{C=O}{|}}}{\overset{\overset{CH_3}{|}}{C}}-)_n-$$

Figure 4.33 Repeating unit of poly(2-hydroxypropylmethacrylamide).

Much experience has been acquired by designing poly(2-hydroxypropyl-methacrylamide) (PHPMA; Figure 4.33) copolymers. Such copolymers were the first synthetic polymer–drug conjugates to be entered in human clinical trials. They are composed of a linear polymer backbone of PHPMA in which several of the hydroxypropyl groups serve as anchor either for the grafting of the drug through a spacer or for the grafting of the targeting ligand. These copolymers have been designed as lysosomotropic drug carriers for most of the first-line anticancer agents, including doxorubicin, paclitaxel and platinates (carboplatinate, 1,2-diaminocyclohexane platinate).

Another polymer candidate identified as a potential carrier is poly(glutamic acid). These polymer–drug conjugates were shown to highly enhance the therapeutic value of the drugs coupled to the polymer carrier. At the same time, they reduced drug toxicity thanks to better control of the biodistribution.

Polymer–drug conjugates can be designed as drug-delivery platforms to carry a cocktail of drugs in a single cell. In this case, at least two types of drug are grafted on a single polymer molecule. A straightforward application of such a drug-carrier system would be therapy of resistant cancer cells. Indeed, the different drugs carried on a single polymer chain would reach the same cells, where they could act in a synergistic manner to counteract the multicellular resistant pathways.

It is noteworthy that the first polymer–drug conjugates developed involved simple structures, i.e. linear polymers. Now it is possible to design polymers with more sophisticated architectures such as star-like or dendrimeric structures. Some of these novel architectures display interesting new properties, including stimuli-responsive abilities that could be integrated into polymer–drug conjugates. However, efforts are still needed to develop such architectures with polymers with suitable toxicological profiles for in vivo applications.

Polymer–protein conjugates

Polymer–protein conjugates constitute the class of drug conjugates that is the most advanced in terms of clinical development and applications. Several such compounds are marketed and used routinely in oncology. In addition, the number of peptide-, protein- and antibody-based drugs entering into use in clinics is growing rapidly, giving new opportunities to develop conjugates to enhance the performance of the drugs. In fact, the main limitations of these drugs are their short half-life because of their poor stability in biological fluids and the immunogenicity of the large proteins. Conjugation to a polymer was suggested to form a shield around the molecule, preventing the action of proteases and hence prolonging the half-life in the blood. Historically, the first polymer–protein conjugate consisted of an antitumor protein, neocarzinostatin (NCS), on which two chains of (styrene-alt-maleic anhydride) copolymer (SMA) were grafted. The resulting conjugate, SMANCS, was brought to market in 1990 to treat patients with primary liver cancer (hepatocellular carcinoma). The concept of building a shield around the protein with a synthetic polymer to protect it from degradation has been found to be very efficient.

The technology developed with SMA was not pursued but evolved towards the use of PEG for more convenient and safer protein therapeutics. The use of PEG presents several advantages. PEG is very well tolerated by the organism after intravenous administration. PEG has been found to reduce and even suppress the immunogenicity of proteins by shielding epitopes. Another interesting property brought by PEGylation is that it increases the solubility of the modified proteins in biological fluids. Finally, the pharmacokinetics of PEGylated proteins are highly modified compared with the pharmacokinetics of the corresponding native protein thanks to efficient protection of the protein drugs against degradation by proteases. All of these advantages place PEG in the first line of polymers used to design polymer–protein drug conjugates. The main applications are concerned with improvement of therapy with enzymes and cytokines.

In practice, there are many possibilities for attaching a PEG molecule to proteins and peptides. In general, a specific group is attached on the terminal hydroxyl group of the PEG chain, allowing chemical grafting on free amine, carboxylic, hydroxyl or thiol groups of the protein. It is noteworthy that only a few reactions can be applied for preserving the biological activity of the protein. The most used methods relied on chemical conjugation through reactive side-chain groups on the amino acids of the peptidic chains. This allowed selective grafting of the PEG chain on to defined amino acids of the protein. To improve the selectivity of the grafting method, it was suggested to use recombinant proteins in which a mutation was introduced on a much more defined amino acid in order to make attachment of the PEG chain possible. Although this method increased control of the grafting method, it required selection of a recombinant protein with the proper mutation for each therapeutic protein to be modified.

Alternative methods of highly selective coupling reactions were developed using enzymes. These methods were easier to develop on a large number of proteins with little effort. In the first example, the PEG chain can be transferred on an O-glycosylated site of glycosylated native proteins. The reaction can be catalysed by a specific enzyme, a glycosyl transferase, which confers a high specificity of the coupling reaction. The PEG chains are positioned exactly on the O-glycosylation site of the protein. This method of grafting was applied for PEGylation of three clinically used proteins – granulocyte colony-stimulating factor (G-CSF), interferon alpha2b (INF-α2b), and granulocyte/macrophage colony-stimulating factor (GM-CSF).

In recent years, another enzymatic mediated modification was applied with success to bind PEG on proteins of clinical interest. The enzyme, a transglutaminase, allowed the transfer of an amino derivative of PEG, PEG-NH$_2$, on a glutamine residue of the protein located in a flexible or unfolded region of the peptidic chain. Specificity of the enzyme was high and led to a very high degree of specificity for the PEGylation of the protein. This method of protein PEGylation has already been used successfully to produce several PEGylated proteins of clinical interest, including human growth hormone and interleukin 2. A promising development for the PEGylation of therapeutic peptides and proteins is expected in the future. Indeed, recent work has opened up the possibility of predicting sites of transglutaminase-mediated PEGylation of therapeutic proteins. This discovery has paved the road towards predicting the possible effects caused by the modification of the physicochemical and functional properties of the protein and will be very useful in the design of proper strategies for the modification of proteins.

Polymeric nanoparticles for drug delivery

Nanoparticles, i.e. particles with a size usually in the range 50–1000 nm, have drawn the attention of researchers designing drug-delivery systems that can be injected intravenously owing to their small size. Nanoparticle is a general name for nanospheres and nanocapsules. Nanospheres have a matrix-type structure, whereas nanocapsules are hollow and have a liquid core surrounded by a polymeric wall, as illustrated in Figure 4.34.

Several methods have been developed for preparing nanoparticles. They can be classified into two main categories according to whether the formation of nanoparticles occurs during a polymerisation reaction or whether it is achieved directly from already prepared macromolecules.

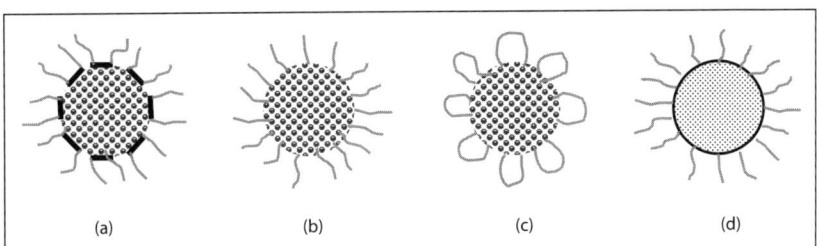

(a)   (b)   (c)   (d)

Figure 4.34 Different types of nanoparticle: (a) nanosphere stabilised by an adsorbed non-ionic surfactant; (b) core-shell nanosphere with a brush shell structure; (c) core-shell nanosphere with a loop shell structure; (d) core-shell nanocapsule with a brush shell structure.

In the biomedical field, polymeric colloidal systems have been proposed for years as supporting surfaces for diagnostic tests, owing to their high specific surface area, high stability and ease of handling. Such nanoparticles can be easily prepared from several monomers by free radical emulsion polymerisation (see Section 3.7.2). In the pharmaceutical field, nanoparticles made of non-biodegradable polymers such as polyacrylamide or poly(methylmethacrylate) were proposed during the 1970s as adjuvants for vaccines. Since then, the technology for making polymeric nanoparticles has been adapted to the many requirements for a drug carrier, including biocompatibility, biodegradability, compatibility with the drug to be carried, drug-loading efficacy, defined drug-releasing properties and in vivo targeting.

Anionic emulsion polymerisation of alkylcyanoacrylates (ACA) was introduced to design bioerodible polymeric nanospheres or nanocapsules suitable for in vivo delivery of drugs. Emulsions formulated to prepare poly(alkylcyanoacrylates) (PACA) nanospheres to be used as drug carriers were rather complex. The monomer ACA is dispersed in acidified water containing a surfactant or a stabilising agent and the drug. This system is left to polymerise spontaneously for a few hours. The resulting colloidal polymeric particles have a diameter ranging from 50 nm to 300 nm. Nanocapsules can be prepared by interfacial polymerisation of ACA performed in micro-emulsion. Oil-containing nanocapsules are obtained by polymerisation of ACA at the oil/water interface of a very fine oil-in-water emulsion. In practice, the oil, the monomer and the drug are dissolved in a water-miscible organic solvent to prepare the organic phase. This organic phase is injected in the aqueous phase containing a surfactant through a fine needle and under strong magnetic stirring. A milky suspension of nanocapsules forms immediately. The organic phase is then removed under reduced pressure. Preparation of oil-containing nanocapsules is illustrated in Figure 4.35.

Water-containing nanocapsules can be obtained by interfacial polymerisation of ACA in water-in-oil micro-emulsion. In such a system, water-swollen micelles of surfactants of small and uniform size are dispersed in

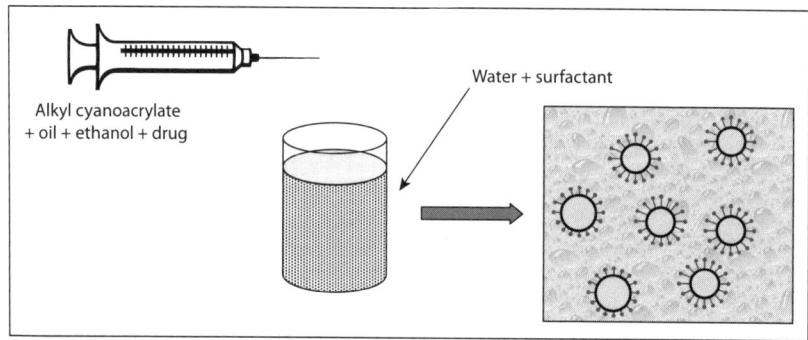

Alkyl cyanoacrylate
+ oil + ethanol + drug

Water + surfactant

Figure 4.35 Formation of nanocapsules by interfacial polymerisation.

an organic phase. The monomer is added to the oily phase once the micro-emulsion has formed and the anionic polymerisation is initiated at the surface of the water swollen micelles. The polymer that forms locally at the water/oil interface precipitates, allowing formation of the nanocapsule shell. Nanocapsules obtained by this method are of special interest for the encapsulation of water-soluble molecules such as peptides.

Nanoparticles can also be obtained from a polymer that has previously been prepared according to a totally independent method. The general principle is based on the solubility properties of the polymer. A diluted solution of the polymer is prepared and a phase separation is induced by addition of a non-solvent or by a salting-out effect. Once the proper conditions to form polymeric colloids are identified, the particles can be stabilised either by elimination of the polymer solvent by evaporation or by chemical cross-linking of the polymer.

Nanospheres and nanocapsules can also be prepared by the same methods as those described for microparticles, except that manufacturing parameters have to be adjusted in order to obtain nanometre-size droplets. Micro-encapsulation techniques adapted for making nanoparticles require formation of an emulsion as a first step of the procedure. Special equipment is needed to reduce the droplet size of the emulsion during dispersion of the polymer solution into the continuous aqueous phase. This equipment is a high-pressure homogeniser and a micro-fluidiser in which a very high energy input is produced. The drug is usually dispersed in the matrix of the nanospheres or dissolved in the core of the nanocapsules. The drug can also be adsorbed on the surface of the nanoparticles.

The main advantage of colloidal drug carrier systems is their submicronic size range. Provided that they do not aggregate, nanoparticles can be administered intravenously without any risk of embolisation and can diffuse through capillary vessels and mucosae. Despite the small size of nanoparticles, it has been shown that they are quickly removed from the circulation after intravenous administration. The uptake by macrophages located in the organs of the mononuclear phagocytic system (MPS) is mediated by particle interaction with opsonins, mainly the complement system, which plays a key role in the non-specific recognition and uptake of foreign bodies. Thus, delivery of drugs carried by nanoparticles to these organs is facilitated, and advantage can be taken of the uptake for delivering drugs, for instance inside infected phagocytes. Indeed, the low efficacy of some drugs is often related to a low uptake of the free drug. Some drugs are also cardiotoxic and can not be administered free. In both cases, delivering such drugs mainly to phagocytes has been shown to be of great interest. Delivery of cytotoxic drugs incorporated into some nanoparticles to multidrug-resistant cancer cells has also been shown to reverse resistance.

Such a particle size range and the associated large specific surface area are also desirable for the oral, lymphatic and pulmonary routes, and for ocular, subcutaneous and intramuscular administration, offering new functions such as increased duration of contact and adhesion to tissues. A lot of work has been done on vaccine delivery by nanoparticles through different routes, and the large specific surface area of such systems has increased the adjuvant properties. Many reviews are available on such applications of nanoparticles.

Despite these already cited uses, site-specific delivery of drugs to tissues and organs other than MPS through intravenous injection has been hindered by the uptake by phagocytes. In an attempt to reduce opsonisation followed by fast uptake by phagocytes, the concept of steric stabilisation of particles has been introduced. To this end, nanoparticles with prolonged blood circulation times have been designed. These nanoparticles usually comprise a hydrophobic biodegradable core stabilised by a hydrophilic shell. They are spontaneously formed in aqueous phase from amphiphilic block copolymers, i.e. polymeric surfactants, in which a long enough hydrophobic block is bound to the hydrophilic block by a covalent linkage. The most popular systems designed for human use have been obtained by preparing block copolymers in which poly(ethylene oxide) (PEO) or PEG are introduced as the hydrophilic blocks of the copolymers. The hydrophobic blocks associated with PEO and PEG are composed of PLA, PLGA or PACA. Biblock, triblock and graft copolymers have been obtained and are illustrated in Figure 4.36.

Special attention should be devoted to nanoparticles obtained from copolymers containing sugars or polysaccharides as constituents of the

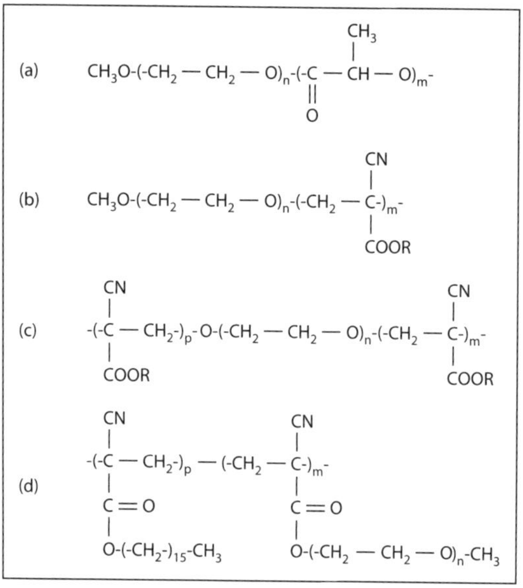

Figure 4.36 Block and graft amphiphilic copolymers leading to core-shell nanoparticles in aqueous solutions: (a) PEO-PLA biblock copolymer, (b) PEO-PACA biblock copolymer, (c) PACA-PEG-PACA triblock copolymer, and (d) Poly[hexadecyl cyanoacrylate-graft-(PEO)-] copolymer.

hydrophilic shell. Sugars are present on the surface of cells and are involved in many surface properties of the cells. Therefore, biomimetic strategies could be developed that take advantage of the presence of polysaccharides on the surface of the nanoparticles. A few polysaccharides are already administered to humans, for instance dextran and heparin. Heparin is well known for its anticoagulant activity and has been shown to act as a physiological inhibitor of complement activation. In order to mimic the behaviour of cells and pathogens that normally escape recognition by complement and phagocytes, block copolymers of heparin and poly(methylmethacrylate) or PACA have been produced and heparin-coated nanospheres have been prepared. These nanospheres have been shown to be non-activators of complement in vitro. In vivo, after intravenous administration to mice, these nanospheres could remain in the bloodstream and show long circulating properties. In addition, it has been shown that the conformation of the polysaccharide chains grafted on the nanosphere surface could play a very important role in defining the fate of the colloidal particle after intravenous administration. Indeed, a long enough dextran bound to nanospheres by one end, i.e. in brush conformation (Figure 4.34b), has been shown to be as low an activator of complement as soluble dextran, whereas the same dextran bound by several bonds, i.e. in loops and train conformation (Figure 4.34c), is as strong an activator as cross-linked dextran, i.e. Sephadex. Block copolymers obtained from other poly-saccharides and PACA could be obtained in brush conformation. Provided that the polysaccharide chains are long enough, they could be low activators of complement and have been developed for purposes in which at least long-circulating properties are required.

Core-shell nanoparticles with a heparin and/or dextran shell in brush conformation have been shown to be able to carry functional haemoglobin and to protect it from degradation. Similarly, core-shell nanoparticles with a chitosan shell in brush conformation have been shown able to carry siRNA active against cancer in a mice model after intravenous administration.

4.4.7 Safety and recognition of new polymers as excipients

Pharmaceutical excipients have a vital role in drug formulations. However, the development of new excipients is often neglected because of a lack of mechanisms to assess the safety of excipients outside a new drug application process. Existing regulations and guidelines state that new excipients should be treated as new chemical entities with full toxicological evaluation. Therefore, successful development of new polymeric excipients depends on obtaining appropriate toxicological data on the safety and biocompatibility of such excipients. There exist specific relevant guidelines for specific delivery systems, such as implant applications, which have been developed by the United States Pharmacopoeia (USP) for testing of the polymer safety and tissue irritability. One example of such a test is the USP Biological Reactivity Test, in vivo, which includes the systemic injection test, the intracutaneous test and the implantation test. Such guidelines may be of relevance when developing a polymer excipient for parenteral controlled-release applications. Other guidelines from the European Medicines Evaluation Agency (EMEA) and the FDA describe the type of data package required in the preclinical development of a new excipient.

Bibliography

Polymeric biomaterials

Arshady R, ed. (1999). *Microspheres, Microcapsules and Liposomes. Vol. 2: Medical and Biotechnology Applications.* London: Citus Books.
Barbucci R, ed. (2002). *Integrated Biomaterials Science.* New York: Kluwer Academic/Plenum.
Dumitriu S, ed. (2001). *Polymeric Biomaterials*, 2nd edn. New York: Marcel Dekker.
Vert M (2007). Polymeric biomaterials: strategies of the past vs. strategies of the future. *Prog Polym Sci* 32: 755–761.
Williams DF, ed. (1987). *Definitions in Biomaterials.* Oxford: Elsevier.

Excipients for formulation of conventional dosage forms

American Pharmaceutical Association and the Pharmaceutical Society of Great Britain, eds (2006). *Handbook of Pharmaceutical Excipients*, 5th edn. London: Pharmaceutical Press.
Robyt JF, ed. (1998). *Essentials of Carbohydrate Chemistry.* New York: Springer.
Dumitriu S, ed. (2004). *Polysaccharides: Structural Diversity and Functional Versatility*, 2nd edn. Hoboken: CRC Press.

Polymers as excipients for controlled release by the oral route

Gupta P, Vermani K, Garg S (2002). Hydrogels: from controlled release to pH-responsive drug delivery. *Drug Discov Today* 7: 569–579.
Ponchel G, Irache JM (1998). Specific and non-specific bioadhesive particulate systems for oral delivery to the gastrointestinal tract. *Adv Drug Deliv Rev* 34: 191–219.

Polymers for coating applications

American Society for Testing and Materials (ASTM) (2001). Monograph F 372–99. Standard test method for water vapor transmission rate through plastic film and sheeting using a modulated infrared sensor. West Conshohocken, PA: American Society for Testing and Materials.
Ginity JW, ed. (1996). *Aqueous Polymeric Coatings for Pharmaceutical Dosage Forms*, 2nd rev. expanded edn. New York: Marcel Dekker.
Hercules Technical Bulletin. VC-556C. FMC's excipients for pharmaceutical tablets, capsules and suspensions. The use of Klucel® Pharm hydroxypropylcellulose to increase the utility of hydroxypropyl methylcellulose in aqueous film coating.
Hercules Technical Bulletin. VC-598A. Klucel® EF Pharm hydroxypropylcellulose use in plasticizer-free aqueous film coating.
International Organization for Standardization (ISO) (1995). ISO 2528. Sheet materials. Determination of water vapour transmission rate by the gravimetric (dish) method. Geneva: International Organization for Standardization.

Siepmann F, Siepmann J, Walther M, MacRae RJ, Bodmeier R (2008). Polymer blends for controlled release coatings. *J Control Release* 125: 1–15.

Wood RW, Mulski MJ (1989). Methodology for the determination of water vapor transport across plastic films. *Int J Pharmaceutics* 50: 61–66.

Adhesive polymers for skin delivery

Benedek I, Feldstein MM, eds (2008). *Applications of Pressure-Sensitive Products*. Hoboken: CRC Press.

Satas D (1991). Pressure-sensitive adhesives. In: Szycher M, ed. *High Performance Biomaterials: A Comprehensive Guide to Medical and Pharmaceutical Applications*. Hoboken: CRC Press.

Webster I (1997). Recent developments in pressure sensitive adhesives for medical applications. *Int J Adhesion Adhesives* 17: 69–73.

Polymer–drug conjugates and targeting by water-soluble polymeric conjugates

Chari RVJ (2008). Target cancer therapy: conferring specificity to cytotoxic drugs. *Acc Chem Res* 41: 98–107.

Duncan R (2007). Designing polymer conjugates as lysosomotropic nanomedicines. *Biochem Soc Trans* 35: 56–59.

Duncan R, Ringsdorf H, Satchi-Fainaro R (2006). Polymer therapeutics: polymers as drugs, drug and protein conjugates and gene delivery systems. Past, present and future opportunities. *J Drug Target* 14: 337–341.

Fontana A, Spolaore B, Mero A, Veronese FM (2008). Site specific modification and PEGylation of pharmaceutical proteins mediated by transglutaminase. *Adv Drug Delivery Rev* 60: 13–28.

Kratz F, Ajai KA, Warnecke A (2007). Anticancer carrier-linked prodrugs in clinical trials. *Expert Opin Investig Drugs* 17: 1037–1058.

Polymeric nanoparticles for drug delivery

Arshady R, ed. (2006). *Microspheres, Microcapsules and Liposomes. Vol. 8: Smart Nanoparticles in Nanomedicine*. London: Kentus Books.

Chauvierre C, Vauthier C, Labarre D, Couvreur P, Marden MC, Leclerc L (2004). A new generation of polymer nanoparticles for drug delivery. *Cell Mol Biol* 50: 233–239.

Uchegbu I, Schätzlein A, eds (2006). *Polymers in Drug Delivery*. Boca Raton, FL: CRC Taylor & Francis.

Vauthier C, Labarre D (2008). Modular biomimetic drug delivery systems. *J Drug Deliv Sci Technol* 18: 59–68.

Glossary

Amphiphilic copolymer	Copolymer with hydrophilic and hydrophobic blocks
Biocompatibility	Ability of a material to perform with an appropriate host response in a specific application
Biodegradable polymer	Polymer that can be degraded in vivo into smaller products, i.e. the main chain of the polymer can be cleaved
Biomaterial	Non-viable material used in a medical device, intended to interact with biological systems
Biopolymer	Polymer obtained by biosynthesis
Cohesive energy	For a solid, the energy required to break the atoms of the solid into isolated atomic species. Cohesive energy is related to solubility parameters
Colloid	System in which finely divided particles, approximately 1–1000 nm in size, are dispersed within a continuous medium in a manner that prevents them from being filtered or settled easily
Compliance	In mechanical science (cf. rheology), the inverse of stiffness
Copolymer	Polymer made up of two or more monomers
Critical micelle concentration (CMC)	Concentration above which micelles are spontaneously formed, i.e. above CMC micelles are in equilibrium with single chains
Cross-links	Bonds that link one polymer chain to another
Crystallinity	Degree of structural order in a solid. In a crystal, the atoms or molecules are arranged in a regular, periodic manner. Amorphous materials, such as liquids and glasses, have order over only short distances

Cyclodextrins	Family of cyclic oligosaccharides, composed of α-D-glucopyranoside units linked 1->4, as in amylose. Typical cyclodextrins contain six to eight glucose units in a ring, creating a cone shape
Glass transition temperature (T_g)	Temperature at which the amorphous domains of polymers undergo a second-order phase transition from a rubbery, viscous solid, to a brittle, glassy solid
Hydrogel	Water-insoluble, three-dimensional network of polymeric chains that is capable of swelling substantially in aqueous conditions
Macromolecule	High-molecular-weight molecule
Magnetic resonance imaging (MRI)	Medical imaging technique used to visualise detailed internal structure of the body. MRI uses a magnetic field to align the nuclear magnetisation of hydrogen atoms in water in the body
Medical device	Product used for medical purposes in patients, in diagnosis, therapy or surgery. The effect of the medical device is primarily physical, in contrast to pharmaceutical drugs, which exert a biochemical effect. Complete definition of a medical device can be found in ISO 13485 Standard
Micelle	Submicronic aggregation of molecules, as a droplet in a colloidal system
Monomer	Low-molecular-weight compound that can be connected together to give a polymer
Oligomer	Short polymer chain
PEGylation	Modification by attachment of PEG
Polydispersity	Equivalent to polymolecularity
Poly(ethylene glycol) (PEG) and poly (ethylene oxide) (PEO)	The repeating monomer units are similar in these, but due to different methods of synthesis, both chain ends of PEG are OH, whereas only one chain end of PEO is OH. Chains of PEO can be longer than chains of PEG
Polymer	High-molecular-weight molecule made up of small repeat units (monomer units) connected to each other by covalent bonds
Polymerisation	Process of linking together monomer molecules through chemical reactions
Polymolecularity	Distribution in molecular weight of the population of polymer chains
Polyolefin	Polymer made from olefins (alkenes, e.g. ethylene) monomers

Polypeptide	Polymer composed of amino acids
Polysaccharide	Polymer composed of sugars
Protein	Macromolecule mainly obtained by biosynthesis, composed of either amino acids and sugars (glycoproteins) or amino acids and lipids (lipoproteins)
Rheology	Study of the flow of matter
Solubility parameter (δ)	Parameter used in predicting the solubility of non-electrolytes (including amorphous polymers) in a given solvent. The Hildebrand solubility parameter provides a numerical estimate of the degree of interaction between materials and solvents. The Hildebrand solubility parameter is the square root of the cohesive energy density
Stiffness	Resistance of an elastic body to deformation by an applied force
Swelling	Increase in volume, due to interactions between solvent and polymer chains, resulting in increasing polymeric chain mobility, which can lead to possible solubilisation
Vulcanisation	Process in which rubber is slightly cross-linked by reaction with sulphur

Index